Side-Effects
of Anti-Inflammatory Drugs
3

INFLAMMATION AND DRUG THERAPY SERIES

Volume I: *Side-Effects of Anti-Inflammatory Drugs 1: Clinical and Epidemiological Aspects.* Rainsford KD, Velo GP, eds. Lancaster: MTP Press Ltd; 1987.

Volume II: *Side-Effects of Anti-Inflammatory Drugs 2: Studies in Major Organ Systems.* Rainsford KD, Velo GP, eds. Lancaster: MTP Press Ltd; 1987

Volume III: *New Developments in Antirheumatic Therapy.* Rainsford KD, Velo GP, eds. Lancaster: Kluwer Academic Publishers; 1989.

Volume IV: *Copper and Zinc in Inflammation.* Milanino R, Rainsford KD, Velo GP, eds. Lancaster: Kluwer Academic Publishers; 1989.

Volume V: *Side-Effects of Anti-Inflammatory Drugs 3.* Rainsford KD, Velo GP, eds. Lancaster: Kluwer Academic Publishers; 1992.

INFLAMMATION AND DRUG THERAPY SERIES
VOLUME V

Side-Effects of Anti-Inflammatory Drugs 3

Edited by

K.D. Rainsford
Department of Biomedical Sciences
McMaster University Faculty of Health Sciences
Hamilton, Ontario
Canada

G.P. Velo
Institute of Pharmacology
University of Verona
Italy

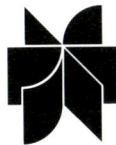

KLUWER ACADEMIC PUBLISHERS
DORDRECHT / BOSTON / LONDON

1992

Distributors

for the United States and Canada: Kluwer Academic Publishers, PO Box 358, Accord Station, Hingham, MA 02018-0358, USA
for all other countries: Kluwer Academic Publishers Group, Distribution Center, PO Box 322, 3300 AH Dordrecht, The Netherlands

British Library Cataloguing in Publication Data

Side-effects of anti-inflammatory drugs 3. – (Inflammation and drug therapy; 5)
    I. Rainsford. K.D. (Kim D), *1941–*   II. Velo, G.P. (Giampaolo P), *1943–* III. Series
    615.7042

    ISBN 0-7923-8966-2

Library of Congress Cataloging-in-Publication Data

Side-effects of anti-inflammatory drugs 3 / edited by K.D. Rainsford, G.P. Velo
       p.   cm. – (Inflammation and drug therapy series ; v. 5)
    Based on the Third International Meeting on the Side-Effects of Anti-Inflammatory and Analgesic Drugs held under the auspices of the University of Verona on May 8–11, 1991, and held in conjunction with the 13th European Workshop on Inflammation.
    Includes bibliographical references and index.
    ISBN 0-7923-8966-2 (casebound)
    1. Anti-inflammatory agents – Side effects – Congresses.
    I. Rainsford, K.D., 1941– . II. Velo, G.P. (Giampaolo P.) III. Università di Verona. Institute of Pharmacology. IV. International Meeting on the Side-effects of Anti-Inflammatory and Analgesic Drugs (3rd : 1991 : Verona, Italy) V. European Workshop on Inflammation (13th : 1991 : Verona, Italy) VI. Title: Side-effects of anti-inflammatory drugs, three. VII. Series.
    [DNLM: 1. Anti-Inflammatory Agents – adverse effects – congresses. 2. Anti-Inflammatory, Non-Steroidal – adverse effects – congresses. QV 247 S5683 1991]
    RM405.S54   1992
    DNLM/DLC
    for Library of Congress   91-35335
                                                       CIP

Published in the United Kingdom by Kluwer Academic Publishers, PO Box 55, Lancaster.

Kluwer Academic Publishers BV incorporates the publishing programmes of D. Reidel, Martinus Nijhoff, Dr W. Junk and MTP Press.

Printed and bound in Great Britain by Hartnolls Limited, Bodmin, Cornwall.

Contents

Section III: GASTROINTESINAL TRACT: PREVENTION OF ADVERSE EFFECTS

Section VIII: EXTENDED POSTER PRESENTATIONS

List of Contributors

C. ACKERMAN
Department of Rheumatology
Ghent University Hospital
Ghent
Belgium

Z. ACKERMAN
Department of Medicine
Hadassah University Hospital
Jerusalem 91 120
Israel

S. ARDIZZONE
Gastroenterology Unit
L. Sacco Hospital
Milan
Italy

P. BACCHINI
S. Orsola Malpighi Hospital
Bologna
Italy

L.M. BAMBARA
Istituto di Patologia Medica
Università di Verona
Policlinico Borgo Roma
Verona
37134 Italy

D. BIASI
Istituto di Patologia Medica
Università di Verona
Policlinico Borgo Roma
Verona
37134 Italy

I.L. BONTA
Department of Pharmacology
Faculty of Medicine
Erasmus University Rotterdam
POB 1738
3000 DR Rotterdam
The Netherlands

K. BRUNE
Department of Pharmacology and Toxicology
University of Erlangen-Nürnberg
Universitätsstrasse 22
8520 Erlangen
Germany

W.W. BUCHANAN
Rheumatology Unit
Department of Medicine
McMaster University Faculty of Health Sciences
1200 Main Street West
Hamilton
Ontario, L8N 3Z5
Canada

X. CARNÉ
Servei de Farmacologia Clínica
CS Vall d'Hebron i Universitat Autónoma de
Barcelona
08035 Barcelona
Spain

J.L. CARSON
Division of General Internal Medicine
Department of Medicine
University of Medicine and Dentistry of New
Jersey
Robert Wood Johnson Medical School
New Brunswick
New Jersey
USA

J.S.A. COLLINS
Royal Victoria Hospital
Grosvenor Road
Belfast
Northern Ireland BT12 6BA
UK

F. COMINELLI
Department of Medicine
Division of Gastrointestinal and Liver Diseases
University of Southern California
School of Medicine
Los Angeles CA 90033
USA

M. COVELLI
Chair of Rheumatology
University of Bari
Bari
Italy

E. COZZI
Institute of Internal Medicine
University of Padua
Padua
Italy

L. COZZI
Division of Rheumatology
University of Padua
Padua
Italy

C. CUVELIER
Department of Rheumatology
Ghent University Hospital
Ghent
Belgium

N. DEBBAS
Charterhouse Clinical Research Unit Ltd.
91 Charterhouse St.
London EC1
UK

M. DE VOS
Department of Rheumatology
Ghent University Hospital
Ghent
Belgium

A. DEL FAVERO
Istituto di Clinica Medica I
Policlinico Monteluce
Università degli Studi di Perugia
06100 Perugia
Italy

J.T. DINGLE
Strangeways Research Laboratory
Wort's Causeway
Cambridge CB1 4RN
UK

J.S. DIXON
Division of Gastroenterology
Glaxo Group Research Limited
Greenford Road
Greenford
Middlesex UB6 OHE
UK

R. DIXON
Merck Frosst Centre for Therapeutic Research
Kirkland
PO Box 1005
Pointe Claire-Dorval
Québec, H9R 4P8
Canada

G.E. EHRLICH
Department of Medicine (Rheumatology)
School of Medicine
University of Pennsylvania
Philadelphia
USA

R. ELIAKIM
Department of Medicine
Hadassah University Hospital
Mount Scopus
Jerusalem
Israel

G.R. ELLIOT
Department of Pharmacology
Faculty of Medicine
Erasmus University Rotterdam
POB 1738
3000 DR Rotterdam
The Netherlands

I. ERBETTI
Istituto di Farmacologia
Università di Verona
Policlinico Borgo Roma
Verona
37134 Italy

D. ETHIER
Merck Frosst Centre for Therapeutic Research
Kirkland
PO Box 1005
Pointe Claire-Dorval
Québec, H9R 4P8
Canada

J. EVANS
Merck Frosst Centre for Therapeutic Research
Kirkland
PO Box 1005
Pointe Claire-Dorval
Québec, H9R 4P8
Canada

U. FAGIOLO
Institute of Internal Medicine
University of Padua
Padua
Italy

M. FARTHING
St Bartholomew's Hospital
London
UK

H. FENNER
Department of Pharmacology and Toxicology
University of Erlangen-Nürnberg
Universitätsstrasse 22
8520 Erlangen
Germany

A. FIGUERAS
Servei de Farmacologia Clínica
CS Vall d'Hebron i Universitat Autónoma de
Barcelona
08035 Barcelona
Spain

U. FIOCCO
Division of Rheumatology
University of Padua
Padua
Italy

A.W. FORD-HUTCHINSON
Merck Frosst Centre for Therapeutic Research
Kirkland
PO Box 1005
Pointe Claire-Dorval
Québec, H9R 4P8
Canada

R. FORTIN
Merck Frosst Centre for Therapeutic Research
Kirkland
PO Box 1005
Pointe Claire-Dorval
Québec, H9R 4P8
Canada

M.E. FRACASSO
Istituto di Farmacologia
Università di Verona
Policlinico Borgo Roma
Verona
37134 Italy

L. FRANCO
Istituto di Farmacologia
Università di Verona
Policlinico Borgo Roma
Verona
37134 Italy

A. FRIGO
Istituto di Patologia Medica
Università di Verona
Policlinico Borgo Roma
Verona
37134 Italy

R. GASPERINI
Institute of Pharmacology
University of Policlinico Borgo Roma
Verona
37134 Policlinico Borgo Roma
Verona
37134 Italy

J.W. GILLARD
Merck Frosst Centre for Therapeutic Research
Kirkland
PO Box 1005
Pointe Claire-Dorval
Québec, H9R 4P8
Canada

Y. GIRARD
Merck Frosst Centre for Therapeutic Research
Kirkland
PO Box 1005
Pointe Claire-Dorval
Québec, H9R 4P8
Canada

S. GOEMAERE
Department of Rheumatology
Ghent University Hospital
Ghent
Belgium

Y. GUINDON
Merck Frosst Centre for Therapeutic Research
Kirkland
PO Box 1005
Pointe Claire-Dorval
Québec, H9R 4P8
Canada

K. GYIRES
Department of Pharmacology
Semmelweis University of Medicine
Nagyvárad tér 4
POB 370
H-1445 Budapest
Hungary

E. GYOMBER
Chemical Pathology Research Division
Department of Pathology
Brigham and Women's Hospital
Harvard Medical School
Boston, MA 02115
USA

P. HAMEL
Merck Frosst Centre for Therapeutic Research
Kirkland
PO Box 1005
Pointe Claire-Dorval
Québec, H9R 4P8
Canada

C.J. HAWKEY
Department of Therapeutics
University Hospital
Nottingham NG7 2UH
UK

M.G. HOGAN
Rheumatic Disease Unit and Laboratories for
Inorganic Medicine
McMaster University
Hamilton
Ontario, L8S 4L8
Canada

M. HORTON
St Bartholomew's Hospital
London
UK

H. HOWARD-LOCK
Rheumatic Disease Unit and Laboratories for
Inorganic Medicine
McMaster University
Hamilton
Ontario, L8S 4L8
Canada

J. JUAN
Servei de Farmacologia Clínica
CS Vall d'Hebron i Universitat Autónoma de
Barcelona
08035 Barcelona
Spain

T. JONES
Merck Frosst Centre for Therapeutic Research
Kirkland
PO Box 1005
Pointe Claire-Dorval
Québec, H9R 4P8
Canada

F. KARMELI
Department of Medicine
Hadassah University Hospital
Mount Scopus
Jerusalem
Israel

W.F. KEAN
Rheumatology Unit
Department of Medicine
McMaster University Faculty of Health Sciences
1200 Main Street West
Hamilton
Ontario L8N 3Z5
Canada

M. KUROWSKI
Department of Pharmacology and Toxicology
University of Erlangen-Nürnberg
Universitätsstrasse 22
8520 Erlangen
Germany

M. LAMA
Institute of Internal Medicine
University of Padua
Padua
Italy

C.B.H.W. LAMERS
Department of Gastroenterology-Hepatology
University Hospital Leiden
Leiden
The Netherlands

R. LANZ
Department of Pharmacology and Toxicology
University of Erlangen-Nürnberg
Universitätsstrasse 22
8520 Erlangen
Germany

F.L. LANZA
Clinical Professor of Medicine
Section of Gastroenterology
Baylor College of Medicine
Houston
Texas
USA

G. LAPADULA
Chair of Rheumatology
University of Bari
Bari
Italy

J.R. LAPORTE
Servei de Farmacologia Clínica
CS Vall d'Hebron i Universitat Autónoma de
Barcelona
08035 Barcelona
Spain

C. LEVEILLÉ
Merck Frosst Centre for Therapeutic Research
Kirkland
PO Box 1005
Pointe Claire-Dorval
Québec, H9R 4P8
Canada

M.LEVY
Department of Medicine
Hadassah University Hospital
Jerusalem 91 120
ISRAEL

J. LINDNER
Department of Pharmacology and Toxicology
University of Erlangen-Nürnberg
Universitätsstrasse 22
8520 Erlangen
Germany

C.J.L. LOCK
Rheumatic Disease Unit and Laboratories for
Inorganic Medicine
McMaster University
Hamilton
Ontario, L8S 4L8
Canada

A. LORD
Merck Frosst Centre for Therapeutic Research
Kirkland
PO Box 1005
Pointe Claire-Dorval
Québec, H9R 4P8
Canada

M. MAERTENS
Department of Rheumatology
Ghent University Hospital
Ghent
Belgium

L. MAINENTI
Istituto di Farmacologia
Università di Verona
Policlinico Borgo Roma
Verona
37134 Italy

A. MALCHOW-MØLLER
The Department of Internal Medicine
Svendborg Hospital
DK-5700 Svendborg
Denmark

M. MARRELLA
Istituto di Farmacologia
Università di Verona
Policlinico Borgo Roma
Verona
37134 Italy

U. MARTIN
University Department of Clinical Pharmacology
The Royal Infirmary
Edinburgh EH3 9YW
UK

F. MARUMO
Second Department of Internal Medicine
Faculty of Medicine
Tokyo Medical and Dental University
Tokyo
Japan

H. MIELANTS
Department of Rheumatology
Ghent University Hospital
Ghent
Belgium

R. MILANINO
Istituto di Farmacologia
Università di Verona
Policlinico Borgo Roma
Verona
37134 Italy

D. MILLER
Merck Frosst Centre for Therapeutic Research
Kirkland
PO Box 1005
Pointe Claire-Dorval
Québec, H9R 4P8
Canada

R.E. MORALES
Chemical Pathology Research Division
Department of Pathology
Brigham and Women's Hospital
Harvard Medical School
Boston, MA 02115
USA

U. MORETTI
Istituto di Farmacologia
Università di Verona
Policlinico Borgo Roma
Verona
37134 Italy

H. MORTON
Merck Frosst Centre for Therapeutic Research
Kirkland
PO Box 1005
Pointe Claire-Dorval
Québec, H9R 4P8
Canada

K.G. MUGRIDGE
Sclavo Research Centre
via Fiorentina 1
53100 Siena
Italy

L. NAGY
Chemical Pathology Research Division
Department of Pathology
Brigham and Women's Hospital
Harvard Medical School
Boston, MA 02115
USA

P.A. NICHOLSON
G.D. Searle
4901 Searle Parkway
Skokie, IL 60077
USA
Now at: SmithKline Beecham Pharmaceuticals
PO Box 1510
King of Prussia, PA 19406
USA

R. NUMO
Centre for Rheumatic Diseases
Policlinico
Bari
Italy

W.M. O'BRIEN
Professor of Internal Medicine Emeritus
c/o Department of Internal Medicine
Section of Rheumatology
The University of Virginia
Charlottesville, Virginia
USA

R. PAGANELLI
Department of Allergy and Clinical Immunology
University La Sapienza
Rome
Italy

M.C. PAGE
Rheumatic Disease Unit and Laboratories for
Inorganic Medicine
McMaster University
Hamilton
Ontario, L8S 4L8
Canada

L. PARENTE
Sclavo Research Centre
via Fiorentina 1
53100 Siena
Italy

M. PASQUALICCHIO
Istituto di Farmacologia
Università di Verona
Policlinico Borgo Roma
Verona
37134 Italy

L. PATOIA
Istituto di Clinica Medica I
Policlinico Monteluce
Università degli Studi di Perugia
06100 Perugia
Italy

M. PERRETTI
Sclavo Research Centre
via Fiorentina 1
53100 Siena
Italy

G.B. PORRO
Gastroenterology Unit
L. Sacco Hospital
Milan
Italy

L.F. PRESCOTT
University Department of Clinical Pharmacology
The Royal Infirmary
Edinburgh EH3 9YW
UK

D. RACHMILEWITZ
Department of Medicine
Hadassah University Hospital
Mount Scopus
Jerusalem
Israel

K. D RAINSFORD
Departments of Biomedical Sciences and
Pathology
McMaster University Faculty of Health Sciences
Hamilton
Ontario L8N 3Z5
Canada

P.J. RANLØV
The Division of Medical Gastroenterology
Department of Internal Medicine B
Central Hospital
DK-3400 Hillerød
Denmark

M. ROSADA
Division of Rheumatology
University of Padua
Padua
Italy

C. ROUZER
Merck Frosst Centre for Therapeutic Research
Kirkland
PO Box 1005
Pointe Claire-Dorval
Québec, H9R 4P8
Canada

L. SANTUCCI
Istituto di Gastroenterologia ed Endoscopia
Digestiva
Policlinico Monteluce
Università degli Studi di Perugia
06100 Perugia
Italy

C. SATO
Division of Health Science
Faculty of Medicine
Tokyo Medical and Dental University
Tokyo
Japan

R. SCHINNAR
Clinical Epidemiology Unit
Section of General Internal Medicine
Department of Medicine
University of Pennsylvania School of Medicine
Philadelphia
Pennsylvania

E.S. SNYDER
Clinical Epidemiology Unit
Section of General Internal Medicine
Department of Medicine
University of Pennsylvania School of Medicine
Philadelphia
Pennsylvania

B.L. STROM
Clinical Edpidemiology Unit
Section of General Internal Medicine
Department of Medicine
University of Pennsylvania School of Medicine
Philadelphia
Pennsylvania
USA

S. SZABO
Chemical Pathology Research Division
Department of Pathology
Brigham and Women's Hospital
Harvard Medical School
Boston, MA 02115
USA

A. THILLAINAYAGAM
St Bartholomew's Hospital
London EC1
UK

S. TODESCO
Division of Rheumatology
University of Padua
Padua
Italy

A. UMILE
Medical Department
Chiesi Farmaceutici SpA
Parma
Italy

P. VATTAY
Chemical Pathology Research Division
Department of Pathology
Brigham and Women's Hospital
Harvard Medical School
Boston, MA 02115
USA

G.P. VELO
Istituto di Farmacologia
Università di Verona
Policlinico Borgo Roma
Verona
37134 Italy

E.M. VEYS
Department of Rheumatology
Ghent University Hospital
Ghent
Belgium

X. VIDAL
Servei de Farmacologia Clínica
CS Vall d'Hebron i Universitat Autónoma de Barcelona
08035 Barcelona
Spain

J.L. WALLACE
Gastrointestinal Research Group
University of Calgary
Alberta, TN2 4NI
Canada

S. WARRINGTON
Charterhouse Clinical Research Unit Ltd.
91 Charterhouse St.
London EC1
UK

S. WEST
Clinical Epidemiology Unit
Section of General Internal Medicine
Department of Medicine
University of Pennsylvania School of Medicine
Philadelphia
Pennsylvania

C. YOAKIM
Merck Frosst Centre for Therapeutic Research
Kirkland
PO Box 1005
Pointe Claire-Dorval
Québec, H9R 4P8
Canada

Preface

The contents of this book represent papers which were presented at the Third International Meeting on "Side-Effects of Anti-Inflammatory and Analgesic Drugs" which was held under the auspices of the University of Verona, Institute of Pharmacology in Verona on 8–11 May 1991. This meeting was held in conjunction with the 13th European Workshop on Inflammation and although publications from this part of the meeting are not published here (they appear in *Agents and Actions*), we were fortunate in having a group of people interested in inflammation from varying backgrounds. The success of the third meeting followed previous meetings held in Cambridge and Verona respectively and continue a tradition which has now become well established. The meeting brought together physicians, scientists and those concerned with the production and use of anti-inflammatory drugs to a very stimulating conference to discuss basic issues affecting all aspects of side-effects of anti-inflammatory and analgesic drugs as well as their detection and treatment.

The meeting was held in the Auditorium of Glaxo Italy and we are very grateful to that company for use of their facilities as well as to the University of Verona, Institute of Pharmacology, for valuable secretarial and administrative help. The success of the conference would not have been possible without valuable financial assistance of the companies listed separately (under Acknowledgements) as well as to the organizers of the 13th European Workshop on Inflammation who collaborated with us.

We would also like to express our grateful appreciation to secretarial staff at McMaster University, Department of Biomedical Sciences and Rheumatic Diseases Unit for their help and arrangements for the meeting.

The papers in this book cover a wide variety of topics including the epidemiology, clinical and experimental aspects of side-effects in the gastrointestinal tract, liver, kidney, cartilage, bone and skin as well as the problems associated with the newer range of disease-modifying anti-rheumatic drugs (DMARDs) such as methotrexate and cyclosporin. Much of the emphasis has been placed on side-effects in the gastrointestinal tract with the increasing recognition of the importance of this side-effect. This should not, of course, detract from the importance of other severe

Side-effects of Anti-inflammatory Drugs 3. Rainsford KD, Velo GP (eds), Inflammation and Drug Therapy Series, Volume V.

conditions. It is an inevitable consequence of interest in a particular field that publications come from that which receives greatest attention. It was notable that progress in the prevention and analysis of many side-effects such as in the haematopoietic and immunological systems as well as in the skin, liver and kidney have not received so much attention in recent years. Clearly there are important developments which are wanting and the papers here at least have highlighted the need for these and made specific suggestions as well as giving full coverage of the current status of side-effects in most of the major organ systems.

K D Rainsford, *McMaster University, Hamilton, Ontario*
G P Velo, *University of Verona, Verona, Italy*

Acknowledgements

We are most grateful to the following Companies for their financial assistance in conducting the meeting:

Hoffman–La Roche (Switzerland)
Master Pharma (Italy)
Boehringer Ingelheim (Germany)
Boehringer Ingelheim (Italy)
Gentili (Italy)
Roche (Italy)
Corvi (Italy)
Rhone-Poulenc Rorer (Italy)
Glaxo (Canada)
Alfa Wassermann (Italy)
Bristol-Myers Squibb (Italy)
Dompé (Italy)
Rottapharm (Italy)
Merck Frosst (Canada)
Hoffmann–La Roche (Canada)
Thomae (Germany)
Tropon (Germany)
Bayer (Italy)
Kabi Pharmacia (Sweden)
ICI Pharmaceuticals (UK)
Du Pont (USA)
Hafslund Nycomed Pharma (Austria)

Chiesi (Italy)
Upjohn (Italy)
Glaxo (Italy)
Fidia (Italy)
Recordati (Italy)
Boehringer Mannheim (Italy)
Italfarmaco (Italy)
Sigma Tau (Italy)
Searle (International)
Boots (Italy)
Ciba-Geigy (Italy)
Formenti (Italy)
Ciba-Geigy (Switzerland)
Pfizer (Italy)
Roussel Pharma (Italy)
Sandoz (Switzerland)
Glaxo (UK)
Lusofarmaco (Italy)
Asta Pharma (Germany)
Abbott (USA)
Hoffmann–La Roche (USA)

1

The gastrointestinal toxicity of the non-steroidal anti-inflammatory drugs

Jeffrey L. Carson and Brian L. Strom

Division of General Internal Medicine, Department of Medicine,
University of Medicine and Dentistry of New Jersey, Robert Wood
Johnson Medical School, New Brunswick, New Jersey, USA;
and Clinical Epidemiology Unit, Section of General Internal Medicine,
Department of Medicine, University of Pennsylvania School of
Medicine, Philadelphia, Pennsylvania, USA

Non-steroidal anti-inflammatory drugs (NSAIDs) are drugs widely prescribed throughout the world. In the United States, these drugs were prescribed to 44 million patients in 1984 [1]. The utility of these drugs is, in part, due to the high frequency of gastric intolerance to aspirin. Unfortunately, gastrointestinal (GI) side-effects are also the most frequent adverse reactions to NSAIDs [2]. The GI problems reported vary from mild symptoms, such as indigestion, to serious events, including GI bleeding, peptic ulcer disease, and intestinal perforation.

In this paper we describe the recent pharmacoepidemiological research on the GI risks associated with the use of NSAIDs. We begin with a review of the evidence which establishes an association between NSAIDs and serious GI toxicity. We then present the data from studies which compare the GI toxicity of the different NSAIDs. Since there are many studies which have evaluated the association between GI toxicity and NSAIDs as a class, we only present selected studies which are representative of the best literature in this area. The reader is referred to other recent comprehensive reviews [3–5].

Our epidemiological analysis will focus on case–control studies, and cohort studies, since case reports and case series suffer from the absence of a control group, making any causal statements impossible [6]. Randomized clinical trials have been used very infrequently to evaluate these serious side-effects.

Side-effects of Anti-inflammatory Drugs 3. Rainsford KD, Velo GP (eds),
Inflammation and Drug Therapy Series, Volume V.

NON-STEROIDAL ANTI-INFLAMMATORY DRUGS AND GI TOXICITY

In 1986, Somerville et al. were the first to provide good epidemiological evidence for an association between NSAIDs and bleeding from peptic ulcer disease [7]. A case–control design was used for this study of hospitalized patients in London, England. Cases were defined as patients over age 60 with a diagnosis of bleeding gastric or duodenal ulcer. A hospital control group consisted of age- and sex-matched hospitalized patients without duodenal or gastric ulcer, taken from the same medical intake. A separate community control group was chosen by selecting the next age- and sex-matched patient from an alphabetical list of patients treated by the same general practitioner. All patients were directly questioned by a trained interviewer using a standardized questionnaire. Patients with a bleeding peptic ulcer were 2.7 to 3.8 times more likely to be exposed to NSAIDs than the control group (Table 1). One limitation of this study is the possibility of recall bias, i.e., patients' suspicion that NSAIDs are ulcerogenic drugs, either independently or due to previous questioning by physicians, leading to better recall of any exposures to NSAIDs. Another limitation of this study was incomplete control of some potentially confounding variables, such as anti-ulcer medications, alcohol, and pre-existing disease.

These results were confirmed by Carson et al. using a retrospective cohort study design [8]. The study was performed using 1980 billing data from all Medicaid patients from the states of Michigan and Minnesota.

Table 1. Association between non-steroidal anti-inflammatory drugs and GI toxicity in selected studies

Author, year	Study outcome	Odds ratio or relative risk (95% confidence interval)
Case–control studies		
Somerville [7]	Bleeding peptic ulcer	2.7 (1.7–4.4)[a]
		3.8 (22–64)[b]
Griffin et al. [10]	Fatal peptic ulcer	4.7 (3.1–7.2)
Laporte et al. [11]	UGI bleeding	17.4 (7.9–38.6)[c]
		7.7 (3.8–15.4)[d]
Griffin et al. [12]	Peptic ulcer	4.1 (3.5–4.7)
Cohort studies		
Carson et al. [8]	UGI bleeding	1.5 (1.2–2.0)
Beard et al. [9]	UGI bleeding	1.4 (0.9–2.1)
Jick et al. 1987	Perforation	1.6 (0.7–3.7)

[a] Hospital control group
[b] Outpatient control group
[c] Men < 60. Risk similar in women < 60
[d] Men ≥ 60. Risk similar in women ≥ 60

2

The risk of upper GI bleeding was compared in 47 136 patients exposed to NSAIDs and 44 634 unexposed patients. Patients exposed to NSAIDs had 1.5 (95% confidence interval, 1.2–1.9) times the risk of developing upper GI bleeding than the unexposed control group. A linear dose–response relationship was demonstrated, as well as a quadratic duration–response relationship. The limitations of this study include the potential for misclassification bias due to the uncertain validity of the diagnosis data; possible detection bias due to exposed patients being followed more closely; incomplete control of exposure to aspirin and alcohol; and questionable generalizability, since the study was performed in an indigent population.

Beard et al. examined the risk of upper GI bleeding in 21 600 patients over the age of 64 from a Health Maintenance Organization from the Seattle metropolitan area [9]. Patients taking NSAIDs were 1.4 times more likely (0.9–2.1) to develop upper GI bleeding than an age and sex matched group of patients unexposed to NSAIDs. This study used a 90 day follow-up period after NSAID exposure which may have diluted an association. While it just missed conventional statistical significance, this may be because the study had inadequate power.

Griffin et al. studied the association of NSAID use and fatal upper gastrointestinal haemorrhage in a case–control study of Medicaid patients over 60 years old [10]. Cases were defined as patients who died from upper GI bleeding. Controls were matched for age, sex, race, calender year, and nursing home status. Cases were 4.7 (3.1–7.2) times more likely to have filled an NSAID prescription than the controls. However, it is unclear whether there was adequate adjustment for severity of illness and alcohol use. Also, it is likely that many cases were missed, since cases were identified via death certificates.

Laporte et al. recently published a multicenter case–control study which assessed the risk of upper GI bleeding associated with NSAIDs [11]. Cases were patients admitted to one of three Spanish hospitals with haematemesis or melaena. Endoscopy was performed to confirm a diagnosis of benign gastric ulcer, duodenal ulcer, acute lesions of the gastric mucosa and erosive duodenitis. Up to four hospital controls were selected matched to hospital, time from admission, age, and sex. Controls included patients with admission diagnoses thought to be unrelated to NSAID use. Patients were interviewed using a structured questionnaire within 14 days of admission to the hospital. The odds ratio for all upper GI bleeding in men ⩽ 60 was 17.4 (7.9–38.6); in men > 60 it was 7.7 (3.8–15.4); in women ⩽ 60 it was 17.4 (6.2–48.6); and in women > 60 it was 7.6 (4.1–14.2). This study is limited by the possibility of recall bias, and the use of a hospitalized control group.

3

Finally, Griffin et al. recently published the largest case–control study yet to evaluate this association [12]. Medicaid enrollees from the state of Tennessee over the age of 65 hospitalized for confirmed peptic ulcer disease were identified through computerized claims data. A total of 1415 cases, and 7063 age, sex, race, and nursing home status matched controls were identified. NSAID exposure was determined by the presence of a bill to Medicaid for a NSAID with a supply that ended the day of or after the index date for the bleed. Overall, the odds ratio was 4.1 (3.5–4.7) for current users of a NSAID. The odds ratios were 5.5 (4.4–6.9) for gastric ulcer, 4.3 (3.5–5.2) for duodenal ulcer, and 2.4 (1.8–3.2) for upper GI bleeding. A dose and duration response were noted. This study suffers from incomplete control of aspirin and alcohol use since these variables were only measured in the cases. Limited generalizability is also possible since the study was performed in a Medicaid population. However, an important strength of this study is that it is not subject to recall bias because NSAID exposure was determined using computerized billing data.

Summary

While there are problems and/or limitations inherent in each of the studies, their results show a consistent association between NSAIDs and both upper GI bleeding and peptic ulcer disease. Dose– and duration–response relationships were documented in two studies. In general, the case–control studies detected a higher relative risk than the cohort studies. Furthermore, the studies that assessed NSAID exposure using interviews of patients had a higher relative risk than those studies that used computerized data to determine NSAID exposure. This is consistent with the presence of a recall bias associated with the assessment of NSAID exposure by interview. Finally, the relative risks associated with NSAID exposure were usually highest with gastric ulcer, and lowest with upper GI bleeding. The association between NSAIDs and serious GI toxicity has been convincingly shown.

RELATIVE TOXICITY OF THE NON-STEROIDAL ANTI-INFLAMMATORY DRUGS

Determining the comparative GI toxicity of the different NSAIDs could be very important clinically, as if one or more drug(s) is shown to be safer or more toxic than other drugs of the class, this drug is clearly preferable for many patients. However, this has proven to be difficult to investigate, because very large sample sizes are needed, as the differences among drugs is likely to be small. Recall bias should not be a problem in these studies, since it is unlikely that the different NSAIDs would be remembered differently. However, selection bias remains a major potential problem, since patients taking different NSAIDs may not be at equal risk of peptic ulcer disease, independent of any effect of the NSAIDs.

Carson et al. were the first to perform a study large enough to examine the relative toxicity of the NSAIDs [13]. They performed a retrospective cohort study on 88 034 Medicaid patients dispensed one of seven NSAIDs. There was a highly significant difference among the rates of upper GI bleeding associated with the use of the different NSAIDs (Table 2). Interdrug comparisons revealed that only sulindac, when compared to the reference drug ibuprofen, had an elevated relative risk [1.7 (1.3–2.3)]. When the analysis was restricted to hospitalizations for upper GI bleeding, the risk associated with sulindac increased to 2.7 (1.7–4.4). The analysis of the average daily dose of drug suggested that sulindac was used in higher doses than the other drugs which might explain the greater rate of side-effects. As before, this study suffers from concerns about diagnostic validity, generalizability, and lack of information about smoking and aspirin use.

Laporte et al. also examined the risk of upper GI bleeding associated with four separate NSAIDs in their case–control study described above (Table 3) [11]. Data are presented on four individual NSAIDs: indomethacin, diclofenac, naproxen and piroxicam. Indomethacin,

Table 2. Comparison of non-steroidal anti-inflammatory drugs in study by Carson et al. [13]

Drug	Relative risk (95% confidence interval)
Phenylbutazone	1.0 (0.5–2.2)
Fenoprofen	1.0 (0.4–3.0)
Indomethacin	1.1 (0.5–2.2)
Ibuprofen	Reference
Naproxen	1.5 (0.7–2.9)
Tolmetin	2.2 (1.0–4.6)
Sulindac	2.7 (1.7–4.4)

Analysis repeated in data from two years later which revealed sulindac with the highest rate of bleeding. Piroxicam had rate of bleeding similar to ibuprofen

Table 3. Comparison of non-steroidal anti-inflammatory drugs in study by Laporte et al. [11]

Drug	Relative risk (95% confidence interval)
Indomethacin	4.9 (2.0–12.2)
Naproxen	6.5 (2.2–19.6)
Diclofenac	7.9 (4.3–14.6)
Piroxicam	19.1 (8.2–44.3)

diclofenac and naproxen had odds ratios which were elevated between 4.9 to 7.9. The relative risk for piroxicam was much higher: 19.1. However, the 95% confidence intervals for each drug overlap, and therefore the odds ratios were not significantly different from one another. However, the very high odds ratio associated with piroxicam, does raise again the question about whether this drug may be more GI toxic than the others. The potential for recall bias is not an issue with this analysis, although selection bias may be present. In addition, this finding could be due to use of the drugs in daily doses which are not equipotent.

Griffin et al. also examined the risk among eight different NSAIDs in their case–control study (Table 4) [12]. Ibuprofen had the lowest relative risk at 2.3 and tolmetin and meclofenamate had the highest relative risks: 8.5 and 8.7, respectively. The risk of peptic ulcer disease was statistically significantly higher in patients exposed to naproxen, piroxicam, tolmetin, and meclofenamate than in patients exposed to ibuprofen. However, it is unclear that the adjustment for dose was appropriate. The use of a daily dose of 1200 mg of ibuprofen as the baseline dose may be problematic, since this dose is lower than that usually used.

Table 4. Comparison of non-steroidal anti-inflammatory drugs in study by Griffin et al. [12]

Drug	Relative risk (95% confidence interval)
Ibuprofen	2.3 (1.8–3.0)
Indomethacin	3.8 (2.4–6.0)
Sulindac	4.2 (2.8–6.3)
Naproxen	4.3 (3.4–5.4)
Fenoprofen	4.3 (2.8–6.6)
Piroxicam	6.4 (4.8–8.4)
Tolmetin	8.5 (4.5–16.1)
Meclofenamate	8.7 (4.6–16.4)

Summary

The data on the relative toxicity of the NSAIDs are inconsistent. The earliest study, performed by Carson et al., suggested that sulindac had the highest risk of upper GI bleeding, possibly due to its more common use in its maximum recommended daily dose. While this was confirmed in the same dataset two years later, Griffin et al., many years later, found the risk associated with sulindac was similar to the other drugs evaluated. Laporte et al. did not present data on sulindac.

The data presented by Laporte et al. raise the possibility that piroxicam is associated with the highest risk of upper GI bleeding. Other observational data had also suggested that the risk of serious GI toxicity was highest for piroxicam, although most of those data have serious problems [14,15]. However, both Carson et al. and Griffin et al. found that the risk associated with piroxicam was similar to other NSAIDs.

Finally, Griffin et al. found that the risk was lowest for ibuprofen. Laporte et al. did not present data on the risk of ibuprofen. Carson et al. found that the risk of upper GI bleeding associated with the use of ibuprofen was similar to that associated with the use of most of the other drugs.

Thus, it is hard to reconcile the differences in these studies. It is possible that selection bias (the patients receiving different drugs had different risks of bleeding that could not be controlled in the analysis) explains the differences found. The differences also could be a function of dose and pattern of drug utilization. Since these studies were performed at different times and in different populations of patients, prescribing patterns may have been different among the studies. Attempts at controlling for other patient characteristics may have been inadequate.

Several other studies are now underway which hopefully will clarify the relative toxicity of the NSAIDs. If consistent results emerge, then it may be possible to develop a consensus on the comparative GI risk of these drugs. However, it is likely the problems noted here will remain. This could be overcome by performing a randomized clinical trial. However, it would require an extremely large number of patients and would be prohibitively expensive. Thus, it is quite possible that a definitive answer regarding the relative GI toxicity of these drugs will remain elusive.

REFERENCES

1. The National Disease and Therapeutic Index, 1981–1984. IMS America Ltd., Ambler, Pennsylvania.
2. Coles SI, Fries JF, Krainers RG et al. From experiment to experience: Side effects of non-steroidal anti-inflammatory drugs. Am J Med. 1983;74:820–827.
3. Langman MJS. Epidemiologic evidence on the association between peptic ulceration and antiinflammatory drug use. Gastroenterology. 1989;96:640–646.
4. Fries JF, Miller SR, Spitz PW, Williams CA, Hubert HB, Bloch DA. Toward an epidemiology of gastropathy associated with non-steroidal antiinflammatory drug use. Gastroenterology. 1989;96:646–655.
5. Soll AH, Weinstein WM, Kurata J, McCarthy D. Nonsteroidal anti-inflammatory drugs and peptic ulcer disease. Ann Intern Med. 1991;114:307–319.
6. Carson JL, Strom BL. Techniques of postmarketing surveillance: An overview. Med Toxicol. 1986;1:237–246.
7. Somerville K, Faulkner G, Langman M. Nonsteroidal anti-inflammatory drugs and bleeding peptic ulcer. Lancet. 1986;1:462–464.

8. Carson JL, Strom BL, Soper KA, West SL, Morse ML. The association of non-steroidal anti-inflammatory drugs with upper gastrointestinal tract bleeding. Arch Intern Med. 1987;147:85–88.
9. Beard K, Walker AM, Perera DR, Jick H. Nonsteroidal anti-inflammatory drugs and hospitalization for gastroesophageal bleeding in the elderly. Arch Intern Med. 1987;147:1621–1623.
10. Griffin MR, Ray WA, Schaffner W. Non-steroidal anti-inflammatory drug use and death from peptic ulcer in elderly persons. Ann Intern Med. 1988;109:359–363.
11. Laporte JR, Carne X, Vidal X, Moreno V, Jauan J. Upper gastrointestinal bleeding in relation to previous use of analgesics and non-steroidal anti-inflammatory drugs. Lancet. 1991;337:85–89.
12. Griffin MR, Piper JM, Daugherty JR, Snowden M, Ray W. Nonsteroidal anti-inflammatory drug use and increased risk for peptic ulcer disease in elderly persons. Ann Intern Med. 1991;114:257–263.
13. Carson JL, Strom BL, Morse ML. The relative gastrointestinal toxicity of the non-steroidal anti-inflammatory drugs. Arch Intern Med. 1987;147:1054–1059.
14. Rossi AD, Hsu JP, Faich GA. Ulcerogenicity of piroxicam: An analysis of spontaneously reported data. Br Med J. 1987;294:147–150.
15. Collier DStJ, Pain JA. Ulcer perforation in the elderly and non-steroidal anti-inflammatory drugs. Lancet. 1986;1:971.

2

The value of the case–control approach for the evaluation of the risk of upper gastrointestinal bleeding associated with the previous use of non-steroidal anti-inflammatory drugs

J.R. Laporte, X. Carné, A. Figueras, X. Vidal and J. Juan

Servei de Farmacologia Clínica, CS Vall d'Hebron i Universitat Autònoma de Barcelona, 08035 Barcelona, Spain

Several studies have reported an association between upper gastrointestinal bleeding (UGIB) and the previous use of acetylsalicylic acid (ASA) [1–11] or non-steroidal anti-inflammatory drugs (NSAIDs) as a whole [12–14]. However, specific estimates for individual drugs are not available because the lower prevalence of use of each individual NSAID – compared with that of ASA – limits the statistical power of any analytical study designed to quantify individual risks.

To address this issue, we performed a multicentre case–control study in three hospitals in Catalonia and Mallorca. We also measured the incidence of UGIB attributable to peptic ulcer or acute lesions of the gastric mucosa over a 2-month period in the resident population of the island of Mallorca.

POPULATION AND METHODS

We identified all patients presenting at the participating hospitals (Hospital Vall d'Hebron, Barcelona; Hospital de Sant Pau, Barcelona; Hospital Son Dureta, Ciutat de Mallorca) between February 1, 1987 and December 31, 1988, with an endoscopy-proven diagnosis of UGIB attributable to benign gastric ulcer, duodenal ulcer, and acute lesions of the gastric or duodenal mucosa. Patients with other endoscopic diagnosis (i.e. oesophageal varices, Mallory–Weiss syndrome, gastric carcinoma, etc.), those with a history of liver cirrhosis or coagulopathy, illiterate people, non-residents, and those who could not be reliably interviewed were excluded.

Side-effects of Anti-inflammatory Drugs 3. Rainsford KD, Velo GP (eds), Inflammation and Drug Therapy Series, Volume V.

Up to 4 controls were randomly selected for each case, matched according to centre, time from admission (within 2 months), age (within 5 years), and sex, among patients admitted to hospital with acute clinical disorders thought to be unrelated to the intake of analgesics and NSAIDs. We applied the same exclusion criteria as for the cases.

Cases and controls were interviewed with a structured questionnaire, by specially trained nurses and physicians. The interview covered: 1) general demographic information; 2) details on the clinical course leading to the present hospitalization; 3) previous medical history, with special emphasis on gastrointestinal, rheumatic and other painful disorders; 4) alcohol, tobacco and coffee intake, and 5) drug history. This included (a) an open question on use of medicines before admission; (b) a list of symptoms commonly leading to drug use, and (c) a list of the names of the most consumed analgesics, NSAIDs, and preparations for the treatment of dyspepsia or ulcer disease. Information on the use of medicines was taken on a daily basis for the 28 days before admission, and it included information about the dose taken. Without knowledge of previous drug use, two investigators defined the 'index day' for cases and controls, as the day on which the first sign or symptom of the disease that caused admission appeared.

By means of a conditional logistic regression model, we calculated the odds ratio estimates and their 95% confidence interval (CI), for ASA, paracetamol, propyphenazone, metamizol (dipyrone), diclofenac, indomethacin, naproxen, piroxicam and the other NSAIDs. The model included all potential confounding factors. Details have been given in a previous publication [15]. Odds ratios and their 95% CI were calculated for all patients, and for the subgroups of gastric and duodenal patients in relation to the use of each analgesic and NSAID during an exposure window of 7 days prior to the index day. The 7-days non-user group was the reference group for all estimations. Odds ratios were calculated for all the patients as well as for patients without a previous history of GI bleeding or ulcer disease [15].

RESULTS

Of 938 eligible cases, 38 were not interviewed because they died (1.1%), could not be found within 14 days (1.8%), had psychological difficulties (1.0%), or refused (0.3%). Nine hundred cases were therefore interviewed. Table 1 shows the probable causes of bleeding.

Of 2719 eligible controls, 10 (0.4%) refused to be interviewed. Twenty-five cases and 27 controls were not included in the case–control analysis because their responses to the questions were judged unreliable by the interviewer, thus leaving 875 cases and 2682 controls for the case control

Table 1. Probable cause of bleeding among 900 consecutive patients admitted with upper gastrointestinal bleeding, evaluated by endoscopy

	Men	Women	Total
Duodenal ulcer	377	88	465
Erosive duodenitis	21	7	28
Gastric ulcer	192	121	313
ALGM[a]	39	30	69
Mixed lesions	19	6	25
Total	648	252	900

[a] Acute lesions of the gastric mucosa

analysis. This was performed for all cases and, separately, for gastric (gastric ulcer plus acute lesions of gastric mucosa) and for duodenal patients (duodenal ulcer plus erosive duodenitis).

Patients with gastric lesions were older than those with duodenal lesions (mean (SD) 63.1 (15.0) vs 55.9 (17.4) years; median 64 vs 56 years). The men/women ratio was fairly constant across the different age categories (4.2) among duodenal patients, but not among gastric patients (4.8 among patients younger than 60 years, and 0.9 among those older than 60 years).

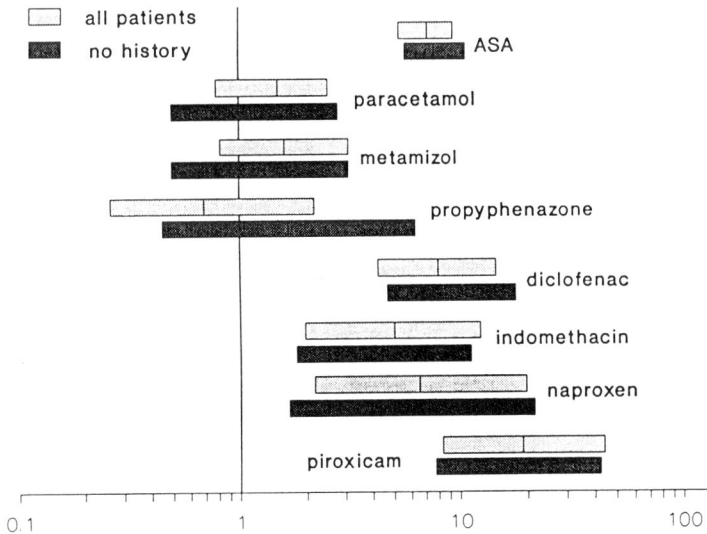

Figure 1. Risk of GI bleeding associated with each one of the most commonly used analgesics and NSAIDs. Odds ratio estimates for all patients with UGIB (darker diagrams), and for patients without a previous history of peptic ulcer or gastrointestinal bleeding. The values of odds ratio are represented as solid vertical lines within each diagram; each diagram represents the 95% confidence interval. The solid vertical line represents an odds ratio of unity (no drug effect)

11

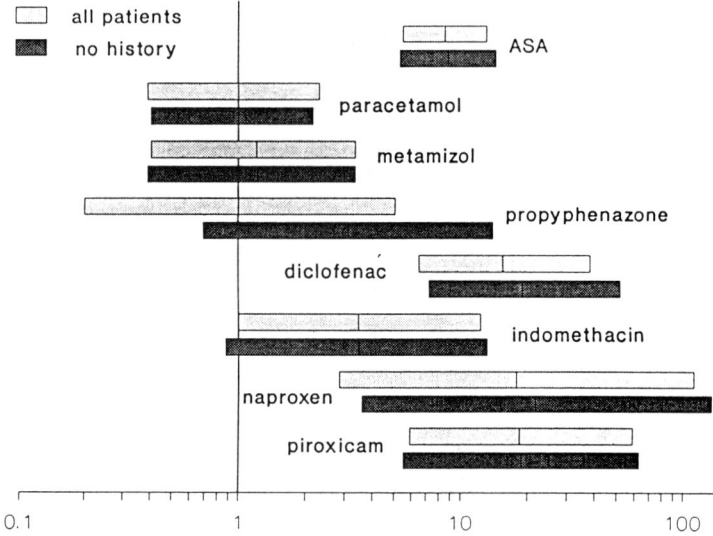

Figure 2. Risk of bleeding from a gastric ulcer associated with each one of the most commonly used analgesics and NSAIDs. Odds ratio estimates for all patients with gastric bleeding (darker diagrams), and for patients without a previous history of peptic ulcer or gastrointestinal bleeding. The values of odds ratio are represented as solid vertical lines within each diagram; each diagram represents the 95% confidence interval. The solid vertical line represents an odds ratio of unity (no drug effect)

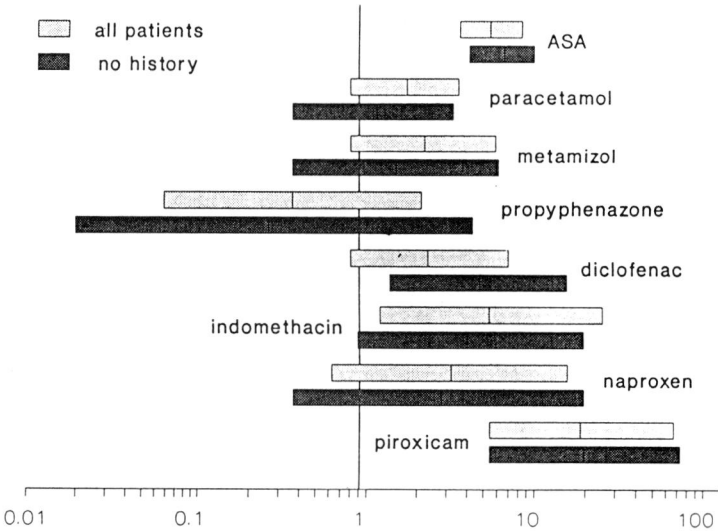

Figure 3. Risk of bleeding from a duodenal ulcer associated with each one of the most commonly used analgesics and NSAIDs. Odds ratio estimates for all patients with duodenal bleeding (darker diagrams), and for patients without a previous history of peptic ulcer or gastrointestinal bleeding. The values of odds ratio are represented as solid vertical lines within each diagram; each diagram represents the 95% confidence interval. The solid vertical line represents an odds ratio of unity (no drug effect)

12

Figure 1 shows the odds ratio estimates and their 95% CI for the most commonly used analgesics and NSAIDs for all patients with UGIB, and separately for the 480 patients (55%) without a previous history of peptic ulcer or gastroduodenal bleeding. Figures 2 and 3 show the same estimates separately for patients with gastric and duodenal bleeding respectively. For the overall, as well as for the subgroup analyses, the OR estimates for paracetamol, metamizol, and propyphenazone included 1.0. In the overall analysis, ASA, diclofenac, naproxen, indomethacin and piroxicam did show an increasing risk of GI bleeding, with OR estimates ranging from 4.9 for indomethacin to 19.1 for piroxicam. Naproxen and diclofenac showed non-significant OR estimates for duodenal bleeding, but these were based on small numbers: 4 exposed cases and 6 exposed controls for naproxen, and 12 and 16 for diclofenac.

Risks of GI bleeding from any origin associated with the use of ASA did not vary greatly within the different age- and sex-categories (Table 2). However, the risks of gastric bleeding associated with non-ASA-NSAIDs varied with age. In fact, they were higher among patients under 60 years than in older ones (78.7 [19.1–325] vs 7.6 [4.0–14.6]; $p < 0.005$) ranges in

Table 2. Use of ASA and NSAIDs and risk of gastric and duodenal bleeding associated with their use, according to age and sex

	Men			Women		
	Cases	Controls	OR (95% CI)	Cases	Controls	OR (95% CI)
ASA						
All						
≤60 y	97	75	8.1 (5.0–13.0)	26	30	7.7 (4.1–14.5)
>60 y	54	45	6.7 (4.0–11.1)	39	57	6.4 (3.8–10.7)
Gastric						
≤60 y	41	14	19.9 (8.0–49.4)	10	16	8.0 (3.0–21.4)
>60 y	27	17	13.0 (5.6–29.9)	28	44	5.3 (2.7–10.1)
Duodenal						
≤60 y	52	57	5.7 (3.1–10.6)	15	14	9.1 (3.4–24.3)
>60 y	25	28	4.7 (2.3–9.6)	9	13	7.5 (1.0–20.8)
Non-ASA-NSAIDs						
All						
≤60 y	66	73	17.4 (7.9–38.6)	23	32	17.4 (6.2–48.6)
>60 y	61	38	7.7 (3.8–15.4)	65	80	7.6 (4.1–14.2)
Gastric						
≤60 y	20	24	152.0 (29.4–783)	15	19	40.9 (7.4–227)
>60 y	30	19	21.4 (6.5–71.1)	41	56	5.8 (2.2–15.4)
Duodenal						
≤60 y	43	8	4.8 (1.6–14.1)	47	12	33.2 (5.1–215)
>60 y	29	22	4.3 (1.6–11.3)	19	21	29.4 (6.5–133)

brackets) and higher in men than in women (40.0 [14.5–111] vs 7.1 [3.4–14.9]; $p < 0.005$). Other subgroup differences were not statistically significant after Bonferroni's adjustment.

The mean daily dose of all the drugs under study in the days of exposure was calculated, for the cases and for the controls. For all drugs, it was higher among the cases. This difference was maximal for propyphenazone (458 mg per day among the cases vs 316 mg among the controls), and minimal for indomethacin (91 mg among the cases vs 84 among the controls).

DISCUSSION

Our study confirms previous reports about the risk of gastrointestinal bleeding associated with the use of ASA and other NSAIDs. The apparent gastrointestinal safety of paracetamol, metamizol, and propyphenazone has been discussed in a previous report [15].

As shown in figures 1 to 3, in our model a previous history of peptic ulcer or gastrointestinal bleeding did not affect the odds ratio estimate for all NSAIDs, which was 7.4 (2.4–23.0) among patients with such a history, and 8.0 (3.8–16.6) among those without it. However, this does not mean that a previous history of peptic ulcer disease does not add any risk. In fact, we found that a previous history of subjective symptoms was associated with an increased risk of subsequent GI bleeding (OR = 2.6, 95% CI 1.9–3.5); a previous confirmed diagnosis of peptic ulcer was strongly associated with GI bleeding (OR = 5.5, 95% CI 2.8–11.0), and the risk of a second bleeding in patients who had already suffered a previous episode was even greater (OR = 14.5, 95% CI 7.5–28.2).

Several issues related to the methodology of our study have also been discussed [15]. An aspect which deserves special attention is the magnitude of the risk found in the different studies carried out up to now on GI bleeding in relation to the use of NSAIDs. As we have previously pointed out, the different risk estimates may be explained by certain methodological weaknesses. Lack of endoscopic diagnosis for some of the cases (4–6,8–10) and inclusion of controls with disorders possibly related to the use of ASA [3] may lead to underestimation of the risk. Inadequate age matching of controls and cases [3] may lead to overestimation of the risk. We have also suggested misclassification of analgesic use [4,6–9] and failure to control for other confounders [3–6,8,16] as other factors which may explain the different results obtained in each study.

The 'time window' when previous drug use is considered in cases and in controls may also strongly affect the magnitude of the risk estimates. One weakness of case–control studies is that they may not have enough statistical power to quantify the magnitude of the risk of adverse effects

Table 3. Case control studies on the relationship between gastrointestinal bleeding and previous use of acetylsalicylic acid (modified from Belcon et al. [17])

Study	Odds ratio	Power $(1-\beta)$
Kelly [2]	11.6 (3.3–50.3)	0.30
Alvarez and Summerskill [3]	5.8 (2.9–11.8)	0.65
Allibone and Flint [1]	1.1 (0.6–1.8)	0.78
Muir and Cossar [4]	6.1 (3.0–12.3)	0.66
Levy [6]	1.7 (1.4–2.2)	0.86
Coggon et al. [9]	4.8 (2.4–10.7)	0.98
Bartle et al. [12]	2.2 (1.0–4.9)	0.69
Levy et al. [10]	5.6 (2.7–12)	0.99
Faulkner et al. [11]	3.1 (1.8–5.8)	0.81

Table 4. Consumption of analgesics and non-steroidal anti-inflammatory drugs in different countries (defined daily doses/1000 inhabitants/day)

	Denmark (20) (1983)	Norway (20) (1983)	Sweden (20) (1983)	Spain (18) (1985)	Finland (19) (1988)
Diclofenac	1.2	–	1.5	3.4	3.7
Flurbiprofen	–	–	–	0.4	–
Ibuprofen	9.2	1.5	3.8	0.6	6.3
Indole derivatives	3.4	2.4	4.0	1.7	3.7
Ketoprofen	–	–	–	0.4	5.9
Naproxen	3.0	9.8	7.3	2.3	5.2
Paracetamol	7.3	2.2	8.3	4.2	–
Phenylbutazone	–	–	–	1.4	0.1
Piroxicam	0.9	4.5	2.6	3.5	2.4
Pyrazolones	12.8	9.0	0.8	10.5	1.2
Salicylates	41.3	17.4	32.6	16.4	23.8
Sulindac	1.1	–	1.9	0.4	–

associated with the use of drugs with a low prevalence of use. Table 3 shows a summary of the results of the case–control studies on the risk of GI bleeding associated with ASA performed up to now, and the statistical power of each one of them. This would be much lower if the risk specifically associated with each one of the different non-ASA-NSAIDs on the market had to be studied, because their prevalence of use is also much lower. Table 4 shows the consumption of different NSAIDs and analgesic drugs in Spain and in the Nordic countries at the time when we started our study. A case–control study aimed at finding an expected relative risk of 5, with 3 controls per case, an α error of 0.05, and a β error of 0.20, would need 172 patients for a drug with a prevalence of use of 0.01, 337 if the prevalence of use is 0.005, and 668 if the prevalence of use is 0.0025 [21]. As a prevalence figure of 0.0025 roughly corresponds to 2.5 defined daily doses per 1000 inhabitants and per day, the latter would be the case of the top ranking NSAIDs (see Table 4). In this context, widening the aetiological time window during which drug exposure is considered gives a higher prevalence of use of the drugs under study, among the cases as well as among the controls. Thus, for example, if a time window of 30 days is considered, the proportions of exposed cases and exposed controls will be higher than considering exposure only during one week before the index day, but this would dilute the true value of the odds ratio. Our present knowledge on the pathophysiology of mucosal damage suggests that one week is a proper latency period to consider in these studies [15].

These considerations raise the problem of the sensitivity and specificity of the different approaches used in drug safety evaluation. Any drug surveillance method should be sensitive enough to quantify severe adverse drug reactions. It should also be specific enough first, to identify ADRs which are clinically, pathologically or biochemically indistinguishable from those which can occur randomly in untreated patients, and second, not to confound random clinical incidents with true ADRs.

To date, assembling series of cases – through voluntary reporting or by any other way – has been the main method for the discovery of ADRs, particularly those which are rare. However, while being simple to carry out, the case approach lacks specificity and its results can be grossly distorted by selective reporting. In contrast, controlled studies suffer from lack of sensitivity: unless very large, the cohort approach cannot identify rare ADRs, and the case–control strategy cannot study the risks associated with drugs with a low prevalence of use. This is especially relevant for recently marketed drugs: during their initial market life less is known about their safety, and their use is generally low.

Selective reporting and under-reporting are the main drawbacks of voluntary reporting. On the other hand, certain clinical events, such as GI bleeding, tend to be referred to the emergency ward of hospitals. Therefore, all the cases of this condition attending the emergency wards of large hospitals with monopoly on care in their own area could be systematically assembled. Selective bias would be unlikely, because the reason for attending the emergency ward is bleeding, rather than the drugs to which the patient has been exposed. If reliable drug utilization data from the same area are available, any excess prevalence of use of a given drug can be checked in patients with GI bleeding. The following steps could be applied:

1. A systematic daily review of the diagnoses at the hospital emergency ward, applying strict clinical criteria;

2. Interview of the selected patients by means of a structured questionnaire to identify previous use of drugs (if any), and

3. Correlation of the number of previously exposed cases with sales figures that are geographically and time specific.

16

We are now evaluating the possibility of developing this new method with the series of 900 patients included in the case–control study on GI bleeding. If it proves useful, it can also be applied to the aetiological study of other conditions, and it may become a rapid and sensitive tool for hypothesis generation and, in some cases, a useful way to gather information for use in public health decisions.

REFERENCES

1. Allibone A, Flint FS. Bronchitis, aspirin, smoking and other factors of the aetiology of peptic ulcer. Lancet. 1958;2:179–182.
2. Kelly J. Salicylate ingestion: a frequent cause of gastric hemorrhage. Am J Med Sci. 1956;232:119–127.
3. Alvarez AS, Summerskill WHJ. Gastrointestinal haemorrhage and salicylates. Lancet. 1958;1:920–925.
4. Muir A, Cossar IA. Aspirin and gastric haemorrhage. Lancet. 1959;1:539–541.
5. Valman HB, Parry DJ, Coghill NF. Lesions associated with gastroduodenal haemorrhage, in relation to aspirin intake. Br Med J. 1968;4:661–663.
6. Levy M. Aspirin use in patients with major upper gastrointestinal bleeding and peptic-ulcer disease. N Engl J Med. 1974;290:1158–1162.
7. Jick H. Effects of aspirin and acetaminophen in gastrointestinal haemorrhage. Results from the Boston Collaborative Drug Surveillance Program. Arch Intern Med. 1981;141:316–321.
8. Jick H, Porter J. Drug-induced gastrointestinal bleeding. Report from the Boston Collaborative Drug Surveillance Program. Boston University Medical Center. Lancet.1978;2:87–89.
9. Coggon D, Langman MJS, Spiegelhalter D. Aspirin, paracetamol and haematemesis and melaena. Gut. 1982;23:340–344.
10. Levy M, Miller DR, Kaufman DW et al. Major upper gastrointestinal tract bleeding. Relation to the use of aspirin and other nonnarcotic analgesics. Arch Intern Med. 1988;148:281–285.
11. Faulkner G, Prichard P, Somerville K, Langman MJS. Aspirin and bleeding peptic ulcers in the elderly. Br Med J. 1988;297:1311–1313.
12. Bartle WR, Gupta AK, Lazor J. Nonsteroidal anti-inflammatory drugs and gastrointestinal bleeding. A Case–control study. Arch Intern Med. 1986;146:2365–2367.
13. Somerville K, Faulkner G, Langman M. Non-steroidal anti-inflammatory drugs and bleeding peptic ulcer. Lancet. 1986;1:462–464.
14. Matthewson K, Pugh S, Northfield TC. Which peptic ulcer patients bleed? Gut. 1988;29:70–74.
15. Laporte JR, Carné X, Vidal X, Moreno V, Juan J and the Catalan Countries Study on Upper Gastrointestinal Bleeding. Upper gastrointestinal bleeding in relation to previous use of analgesics and non-steroidal anti-inflammatory drugs. Lancet. 1991;337:85–89.
16. Griffin MR, Ray WA, Schaffner W. Non-steroidal anti-inflammatory drug use and death from peptic ulcer in elderly persons. Ann Intern Med. 1988;109:359–363.
17. Belcon MC, Rooney PJ, Tugwell P. Aspirin and gastrointestinal bleeding and the use of aspirin and other non-narcotic analgesics. J Chron Dis. 1985;38:101–111.
18. Laporte JR, Carné X, Capellà D. Post-marketing surveillance. In: Burley D, Haward Ch, Mullinger B, eds. The focus for pharmaceutical knowledge. London: Macmillan Press; 1988:136–159.
19. Finnish Committee on Drug Information and Statistics. Finnish Statistics on Medicines. Helsinki: National Board of Health; 1989.
20. Nordic Council on Medicines. Nordic statistics on medicines 1981–1983. Part II. Uppsala: NLN Publications (16); 1986.
21. Schlesselman JJ. Case–control studies. Design, conduct, analysis. New York: Oxford University Press; 1982:144–170.

3

Liver toxicity of antipyretic drugs in conjunction with measles infections

Micha Levy and Zvi Ackerman
Department of Medicine, Hadassah University Hospital,
Jerusalem 91 120, Israel

Hepatic involvement may be a part of many viral infections in addition to the classic 'hepatitis viruses'. These include cytomegalovirus, Epstein–Barr virus, herpes simplex, varicella, adenovirus, yellow fever, coxsackie viruses and measles [1].

In recent years, several clinical entities have been described in which a viral infection and drug exposure seem to interact [2]. A well-known example is Reye's syndrome, in which viral illnesses, notably varicella-zoster and influenza B infection combined with salicylates act in the aetiology of the disease [3].

Recently, during a measles epidemic, we found that hepatic impairment was more common in those treated for the fever with paracetamol compared to those treated with dipyrone [4].

One hundred and eighteen young adults (18–21-years-old) were treated in an in-patient clinic for measles. Eighty-three were men and 35 women. The clinical diagnosis was confirmed by a four-fold increase of the haemagglutinin inhibition antibody titers to measles from the acute stage to up to 4 weeks following clinical recovery.

The clinical hallmarks of the disease were obviously fever and rash. The duration of fever was 8.1 ± 1.6 (SD) days and the maximal temperature was $39.6 \pm 0.5°C$, the duration of rash was 4.4 ± 1.3 days and the total duration of illness 13.6 ± 2.3 days. Ninety-five percent of the patients had cough, 45% nausea, 43% vomiting and 5% hepatomegaly. The most common complications were otitis media (47%) and bronchitis (36%). Five percent had jaundice.

The white cell count was 5638 ± 2169 per mm^3 and the platelets $176\,000 \pm 106\,000$ per mm^3. The serum albumin 40.0 ± 3.4 and the globulin 31.3 ± 4.1 g/l.

Side-effects of Anti-inflammatory Drugs 3. Rainsford KD, Velo GP (eds),
Inflammation and Drug Therapy Series, Volume V.

Fifty-six percent of the patients exhibited some impairment in the liver function tests. The serum bilirubin was increased in 7%, aspartate aminotransferase (AST) in 44%, alanine aminotransferase (ALT) in 53%, alkaline phosphatase in 43%, γ-glutamyl transpeptidase in 50% and lactic dehydrogenase in 56% of the patients.

All patients received antipyretic drugs to alleviate the fever. The drug choice was made by the treating physician at the clinic; at the time no research was envisioned. In retrospect, we identified three treatment groups to alleviate the fever, A – paracetamol only ($n=43$), B – dipyrone only ($n=13$) and C – first paracetamol and later dipyrone ($n=62$). Drug doses were all within the therapeutic range. The total doses were 10.1 ± 5.5 g paracetamol for group A, 3.9 ± 1.7 g dipyrone for group B and 5.1 ± 3.7 g paracetamol and 3.6 ± 2.7 g dipyrone for group C.

The three groups were found to be similar with regard to the duration of fever, maximal temperature, duration of rash, cough, nausea, vomiting and secondary bacterial complications. There were no significant differences between the three groups in the blood count, the serum albumin and globulin concentrations. The bilirubin and AST levels were significantly higher in group A compared to group B (12.0 ± 6.0 vs. 7.0 ± 2.0 μmol/litre and 92 ± 86 vs. $42 \pm$ IU/litre, respectively) ($p < 0.02$). The ALT, LDH, GT and alkaline phosphatase levels did not differ significantly.

The proportion of patients having impaired liver function tests was highest in group A, intermediate in group C and lowest in group B. Twenty-five (58%) and 28 (68%) out of the 45 patients treated with paracetamol had increased levels of AST and ALT respectively, compared with 2 (15%) out of the 13 patients treated with dipyrone ($p > 0.01$). No correlation was found between the drug dose and the liver impairment; however, the cumulative dose of paracetamol in those who developed disturbed liver function tests was higher than in those who did not display these disturbances (11.6 ± 5.8 vs. 7.6 ± 4.2 g; $p = 0.02$).

Hepatotoxicity is a well-known result of paracetamol overdosage; i.e. > 4 g daily in the adult. It has also been described following therapeutic doses in alcoholics and in those receiving drugs such as phenobarbital.

Either induction of the cytochrome P-450 system or impaired synthesis of glutathione may cause increased amounts of the toxic metabolite of paracetamol [5–7]. It is suggested that viral infection, i.e. measles, may act in a similar way. In mice, preinfected with influenza B virus, centrilobular necrosis appeared following lower paracetamol doses than those required to induce such changes in the control animals [8].

Potential biases that could have affected our results must be considered, notably the lack of blinding. Nevertheless, our results support the hypothesis that virus (measles) and drug (paracetamol) have a combined hepatoxic effect. The pathogenic mechanism, possible enhanced formation of toxic metabolite, remains to be elucidated.

19

If true, the present finding adds another example for the adverse virus–drug interactions [9]. Well-known examples are the ampicillin rash in infectious mononucleosis and Reye's syndrome [10,11]. High rates of adverse reactions to trimethoprim/sulphamethoxazole have been reported in AIDS patients treated for *Pneumocystis carinii* pneumonia [12,13]. In the International Agranulocytosis and Aplastic Anemia Study an association was found between antecedent infection and (drug-induced) agranulocytosis, but it proved impossible to determine if these were of viral origin [14]. In the same study, an intriguing association was also found between infectious mononucleosis in the past and agranulocytosis [15].

The pathogenetic mechanisms responsible for the drug–virus combined effect seem to vary. For the ampicillin rash in infectious mononucleosis and for agranulocytosis an immune modulation is plausible. In Reye's syndrome mitochondrial dysfunction is implied [13].

For the association between EBV infection (in the past) and agranulocytosis possible mechanisms include T cell dysfunction, B cell polyclonal activation or cross reactivity of viral and self antigens.

The risk of a combined effect also varies from the very common (for the ampicillin) to the very rare.

Further investigation, laboratory and epidemiological, should be undertaken to provide understanding of the importance and place of the combined effect of viruses and drugs in the aetiology of diseases.

REFERENCES

1. Sherlock S. Virus hepatitis. In: Sherlock S, ed. Diseases of the liver and biliary system, Ed. 7. Oxford: Blackwell Scientific Publications;1985:275–279.
2. Levy M. The combined effect of viruses and drugs in drug-induced diseases. Med Hypoth. 1984;14:293–296.
3. Osterloh J, Cunningham W, Dixon A, Combest D. Biochemical relationships between Reye's and Reye's-like metabolic and toxicological syndromes. Med Toxicol Adverse Drug Exp. 1989;4:272–294.
4. Ackerman Z, Flugelman Y, Wax Y, Shouval D, Levy M. Hepatitis during measles in young adults: possible role of antipyretic drugs. Hepatology. 1989;10:203–206.
5. Black M. Acetaminophen hepatotoxicity. Annu Rev Med. 1984;35:577–593.
6. Seeff LB, Cuccherini BA, Zimmerman HJ, et al. Acetaminophen hepatotoxicity in alcoholics. Ann Intern Med. 1986;104:399–404.
7. Prescott LF. Effect of non-narcotic analgesics on the liver. Drugs. 1986;32(4):129–147.
8. MacDonald MG, McGrath PP, McMartin DN, et al. Potentiation of the toxic effects of acetaminophen in mice by concurrent infection with influenza B virus. A possible mechanism for human Reye's syndrome. Pediatr Res. 1984;18:181–187.
9. Haverkos HW, Drotman DP. Adverse virus-drug interactions. Rev Infect Dis. (in press).
10. Pullen H, Wright N, Murdock JM. Hypersensitivity reactions to antibacterial drugs in infectious mononucleosis. Lancet. 1967;2:1176–1178.
11. Starko KM, Ray G, Dominquez LB, Stromberg WL, Woodall DF. Reye's syndrome and salicylate use. Pediatrics. 1980;66:859–864.
12. Jaffe HS, Abrams DI, Ammann AJ, Lewis BJ, Golden JA. Complications of co-trimoxazole of AIDS-associated pneumocystis carinii pneumonia in homosexual men. Lancet. 1983;11:1109–1111.

13. Glatt AE, Chrigin K. Pneumocystis carinii pneumonia in human immunodeficiency virus-infected patients. Arch Intern Med. 1990;150:270–279.
14. Kaufman DW, Kelly JP, Levy M, Shapiro S. The drug etiology of agranulocytosis and aplastic anemia. In: The International Agranulocytosis and Aplastic Anemia Study. Oxford: Oxford University Press; 1991.
15. Levy M, Kaufman D, Kelly J, Shapiro S. Infectious mononucleosis in the past predisposed to drug induced agranulocytosis. 23rd Congress of the International Society of Hematology/American Society of Hematology Meeting, Boston, December 1990. Blood. 1990;76(suppl):386

4

Non-steroidal anti-inflammatory drugs and hypersensitivity reactions

Brian L. Strom[1], Jeffrey L. Carson[1,2], Rita Schinnar[1], Ellen Sim Snyder[1] and Suzanne West[1]

[1]Clinical Epidemiology Unit, Section of General Internal Medicine of the Department of Medicine, University of Pennsylvania School of Medicine, Philadelphia, Pennsylvania; [2]Division of General Internal Medicine of the Department of Medicine, UMDNJ-Robert Wood Johnson Medical School, New Brunswick, New Jersey, USA

INTRODUCTION

In March 1983, reports of deaths from anaphylactoid reactions resulted in the recall of zomepirac from market. Zomepirac is chemically closely related to tolmetin and, even prior to these results, a disproportionate number of reports of hypersensitivity reactions had been received by the US Food and Drug Administration regarding tolmetin [1]. In response to these initiatives, a pair of studies was undertaken [2,3].

ZOMEPIRAC AND HYPERSENSITIVITY REACTIONS

Design

The objectives of the first study [1] were to evaluate whether there was an elevated risk of hypersensitivity reactions from non-steroidal anti-inflammatory drugs as a class versus all other drugs and to evaluate whether there was an increased risk of hypersensitivity reactions from zomepirac vs. all other non-steroidal anti-inflammatory drugs. The database used for these studies was the Computerized Online Medicaid Pharmaceutical Analysis and Surveillance System (COMPASS®). COMPASS is an automated database containing Medicaid billing data on demographics, outpatient drugs dispensed, inpatient and outpatient diagnoses, procedures, and deaths [4]. Information is available on over-the-counter drugs only when they are prescribed. COMPASS data from a single state was used for the purpose of this first study.

Side-effects of Anti-inflammatory Drugs 3. Rainsford KD, Velo GP (eds), Inflammation and Drug Therapy Series, Volume V.

Table 1. ICD-9-CM codes for hypersensitivity reactions

Code	Reaction
478.75	Laryngeal spasm
478.8	Upper respiratory tract hypersensitivity reactions, site unspecified
693.0	Dermatitis due to drugs
708	Urticaria
708.0	Allergic urticaria
708.9	Urticaria, unspecified
785.5	Shock without mention of trauma
785.50	Shock, unspecified
995.0	Anaphylactic shock
995.1	Angioneurotic edema
995.2	Unspecified adverse effect of a drug, medicinal and biological substance

The disease of primary interest was hypersensitivity reactions, as defined by the ICD-9-CM codes listed in Table 1. In fact, most of the disease which was studied was urticaria.

A retrospective cohort study was performed. 78,749 users of non-steroidal anti-inflammatory drugs were compared to 78,793 age- and sex-matched unexposed controls. The rate of anaphylactoid reactions within seven days after any non-steroidal anti-inflammatory drug exposure was compared to the entire experience of the controls, adjusting for the unequal person-days at risk. The rates of anaphylactoid reactions within seven days of drug exposure were also compared among the cohorts of non-steroidal anti-inflammatory drug users, each exposed to one and only one of the non-steroidal anti-inflammatory drugs.

RESULTS

In the first study, increased risks of hypersensitivity reactions were associated with decreased age, female sex, and the use of penicillin. Nonsteroidal anti-inflammatory drugs, as a class, were associated with no elevated risk of hypersensitivity reactions. After adjustment for potential confounders the risk was increased, however. In particular, in women, after adjusting for age, the relative risk (95% confidence interval) was 2.0 (1.3–2.9). In men the comparable adjusted relative risk was 2.7 (1.1–7.9). However, in women there was an interaction between acute pain as an indication and the effect of non-steroidal anti-inflammatory drugs on hypersensitivity reactions ($p = 0.0002$). This was not seen in men, but the sample sizes in men were much smaller. In individuals who had a diagnosis compatible with acute pain, the relative risk (confidence intervals) in women was 2.5 (1.5–4.1). After adjusting for age, penicillin exposure, salicylate exposure, and osteoarthritis, this relative risk became 4.1 (2.5–6.7). In contrast, in those who did not have a diagnosis compatible with acute pain, the comparable relative risks were 0.6 (0.3–1.1) and 0.9 (0.5–1.8), respectively.

In order to clarify whether this was an effect of acute pain or whether this was because of the use of zomepirac for acute pain, we then performed analyses specifically for each non-steroidal anti-inflammatory drug. Comparing zomepirac to the other non-steroidal anti-inflammatory drugs, we observed a relative risk (95% confidence interval) of 2.55 (1.26–5.17). The comparable adjusted relative risk was 2.0 (1.1–4.7). Restricting the analysis to those who had a diagnosis of acute pain gave a relative risk of 0.2 (0.02–1.6). In other words, when comparing zomepirac used for pain to other non-steroidal anti-inflammatory drugs used for pain, there was no difference in their risk of hypersensitivity reactions. Restricting the analysis to those with a diagnosis of osteoarthritis, and who did not have a diagnosis compatible with acute pain, the result was indeterminate: there were no cases in the numerator or denominator. Examining the risk of non-steroidal anti-inflammatory drugs other than zomepirac vs. unexposed patients, in those with acute pain the adjusted relative risk was 2.6 (1.3–5.4), which was essentially identical to that observed with zomepirac. In those without pain, the adjusted relative risk was 0.7 (0.3–1.5).

In other words, based on the results of our first study, non-steroidal anti-inflammatory drugs as a class appeared to be associated with an increased risk of hypersensitivity reactions. In addition, zomepirac in particular appeared to result in a greater risk of these illnesses than other non-steroidal anti-inflammatory drugs. However, the increased risk from zomepirac appeared to be a function of the primary indication for the drug or, more likely, the regimen associated with that indication, rather than an intrinsic property of the drug.

TOLMETIN AND HYPERSENSITIVITY REACTIONS

However, the above findings are not compatible with the initial signal from the spontaneous reporting system that tolmetin was associated with an increased risk of hypersensitivity reactions [1]. Tolmetin is closely related to zomepirac chemically, yet it is used like the other non-steroidal anti-inflammatory drugs for long-term therapy in chronic conditions. This would imply that there is some unique risk associated with the structure of these drugs, rather than the patterns of use. In order to clarify this, we performed an additional study, very similar to the first [3]. In this study, we used Medicaid claims data from three other, very large US states, in order to achieve much larger sample sizes. Examining users of tolmetin, fenoprofen, meclofenamate, naproxen, piroxicam, and sulindac, we had 128,344 subjects. Examining the relative risk associated with the use of tolmetin vs. the other non-steroidal anti-inflammatory drugs, without adjusting for other potential confounding variables, the relative risk (confidence interval) was 1.1 (0.7–1.8). Controlling for all potential confounding variables simultaneously did not subsequently change the results; the adjusted odds ratio (confidence interval) was 0.9 (0.6–1.2). Thus, despite its structural similarity to zomepirac, tolmetin was associated with a risk of hypersensitivity reactions similar to that of the other chronically used non-steroidal anti-inflammatory drugs.

CONCLUSION

Thus, these data indicate that non-steroidal anti-inflammatory drugs, as a class, are associated with an increased risk of hypersensitivity reactions and that use of zomepirac was associated with a higher risk than use of the other non-steroidal anti-inflammatory drugs. However, the data suggest that intermittent use of zomepirac as an analgesic was probably the reason for the increased risk of hypersensitivity reactions. This is consistent with the data available to the manufacturer from the spontaneous reporting system, in which 75% of the individuals reported with hypersensitivity reactions to zomepirac had previously taken zomepirac on a number of occasions. After varying lengths of time during which the drug was not taken, they restarted the drug and experienced a hypersensitivity reaction. Of this group, over 90% experienced the hypersensitivity reaction after ingesting the very first tablet after restarting the drug. In addition to the mechanistic, pathophysiological, implications of the study, these results are important as we now allow aspirin and other non-steroidal anti-inflammatory drugs to be used over-the-counter as analgesics. While these reactions remain uncommon, the risk should be taken into account in deciding whether or not to use these drugs.

Acknowledgement

Supported by funds from McNeil Pharmaceutical

REFERENCES

1. Rossi AC, Knapp DE. Tolmetin-induced anaphylactoid reactions. N Engl J Med. 1982;307:499–500.
2. Strom BL, Carson JL, Morse ML, West SL, Soper KA. The effect of indication on hypersensitivity reactions associated with zomepirac sodium and other non-steroidal antiinflammatory drugs. Arthritis Rheum. 1987;30:1142–1148.

3.   Strom BL, Carson JL, Schinnar R, Sim E, Morse ML. The effect of indication on the risk of hypersensitivity reactions associated with tolmetin sodium vs. other non-steroidal antiinflammatory drugs. J Rheumatol. 1988;15:695–699.

4.   Strom BL, Carson JL, Morse ML, LeRoy AA. The Computerized On-line Medicaid Pharmaceutical Analysis and Surveillance System: A new resource for postmarketing drug surveillance. Clin Pharmacol Ther. 1985;38:359–364.

5

What can a spontaneous reporting system teach about side-effects of anti-inflammatory drugs?

George E. Ehrlich

Department of Medicine (Rheumatology), School of Medicine, University of Pennsylvania, Philadelphia, USA

The launch of a new anti-inflammatory drug (or any drug, for that matter) is preceded by appropriate defined testing in most industrialized nations. Although the requirements for demonstrating efficacy and safety vary from country to country, they can usually be satisfied by including from a few hundred to 3000 patients in pre-approval testing. In countries without the requisite infrastructure, drugs may be licensed without local testing, accepting data generated elsewhere. These limited studies give considerable insight into the proper use of the drugs in question. They also identify the major frequent untoward events that accompany administration of the drugs, and permit segregation – because of the relatively controlled conditions – of those events causally related from those that are casual interlopers. Generally, it is left to post-marketing studies to delve deeper into specific side-effect liabilities. If, in pre-approval studies, serious side-effects or fatalities occur, and if these can be related to the drug, then approval is placed in jeopardy, depending on the severity of the condition to be treated, the benefits expected and the risks found acceptable. For non-steroidal anti-inflammatory drugs (NSAIDs) the benefit-risk ratio acceptable is more rigorous than for compounds thought capable of altering the disease progression to crippling or death. This assumes that NSAIDs provide no discernable benefits other than pain relief and inflammation suppression, an arguable proposition. Approval by the designated governmental agency permits marketing, and it is expected that the resultant widespread use will signal the rare and unexpected serious and fatal side-effects. To accomplish this aim, spontaneous reporting systems have been created to cumulate the reports of such untoward events.

Side-effects of Anti-inflammatory Drugs 3. Rainsford KD, Velo GP (eds), Inflammation and Drug Therapy Series, Volume V.

Untoward events are generally reported to the manufacturer or distributor of the drug, but often also or instead to the appropriate governmental agency [1]. They are generated by physicians, pharmacists, or other health professionals and rarely by patients themselves (directly, that is). Patients are often quite aware when a change in their health was probably not the consequences of taking a medication, such as diarrhoea shared with other family members after a restaurant visit, but self-monitoring also contributed a higher percentage of purported drug-induced side-effects [2]. In the United States, forms are sent to physicians regularly by the Food and Drug Administration (FDA) to be returned with appropriate data; in the United Kingdom, the yellow card system is in place. Reports are voluntary in the United States, although encouraged. In some countries, as in Scandinavia, they are required by statute. There is thus no direct comparability of data thus generated from country to country, and direct comparison of various drugs cannot be made on the frequency of reports alone.

United States laws mandate reporting of all suspected domestic adverse drug reactions (ADRs) known to the manufacturer or distributor and all international reports as well, in timely fashion. The merging of the data presents a bias in itself. The drugs appear on the market at different times, and can well have reached expiration of patent protection in one country before or shortly after being introduced in another [1]. The drugs may be approved for different indications in different countries or parts of the world, or their use may differ widely (e.g. some drugs perceived as safer may be given predominantly to those with mild problems, or, conversely, to those expected to tolerate drugs less well, depending on local viewpoints). NSAIDs are given to children who have fevers in Latin America and Japan and some other regions, which practice may invoke different types and frequency and severity of adverse reactions. The same NSAID may be sold by different manufacturers in some countries, so that reactions attributed to a generically similar compound will not be reported to the major manufacturer in another country (e.g. United States) whilst a manufacturer responsible for most of a compound marketed internationally may receive a greater number of reports. As the systems and requirements vary, this combines data generated differently and of variable significance. Ascertainment of causality is often made more difficult, yet FDA requires all such events to be reported regardless of causality. More than 75% of reports reaching FDA come from the manufacturers, with fewer than 25% from other sources [3]. Clearly, physicians and others are more likely to report suspected adverse events directly to the manufacturer, in the form of queries or initiated by the sales representative of the company who calls upon the health care provider. The visibility of the company and the frequency of calls by the sales representative, which often bear a relationship to the stage in the life cycle of the drug, also introduce a potential bias [1]. A concerted effort to increase voluntary reporting through education of physicians can generate a flood of reports from one area amid a trickle from others. The Rhode Island project is an example of this [3]. The importance of direct reports to FDA rather than to the manufacturer is emphasized by the statistic that physicians had generated only 1% of direct reports to the agency but that this meagre number identified 24% of all ADRs that resulted in labelling changes' [3]. The reasons so few reports came directly to FDA are many. Among them are fears of increased liability from reporting reactions and, perhaps most commonly, just being busy and assuming that such reactions are already known to the agency. As a result, most physicians tend to report only the most alarming or unusual events.

Without follow-up, such events are only signals. They have been described as numerators in search of their denominators [4] and tend to reflect the recency of the drug's introduction, its labelling, its market share ('widespread use'), and media-generated heightened awareness. Some single events or real or factitious clusters form the basis of case reports in medical journals. These may well represent duplications of reports already filed, but they are often indexed as if they were new cases previously unknown to the agency. However, such reports can prove to be very helpful, as happened after three patients with severe myalgias and marked peripheral eosinophilia were reported to the Centers for Disease Control from New Mexico [5]. The eosinophilia-myalgia syndrome was associated with tryptophan ingestion, and its report prompted a spate of related case reports that not only refined the definition but also enabled identification of a single manufacturer as the source of the offending compound [6–10]. Spontaneous reports thus signaled the problem; epidemiological and other studies clarified it.

Similarly, spontaneous reporting of flank pain in some patients taking suprofen led to the identification of this association [11]. A phenomenon that has little or no background incidence (like the two instances mentioned here, or the metallic facial skin eruption in some patients receiving injectable gold salts or the bluish-silver discoloration of patients receiving an excess of a silver-containing compound, like Argyrol) can be detected readily through spontaneous reports. Only a few hundred patients need to take a medication with such an unusual side-effect for it to be attributed. When, however, there is background incidence, many thousands, up to millions, must take a medication for the association to be noted with reasonable certainty. This applies to the gastropathy attributed to NSAIDs [12]; its prevalence and severity are still in question and the asymptomatic lesions discovered by gastroscopy have been cited as an effect, not a side-effect. Indeed, the asymptomatic lesions would not have been found through a spontaneous reporting system!

Similarly, overt hepatitis, jaundice and liver failure are infrequently reported for most NSAIDs, usually without confirmatory attribution (the background noise: various forms of infectious hepatitis are common), but abnormalities of laboratory tests of liver function are usually gleaned from studies, not spontaneous reports. A purported cluster of serious events was recently reported without assessing the population at risk; a few physicians canvassed a large, densely populated geographic area and discovered seven cases, not all necessarily causally related to the drug in question [13]. In the event, all these patients had previously been reported to FDA and the 'cluster' was artificial. The association between event and drug may well be real, but the magnitude of the association remains undefined.

Eighteen months after diclofenac was first marketed in the United States, the spontaneous reports of ADRs were analysed [14]. This drug had achieved an impressive sales record immediately after launch, becoming one of the five most widely prescribed NSAIDs. Weber had defined the first two years after introduction as the time of maximal spontaneous reporting [15], so a comparison of reports generated between diclofenac and the others (ibuprofen, naproxen, piroxicam, and sulindac) for the same reporting period was possible. An additional factor had to be introduced: the secular trend. Analysis of reporting rates had shown these to be relatively flat, 5 to 10 per million prescriptions, during the 1970s. A number of external environmental factors, including withdrawals of benoxaprofen, suprofen, and zomepirac in the early 1980s, plus some challenges to products by consumer advocates that failed but increased awareness and resulted in communications media-induced notoriety, led to steady increases in reporting rates, to about 30 per million prescriptions by 1987. Thus, if one wanted to compare spontaneous reporting rates for compounds introduced to the United States in the mid-1970s, the early 1980s and the late 1980s, one needed to correct for the reporting rates in the respective years [16]. Uncorrected were the changes in dosage for some of the drugs between the time of introduction and the present. If ADRs reflect in part the dose of the drug, then a significant increase in customary dose between the time of introduction and some later time might result in increased frequency and severity of the dose-related reactions but not be reflected in reporting rates (because of the 'Weber effects' – see ref. 15).

Although such data cannot be used for direct comparisons of drugs, they should signal particular problems that make of the drug an outlier among drugs of its class. The analysis of these five compounds, concentrating on four organ systems (gastro-intestinal, kidney, liver and haematological), suggested safety profiles roughly comparable with each other and raised no special concerns [14]. This is particularly true when the total safety profiles, not just those focused on single body systems, were taken into consideration.

What, then, is the place of the spontaneous reporting systems in understanding anti-inflammatory drugs? They represent a step between the controlled pre-approval studies and the epidemiological and pharmaco-epidemiological studies that determine frequency and excess risks of adverse drug reactions. They identify untoward events, although often without the data and feedback that permit attribution. They signal events so rare that they are difficult or well nigh impossible to study epidemiologically. They are a rapid discovery system for identifying events so rare and distinctive, without background incidence, that a formal study is unnecessary. They identify events that are rare, with no logical clinical relationship to the drug. Spontaneous event reporting is thus an early warning system identifying potential problems to review methodically. If it is codified by statute to achieve a predictable higher reporting rate (as the mandatory system already in place in several countries) it will prove even more useful. As it stands, even in its imperfect state, spontaneous reporting helped identify the eosinophilia–myalgia syndrome and its link to tryptophan, the consequences of diethylstilboestrol ingestion by mothers for their daughters, the phocomelia in the offspring linked to thalidomide ingestion by pregnant women, and even the occurrence, if not the numerical risk, of the less dramatic but still serious events associated with drugs amidst the cacophony of background noise. All recent withdrawals of NSAIDs were initiated by spontaneous reports: hepatorenal consequences of overdosage for benoxaprofen, flank pain for suprofen, hypersensitivity reactions for zomepirac, to name the most obvious.

Spontaneous reports occasionally may be self-serving. The signals they generate lead to regulatory questions but not usually to requests for withdrawal of the drug. The withdrawals of benoxaprofen, suprofen and zomepirac were mainly commercial decisions by the manufacturers, based on questions of ability to market, size of potential remaining sales volume, and risk of malpractice suits (depending on the country; high in USA). Spontaneous reporting should not be used to rank compounds. Spontaneous reporting has other uses: in the case of methotrexate, a current vogue drug for rheumatoid arthritis, the relative infrequency of spontaneous reports of hepatotoxicity has led to the discontinuation by most physicians of pre- and post-administration liver biopsies. Ultimately, spontaneous reports should not be given more importance than warranted, and but for misuse by consumer representatives, media and competitors, should only point to pharmacoepidemiological studies that ought to be done.

REFERENCES

1. Sachs RM, Bortnichak EA. An evaluation of spontaneous adverse drug reaction monitoring systems. Am J Med. 1986;81(suppl 5B):49–55.
2. Fisher S, Bryant SG. Postmarketing surveillance: accuracy of patient drug attribution judgments. Clin Pharmacol Ther. 1990;48:102–107.
3. Scott HD, Thacher-Renshaw A, Rosenbaum SE, et al. Physician reporting of adverse drug reactions. Results of the Rhode Island adverse drug reaction reporting project. JAMA.1990;263:1785–1788.
4. Avorn J. Reporting drug side-effects: signals and noise. JAMA. 1990;263:1823.
5. Centers for Disease Control (CDC). Eosinophilia–myalgia syndrome – New Mexico. MMWR. 1989;38:765–767.
6. Clauw DJ, Nashel D, Umhau A, et al. Tryptophan-associated eosinophilic connective-tissue disease. A new clinical entity? JAMA. 1990;263:1502–1506.
7. CDC. Eosinophilia–myalgia syndrome associated with ingestion of L-tryptophan – United States, through August 24, 1990. JAMA. 1990;264:1655.
8. CDC. Analysis of L-tryptophan for the etiology of eosinophilia–myalgia syndrome. JAMA. 1990;264:1656.
9. Swygert LA, Maes EF, Sewell LER, et al. Eosinophilia–myalgia syndrome. Results of national surveillance. JAMA. 1990;264:1698–1703.
10. Slutsker L, Hoesley FC, Miller L, et al. Eosinophilia–myalgia syndrome associated with exposure to tryptophan from a single manufacturer. JAMA. 1990;264:213–217.
11. Rossi AC, Bosco L, Faich GA, et al. The importance of adverse reaction reporting by physicians: suprofen and the flank pain syndrome. JAMA. 1988;259:1203–1204.
12. Hadler N. There's the forest. The object lesson of NSAID 'gastropathy'. J Rheumatol. 1990;17:280–282.
13. Helfgott SM, Sandberg-Cook J, Zakim D, et al. Diclofenac-associated hepatotoxicity. JAMA. 1990;264:2660–2662.
14. Mason DH, Bernstein J, Bortnichak EA, et al. Spontaneous reporting of adverse drug reactions: diclofenac sodium and four other leading NSAIDs. IM. 1990;11:1–8.
15. Weber JCP. Epidemiology of adverse reactions to non-steroidal anti-inflammatory drugs. In: Rainsford KD, Velo GP, eds. Advances in inflammation research, Vol. 6. New York: Raven Press;1984:1–7.
16. Rossi AC, Hsu JP, Faich GA. Ulcerogenicity of piroxicam. An analysis of spontaneously reported data. Br Med J. 1987;294:147–150.

6

Adverse reactions to NSAIDs: Consecutive evaluation of 30,000 patients in rheumatology

**K. Brune, H. Fenner, M. Kurowski, R. Lanz
and members of the SPALA group**
Department of Pharmacology and Toxicology, University of Erlangen-Nürnberg, Universitätsstrasse 22, D-8520 Erlangen, Germany

INTRODUCTION

Non-steroidal anti-inflammatory drugs (NSAIDs) are among the most widely-used and prescribed drugs world-wide. During the last decade, a number of new compounds have been introduced to the market. Some of them had to be removed because of adverse drug reactions attributed to their use. One lesson learned from these experiences was that the safety of NSAIDs can only be established after introduction and intensive clinical use. In order to estimate adverse reaction frequencies resulting from the use of these drugs, different epidemiological approaches are available: cohort studies, case-control studies and post-marketing surveillance. The analytical capability of the two former methods are clear. They have, however, a couple of drawbacks which are discussed in another chapter of this book.

In the German-speaking world only limited experience with post-marketing surveillance systems has been gathered. In order to further improve that situation, at least in the area of drug treatment of rheumatoid diseases, a non-profit organization 'Verein zur Langzeituntersuchung von Arzneimittelwirkungen auf dem Gebiet der Rheumatologie' (V.L.A.R.) was founded by some physicians and pharmacologists. A pilot project, SPALA, funded by F. Hoffmann La-Roche Ltd., Basel, Switzerland (Table 1) was then developed.

In July 1990, the data-gathering period of this project was terminated and almost 30,000 patients were completely documented and entered into computer files. First results were presented to a small group of experts on the occasion of a symposium held at Berlin on December 10 1991. An

Side-effects of Anti-inflammatory Drugs 3. Rainsford KD, Velo GP (eds), Inflammation and Drug Therapy Series, Volume V.

Table 1. Participating persons and institutions of the SPALA project

Project plan:
R. Lanz, H. Fenner, Basel;
M. Kurowski, K. Brune, Erlangen
Project management:
M. Kurowski, Erlangen
Advisory board:
E. Weber, Heidelberg; K. Brune, Erlangen; M. Franke, Baden-Baden;
H. Kewitz, Berlin; K.H. Kimbel, Koeln; R. Repges, Aachen
In case experts:
M. Schneider, Erlangen (Gastroenterology)
T. Ruzicka, Muenchen (Dermatology)
J. Mann, Nuernberg (Nephrology)
W. Heit, Ulm (Haematology)
Participating centres:
Germany:
U. Botzenhardt, Bremen; D. Jentsch, E. Keck, K. Miehlke, Wiesbaden; G. Josenhans,
Bad Bramstedt; E.-M. Lemmel, Baden-Baden; H. Menninger, Bad Abbach; M.
Schattenkirchner, Muenchen; H. Soerensen, Berlin; T. Stratz, Bad Saeckingen; H.
Zeidler, Hannover
Austria:
R. Eberl, A. Dunky, Wien; G. Kolarz, O. Scherak, N. Thumb, Baden
Switzerland:
P. Mennet, Rheinfelden; W. Mueller, Basel; F.J. Wagenhaeuser, M. Felder, Zürich
Data management:
G. Kiep, K. Szendey, Frankfurt

extended version of the preliminary data extracted and calculated so far on the project is presented in this manuscript cojointly authored by the whole SPALA group.

METHODS

The SPALA (Safety Profile of Antirheumatics in Long-term Administration) project was planned and initiated in 1987–88 (Table 1). It was intended to identify, collect, classify and quantify adverse events (AE) occurring during or following the treatment with non-steroidal anti-inflammatory drugs (NSAIDs). Adverse events were reported directly to the authorities, the manufacturers of the NSAIDs concerned and the Head of a SPALA Advisory Board. The plan, course and evaluation of the project was observed and scrutinized by the Advisory Board consisting of experienced specialists of different medical disciplines.

The project was planned and carried out in accordance with the appropriate laws of Austria, Switzerland and West Germany. The details of the project plan and the methods have been published previously [1,2].

34

In short, the data were collected from a patient population of a substantial size (30,000) who received NSAIDs during hospitalization or ambulatory treatment in the participating rheumatological centres. The centres were in Austria, Switzerland and Germany (German language). The data were collected by trained physicians and nurses exclusively employed for this project. A structured questionnaire consisting of three parts was applied for the documentation of the patient's medical history, the treatment during the observation period and adverse events. Onset and end of the treatment with each prescription including the reason for the discontinuation was registered. Also, application forms and dosage schedules were recorded, but this first evaluation did not take the doses into account. The physicians responsible for the SPALA project in each centre were trained continuously in the recognition and registration of adverse events in order to keep similar standards in the monitoring centres. Despite these efforts, some differences in the sensitivity and accuracy of adverse event recognition and reporting have to be assumed. Once each week, the hospitalized patients were asked whether they had experienced any adverse event. Additional information on the events (if needed) was obtained from physicians, nurses and medical records. A judgement of causality between NSAID use and event was requested from the study physician.

Outpatients were asked the same questions upon every visit. The questionnaires were compiled, mailed to a professional data processing company (PMS, IMS International) and entered into a computer, classified and analysed by PMS. Classification concerned (a) the diseases (according to the International Classification of Diseases by the WHO, 9th Rev.), (b) the adverse events (according to the Adverse Reaction Terminology by the WHO), and (c) the drugs (according to the 'IMS-NDF Product Code').

RESULTS

The presentation of results requires the definition of several applied terms. These definitions were made for practical purposes of the project.

Observation period

The observation period was defined as the period of NSAID treatment at one of the monitoring centres. For hospitalized patients it ended no later than the day of the patient's discharge from the clinic. For ambulatory patients it ended no later than the day of the last visit at the clinic, defined as the visit followed by a period of at least six weeks in which the patient did not attend. Adverse events were collected up to six weeks after the patient left the monitoring programme.

Treatment cases (TC)

Under certain conditions patients could be included and registered more than once, due to:

(a) the start of a new NSAID therapy after the end of an observation period at the same monitoring centre,

(b) the movement between ambulatory and in-hospital status of a patient at the same monitoring centre,

(c) the movement of a patient between different monitoring centres.

The primary data evaluation and the results presented refer to treatment cases. The first step of the further analysis will include the reduction of treatment cases to patients.

Adverse event cases (AE cases)

A treatment case who experienced at least one adverse event is denoted as 'adverse event case'. Obviously, the number of adverse events was higher ($n = 9,480$) than the number of AE cases ($n = 5,457$), which gives an overall ratio of 1.7 AE/AE case.

Table 2 gives an overview of the database on completely documented cases.

Table 2. Overall results

	Male	Female	Total
No. of TC with at least one NSAID-prescription (treatment cases)	10,504	18,560	29,064
No. and percentage of TC with at least one AE (AE cases)	1,439	4,018	5,457
	13.7%	18.1%	16.5%
No. of diagnoses suggesting NSAID treatment	11,050	19,507	30,577
No. of NSAID-prescriptions	12,946	23,201	36,147
No. of adverse events (AE)	2257	7223	9480
Average no. of NSAID-prescriptions per TC	1.2	1.3	1.2
Average no. of AE per AE case	1.6	1.8	1.7
Average no. of NSAID-prescriptions per AE	5.7	3.2	3.8

Description of the centres

The participating centres were in Austria (4), (West) Germany (9), and Switzerland (3). The number of monitored treatment cases per centre ranged from 506 to 4,482. Table 3 illustrates the differences between the

Table 3. Participating centres

City (country code)	Treatment cases (TC) No.	NSAID-prescriptions No.	No./TC	Adverse events (AE) No.	No./TC
Baden (2 centres) (A)	1,061	1447	1.36	439	0.41
Baden (1 centre) (A)	506	795	1.57	121	0.24
Bad Abbach (D)	1,489	1,821	1.22	439	0.29
Bad Bramstedt (D)	4,482	5,668	1.26	1,964	0.44
Bad Saeckingen (D)	547	754	1.38	154	0.28
Baden Baden (D)	3,569	4,422	1.24	1,159	0.32
Basel (CH)	2,115	2,909	1.38	569	0.27
Berlin (D)	1,707	2,225	1.30	1,714	1.00
Bremen (D)	1,495	1,930	1.29	782	0.52
Hannover (D)	1,211	1,358	1.12	190	0.16
Muenchen (D)	1,674	1,907	1.14	452	0.27
Rheinfelden (CH)	938	1,079	1.15	152	0.16
Wien (A)	1,195	1,566	1.31	289	0.24
Wiesbaden (D)	2,597	2,954	1.14	529	0.20
Zürich (CH)	4,478	5,312	1.19	527	0.12
Out-hospital	9,095	10,828	1.19	1,798	0.20
In-hospital	19,969	25,319	1.27	7,682	0.38
Total	29,064	36,147	1.24	9,480	0.33

participating centres indicating no. of TC, no. of NSAID prescriptions, and # of AE and adverse event rates (AE/TC). The differences in the adverse event rates (last column of Table 3) among the participating centres require further analyses and explanations, as the comparability of AE rates is a prerequisite for evaluations of the summarized data. Possible explanations for these differences include different (a) patient populations, (b) diseases, (c) prescription patterns of NSAIDs, (d) intensity of AE monitoring. The reported AE rates of hospitalized patients were approximately twice as high as those of the ambulatory patients, probably due to more intensive monitoring, more comprehensive medical information during hospitalization, and sicker patients in the in-patient group.

Description of the patients

The data have not been assigned to patients so far; the term treatment case (TC) will be used instead in this report. Table 4 illustrates the TC-distribution by sex, country and hospitalization status. The overall sex distribution in the three countries varied considerably with the highest portion of female cases in Austria, a lower one in West Germany and the

Table 4. Treatment cases (TC) by sex, country and hospitalization status

		Male	Female
Countries			
	Austria	854	1,908
	West Germany	6,152	12,619
	Switzerland	3,498	4,033
Status			
	In-hospital	6,645	13,324
	Out-hospital	3,859	5,236
Total		10,504	18,560

lowest in Switzerland. Among hospitalized TC cases a somewhat higher proportion of females were registered than among ambulatory TC. The age distribution for the treatment cases and the AE cases for both genders is given in Table 5.

Diseases

Among rheumatic diseases degenerative disorders generally prevail. The spectrum of diseases treated in the SPALA monitoring centres is clearly different from the overall spectrum. The diagnoses of rheumatic disorders were registered and classified according to the ICD code (see above). A large variety of different diseases is covered by the term 'rheumatic

Table 5. Percentage of different age classes separated by sex and given for treatment cases and AE-cases (fractions of 100% in each line)

Age class (years)	< 20	21–30	31–40	41–50	51–60	61–70	71–80	81–90	> 90
Treatment cases									
Male (%)	2.2	9.8	14.3	22.3	26.6	14.6	8.0	2.2	–
Average age: 50 years									
Female (%)	1.6	5.1	7.9	16.3	22.3	23.8	17.7	5.3	0.1
Average age: 58 years									
Total (%)	1.8	6.8	10.2	18.5	23.8	20.4	14.2	4.2	0.1
Average age: 55 years									
Treatment cases with at least one adverse event (AE-cases)									
Male (%)	2.0	7.1	11.4	22.5	27.0	16.4	10.1	3.4	0.1
Average age: 53 years									
Female (%)	1.7	3.6	6.0	13.7	19.5	25.5	22.1	7.7	0.2
Average age: 61 years									
Total (%)	1.8	4.5	7.4	16.0	21.5	23.1	19.0	6.5	0.1
Average age: 59 years									

disorders'. In order to give an overview of the diagnoses leading to NSAID treatment (30 557 = 100%), a rough classification into four categories was used:

- – primarily inflammatory disorders (48.2%),
- – primarily degenerative disorders (18.2%),
- – other rheumatic disorders (28.8%),
- – other disorders (4.6%).

The latter group comprises diseases which may not be classified as rheumatic but, nevertheless, warranted the prescription of an NSAID.

Treatment with NSAIDs

The number of NSAIDs available varies substantially in the three participating countries. The numbers of prescribed preparations including generic products ranged from 35 (Austria) and 76 (Switzerland) to 182 (West Germany). Due to West German law, no standardization of drug treatment is permitted in this type of study. Thus, the proportions of the drugs prescribed resemble the authentic prescription pattern of the monitoring centres. Despite the variety of drugs available the four most frequently prescribed NSAIDs covered more than 70% of the total number of 36,147 prescriptions. Table 6 shows the ten most frequently prescribed drugs, which amounted to 32,937 or 91% of the total number of prescriptions. The patients were allowed to refuse cooperation with the study physician. The few who did are included in the small (< 2%) group of patients excluded from evaluation due to incomplete data. As in most cases the patients received new prescriptions when entering in- or out-hospital treatment. The average treatment duration was relatively short as compared to the original intention of long-term surveillance and the name of the project. The overall treatment durations with NSAIDs were:

1 day	–1 week	–3 weeks	–6 weeks	> 6 weeks
13.9%	14.3%	30.0%	32.3%	9.5%

Thus, adverse events after long-term administration could not be studied sufficiently.

Adverse events (AE)

A total number of 9,480 adverse events were reported. Some of these related to more than one NSAID: if more than one NSAID was taken for up to six weeks before the onset of an adverse event, they all were defined as linked to the event in this first evaluation. Further evaluation will have to discriminate between events occurring immediately after drug use and those occurring later than 3 days after the last administration. The events were classified according to the WHO Adverse Reaction Terminology

Table 6. NSAID prescriptions

	Drug	Number of prescriptions (of total n = 36,147)	
1.	Diclofenac	14,477	
2.	Ibuprofen	4,037	
3.	Indomethacin	3,896	
4.	Acemetacin	3,633	(a prodrug of indomethacin)
5.	Piroxicam	1,645	
6.	Acetylsalicylic acid	1,211	
7.	Ketoprofen	1,183	
8.	Tenoxicam	1,075	
9.	Naproxen	1,067	
10.	Etofenamate	713	(a prodrug of flufenamic acid)
	Subtotal	32,937	

Table 7. Adverse events and administered NSAIDs

	Drug	No. of AE
1.	Diclofenac	4,891
2.	Indomethacin	1,693
3.	Acemetacin	1,553
4.	Ibuprofen	1,110
5.	Piroxicam	488
6.	Ketoprofen	448
7.	Tenoxicam	359
8.	Naproxen	282
9.	Acetylsalicylic acid	250
10.	Pirprofen	188

under the guidance of an experienced supervisor. In Table 7 the numbers of adverse events reported in users of the 10 most frequently prescribed drugs are given. The proportion and the total number of prescriptions and of adverse events for the four most frequently prescribed NSAIDs can be calculated from Tables 6 and 7.

The drug specific distribution of major adverse events by system organ classes for diclofenac, indomethacin, acemetacin and ibuprofen are given in Table 8. Individual patterns, e.g. the high rate of CNS events with indomethacin, the high rate of GI-tract events with acemetacin, and the high rate of elevated so-called liver enzymes with diclofenac are obvious. The pattern for all NSAIDs shows that the GI-tract is by far the most frequently affected system, followed by the skin, the nervous system, and 'the body as a whole'. It should be mentioned that the WHO category 'body as a whole – general disorders' comprises all forms of oedema, which may be interpreted as effects on the kidneys and the cardiovascular system.

Table 8. Frequencies of adverse events (no. AE/no. prescriptions)

Organ system classes	Diclofenac	Ibuprofen	Indomethacin	Acemetacin
No. of prescriptions	14,477	4,037	3,896	3,633
Gastrointestinal system	14.1%	11.2%	15.9%	19.1%
Skin and appendages	3.5%	3.3%	3.5%	4.5%
Central and peripheral NS	2.5%	3.0%	7.9%	4.8%
Liver and biliary system	2.2%	0.7%	1.8%	1.5%
Body as a whole – general	2.7%	2.2%	3.1%	4.1%

Table 8 also provides frequencies of adverse events in relation to the number of prescriptions. This calculation is a rough estimate of risks and it has to be used and interpreted with great caution as many possible confounders have not yet been examined. It should also be born in mind that the magnitude of 'background' events cannot be subtracted since a 'control group' with rheumatoid patients not treated with NSAIDs is lacking for obvious ethical reasons. Also, the contribution of biases, as e.g. treatment bias, dosage bias etc. are not yet accounted for.

Immediately reportable adverse events (IRAE)

In order to meet the legal requirements for immediate reporting of serious adverse drug reactions in the countries involved and to create a signalling instrument for serious adverse events, the centres had to report such events directly to the project management. According to the project plan, all cases of death, life-threatening or permanently disabling events and events requiring hospitalization or prolongation of hospitalization had to be reported within 24 hours of occurrence to the project manager. Reports were issued for the health authorities, the manufacturers and the Advisory Board. A total number of 220 IRAE were reported in the course of this project (0.8% of all registered treatment cases). Among the IRAE there were 34 cases of death, but none of them was judged to result from NSAID use. A total of 56 IRAE were considered to be associated with the use of NSAIDs. In Table 9 they are summarized by drug and the system organ class according to the WHO. Some of the patients received more than one NSAID either together or in succession within the 6 weeks preceding the IRAE, resulting in a higher number of prescriptions relating to IRAE (70) than IRAE (56).

Table 9. Distribution of 56 IRAE associated with the use of NSAIDs among prescribed NSAIDs and system organ classes

Prescribed NSAIDs	No.	Organ system involved	No.
Diclofenac	21	GI tract	21
Ibuprofen	11	Blood (red, white cells	
Indomethacin	7	and thrombocytes)	18
Acemetacin	5	Urinary tract	5
Piroxicam	5	Respiratory tract	5
Tenoxicam	5	Body as a whole	2
Aspirin	5	CNS	1
Ketoprofen	3	Cardiovascular system	1
Pirprofen	3	Skin and appendages	1
Naproxen	2	Musculoskeletal	1
Tiaprofenic acid	2	Hepatobiliary	1
Benorylate	1		
Diflunisal	1		

CONCLUSIONS

The information given here is extracted from a wealth of details accumulated in the SPALA project. It already shows some distinct patterns of usage and side-effects of NSAIDs. Further evaluation will allow us to establish a complete usage profile of the major drugs in use in the German-speaking part of the world. Moreover, already we have hints that some drugs are specificially associated with e.g. cardiovascular events. This and other information will be detailed in further publications. We are sure that this more detailed information will considerably exceed the data possibly gathered by spontaneous reporting systems [4].

ACKNOWLEDGEMENTS

SPALA was generously funded by a donation from F. Hoffmann-La Roche Ltd (Basel)

REFERENCES

1. The Design of SPALA (Safety Profile of Antirheumatics in Long-Term Administration). Eur J Clin Pharmacol. 1988;34:529–530.
2. Sicherheitsprofil von Antirheumatika bei Langzeitanwendung (SPALA). Muench Med Wschr. 1989;34:103–108.
3. SPALA – Sicherheitsprofil von Antirheumatika bei Langzeitanwendung. Dt Aerztebl. 1990;87:2707–2718.
4. Lasek R, Mathias B, Tiaden JD. Erfassung unerwuenschter Arzneimittelwirkungen. Dt Aerztebl. 1991;88:304–312.
5. Hambleton P, McMahon S. Drug actions on delayed-type hypersensitivity in rats with developing and established adjuvant arthritis. Agents and Actions. 1990;29:328–332.

7

The evaluation of acute gastrointestinal toxicity of NSAIDs in phase I clinical trials: a critical appraisal

A. Del Favero, L. Patoia and L. Santucci*

Istituto di Clinica Medica I, *Istituto di Gastroenterologia ed Endoscopia Digestiva, Policlinico Monteluce, Università degli Studi di Perugia, 06100 Perugia, Italy

Non-steroidal anti-inflammatory drugs (NSAIDs) are among the most widely used drugs and, excluding salicylates, are represented by more than 100 different compounds. Mucosal damage to the upper gastrointestinal (GI) tract is a side-effect common to all NSAIDs. Despite their obvious benefits, the damage they cause in the GI tract is a major health problem in current clinical practice [1]. Although a vast amount of information has accumulated on this topic over many years, only the data published in the very recent past provide convincing evidence that NSAIDs cause severe GI complication and allow the risk to be roughly quantified. Upper GI toxicity occuring after administration of NSAIDs can present a wide spectrum of clinical expressions ranging from relatively mild, but nonetheless discomforting, conditions such as epigastric pain and dyspepsia, to the more serious and potentially life-threatening states, namely GI ulceration and GI bleeding or perforation. Endoscopic evaluation of the upper GI tract in patients treated with NSAIDs reveals a number of lesions that range from simple erythema through diffuse erosions and/or microbleeding to ulceration [2–4]. Roth and Bennett [5] have recently proposed the term 'NSAID gastropathy' to describe those lesions associated with the upper GI tract toxicity that are encountered during NSAID therapy. Damage to the upper GI tract is not limited to the stomach, but can also involve the duodenum and, albeit infrequently, the oesophagus and the intestine.

GI mucosal injury occurring after administration of NSAIDs has been studied in various ways and evidence on the risks of NSAID treatment has mainly been obtained from 4 sources: 1. phase I studies, mainly endoscopic and microbleeding studies, usually conducted in healthy volunteers; 2.

Side-effects of Anti-inflammatory Drugs 3. Rainsford KD, Velo GP (eds), Inflammation and Drug Therapy Series, Volume V.

adverse effects recorded during clinical trials on NSAID therapy; 3. adverse reaction reported to national agencies; 4. *ad hoc* studies, such as case-control or surveillance studies, or as a by-product of data generated through schemes such as prepayment insurance programmes where drug prescriptions can be linked to subsequent events. Each of these sources of information has its merits and limitations, but this paper will deal with phase I trials only.

Clinical investigators and pharmaceutical companies are increasingly faced with the problem of planning phase I clinical trials for investigating new drugs, dosages and/or formulations for their gastrointestinal toxicity. These studies should allow drugs to be identified with lower or greater toxicity than those already on the market and recommendation for continuation in, or withdrawal from, advanced trials.

The aim of this presentation is to highlight the common issues noted in reviewing phase I clinical trials on gastrointestinal toxicity of NSAIDs, to illustrate experience in planning and performing these studies in our Centre and to make a proposal for a consensus on how to perform phase I clinical trials aimed at evaluating NSAID gastrotoxicity.

We reviewed the phase I clinical trials on gastrointestinal toxicity of NSAIDs published in the last 10 years. The Excerpta Medica library was researched, and 42 trials analysed (Table 1).

The problems concerning the study design and methods for assessing gastrointestinal toxicity of NSAIDs will be discussed separately.

Table 1. Phase I studies on gastrointestinal injury from NSAIDs

Total phase I studies	42
Years	1980–1990
Based on	Excerpta Medica
Total number of healthy subjects	946
Total number of patients	206

STUDY DESIGN

Five main characteristics of these studies will be examined: 1. type and number of subjects enrolled; 2. the type of study design; 3. the type of comparator used in comparative studies; 4. the length of the study; 5. the compliance evaluation. These topics have been selected because each of them requires the most careful consideration when planning such phase I trials in order to provide reliable and clinically meaningful results.

Subjects studied

Two main questions should be addressed. Are normal subjects or arthritic patients to be enrolled in this type of phase I trial, and how many subjects have to be studied to provide meaningful results? Most trials (36/42, 85%), not unexpectedly, enrolled young healthy volunteers, usually male. The main reason for utilizing young healthy volunteers is, in our experience, that they are easier to enrol in these studies than arthritic patients. Ethical reasons, for example that the study is not designed to provide evidence of any therapeutic advantage, thus preventing the enrolment of patients, are less convincing. A possible drawback to using healthy volunteers is that this population may not be representative of the one that will be most often prescribed NSAIDs (i.e. elderly, female patients) and toxicity might in consequence be underestimated. However, no evidence in the literature exists that acute toxicity of NSAIDs is greater in elderly patients than in healthy volunteers.

More difficult is the choice of the optimal number of subjects to be enrolled. Most trials (29/42, 70%) have studied 11–20 subjects for each treatment group. This choice is a compromise between the necessity to include a reasonable number of subjects and difficulty in finding volunteers. With this sample size the estimated power of the studies is small and only large differences can be detected (Figure 1). Although this limitation should receive careful consideration when the results are being evaluated, especially when treatments are found to be equivalent, it is not even mentioned in the majority of papers reviewed.

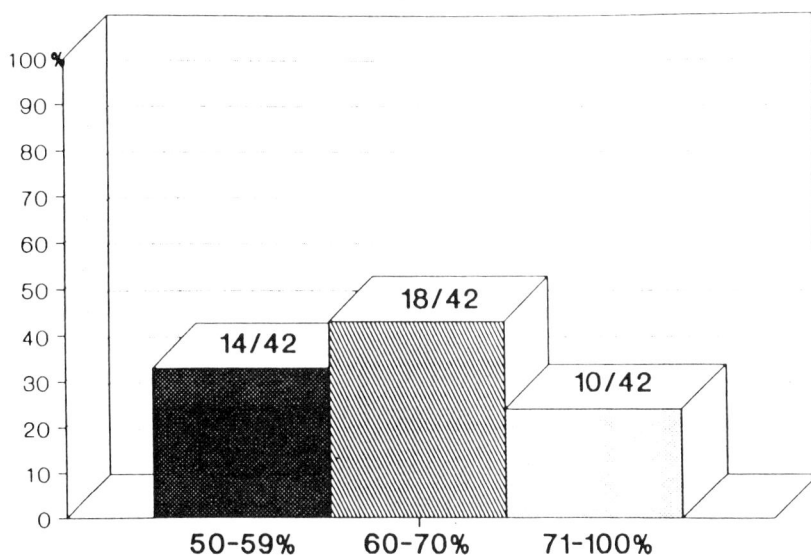

Figure 1. Estimated statistical power of the studies reviewed according to their size ($\alpha = 0.05$; $\beta = 0.2$). Detectable differences as percentages

Study design

Most trials were randomized, double-blind trials, clearly the most appropriate study design (Figure 2). Problems may arise when considering the choice between the parallel or cross-over study design. The parallel group design was adopted for comparing treatments in 59% of the studies, while the other remaining 41% preferred a cross-over design. The advantages and disadvantages of the two methodologies are well known, but their relevance to the type of studies we are interested in should be considered. In our opinion, cross-over design is less likely to offer easily interpreted results, for the following reasons. First, interruption of treatment due to side-effects (not an infrequent occurrence) can nulify the advantage of using the cross-over design; second, assessment and interpretation of carry-over effect can be difficult; in fact the signs of gastric toxicity (i.e. mucosal damage, bleeding and cellular exfoliation) can persist for a long time, even with drugs with a short half-life, and previous exposure to a drug may sensitize the subject to further gastric mucosal damage [6]; last, the necessity to repeat investigations on the same subject limits the number and type of measurements that can be performed. Parallel design is therefore preferable.

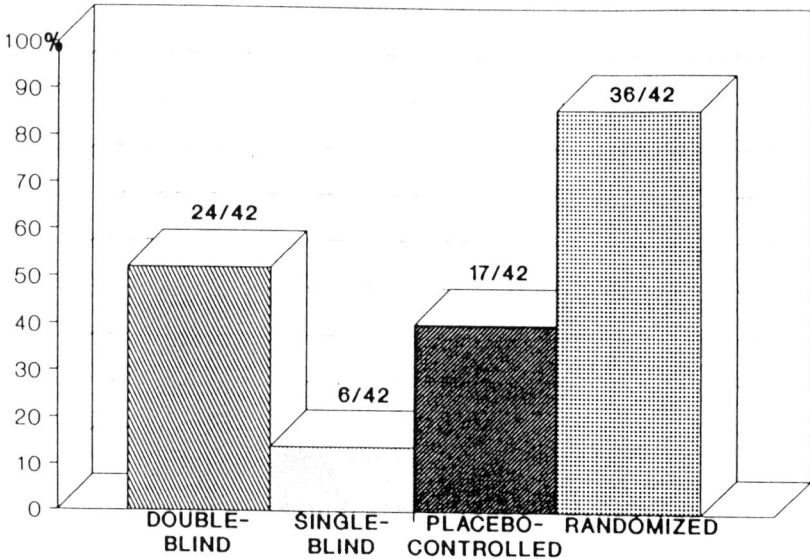

Figure 2. Design of the studies reviewed

46

The comparator

The main issues concern the use of placebo and the choice of the active comparator. Worthy of note is the fact that only 40% of the trials were placebo-controlled (Figure 2). Nonetheless the inclusion of a placebo-group in such studies is important not only for ethical reasons (one can at least offer volunteers the chance of receiving placebo), but also for a correct interpretation of results when the new compound seems to be better tolerated than the active comparator. If not carefully considered, this choice can make the clinical relevance of the study results difficult to interpret. The selection of the type of drug most suitable to become a comparator and the dosage to be chosen is more difficult. Two major considerations may help in making this choice. There is consistent and sufficient evidence that at least two among the most widely used NSAIDs are more gastrotoxic than other compounds in such short term trials: aspirin and indomethacin. Not unexpectedly, they are the most often chosen comparators (18/42), as probably this guarantees a greater chance for a new compound to be shown to be less gastrotoxic. However this may not be the best choice. To achieve clinically meaningful results, any new NSAID should be compared with the best tolerated compound in its class. The most careful consideration should be given to the optimal dose to be employed to avoid introducing a bias in the study, as the gastrotoxicity of the majority of NSAIDs is dose-related. However incomplete knowledge of potency and kinetic characteristics can often make the choice difficult.

Length of treatment

The duration of treatment varied greatly among the studies reviewed, ranging from less than one to four weeks. The choice of the length of treatment should be dictated by the two main variables: the half-life of the compound (long or short) and its indications (short-term analgesic or long-term anti-arthritic drug). Unfortunately, these two aspects are not always considered, and we can see short-term trials with compounds with very long half-life and/or appointed for long-term therapeutic use, making the results of these studies of dubious significance.

Patient compliance

Because poor compliance in clinical trials can result in a new compound being judged less potent (or safer) than it really is, it is now conventional to incorporate some measure of the extent to which patients adhere to the trial protocol in all clinical studies. It is therefore surprising to note that subject or patient compliance was evaluated in only 25% (10/42) of studies. In only one study [7] was it assessed by direct observation of the drug

47

intake (the most appropriate way to assure the best compliance, but surely the most difficult to perform). In the remaining studies compliance was measured by determining the plasma level of the drug at the steady state. Unfortunately, drug plasma levels can vary greatly from one subject to another and this leads to wide standard deviation being accepted as normal, thereby making this method less accurate than generally thought. Even more intriguing are the compliance problems related to some diagnosis techniques such as faecal collection during microbleeding studies, for which no method of monitoring exists.

Although this problem is worthy of more serious consideration, it is probable that non-compliance and its consequences continue to be a problem in these studies.

TYPE AND TECHNIQUES EMPLOYED TO ASSESS NSAID-INDUCED GASTROINTESTINAL DAMAGE

A wide range of diagnostic techniques have been employed in phase I trials to assess the NSAID-related gastrointestinal damage. These techniques have their merits and limitations and when used appropriately can provide useful information. Our attention will be focused mainly on those most often employed.

Endoscopy

Upper gastrointestinal endoscopic evaluation is the technique most frequently used (67% of trials) and has become a must in the evaluation process of any new NSAID as it provides useful data. The most important information derived from endoscopic studies on volunteers can be summarized as follows: 1. subepithelial haemorrhage, erosions and acute ulcers are the most frequent gastroduodenal lesions; 2. the incidence of duodenal injury is usually lower than that of gastric injury and oesophageal damage is even more infrequent; 3. although the dose-response curve for gastrotoxicity of various NSAIDs has not been systematically investigated, endoscopic studies provide evidence for a dose-related effect for some NSAIDs; 4. there is no strict clinical correlation between objective gastroscopic findings and subjective intolerance of medication; 5. non-aspirin NSAIDs cause less gastroduodenal damage than aspirin and the differences between various NSAIDs are usually trivial. However when reviewing the published studies we faced a number of methodological problems that can limit or undermine the information provided by endoscopic studies. First, only 2/28 of these trials evaluated the whole upper gastrointestinal tract (oesophagus plus stomach and duodenum), the remaining studies evaluted only the stomach (11/23, 39%)

or the stomach and duodenum (15/25, 54%), despite the fact that the entire upper gastrointestinal tract can be damaged by NSAIDs, albeit with variable intensity and frequency [8].

Second, because different methods have been applied to defining and quantifying the degree of visualized lesions provoked by NSAIDs, the results of various studies are difficult to compare. The methods most frequently adopted are: a descriptive scale proposed by Lanza [9] (43% of trials) or modifications of this scale (32% of trials) and a visual analogue scale (VAS) (in 14% of the studies). Unfortunately, the Lanza descriptive scale has been modified with time and in some cases VASs incorporated in the line intermediate divisions and/or discrete descriptive terms [10]. This type of analogue scale does not seem to offer any advantage or, even worse, it introduces bias into the measurement provided by the usual VAS and should not be used. The method of scoring the gastrointestinal lesions was not even defined in the remaining 11% of studies.

Last it is worth noting that inter- and intra-observer variability in the endoscopic evaluation of NSAID-related gastrointestinal damage has never been assessed appropriately (i.e. using video-endoscopy). The only study to investigate this problem employed a photographic technique, a debatable choice [9]. It, therefore, remains uncertain whether endoscopy evaluations of NSAID-induced gastrointestinal damage are reproducible. At the very least the repeat endoscopic examination should be performed by the same investigator.

In conclusion, the advantages of endoscopy lie in the direct visualization of mucosal lesions of the oesophagus, stomach and duodenum, even asymptomatic, and the possibility of quantifying the damage by an appropriate scale. However, limitations to be considered are that: the lesions below the Treitz ligament are not visualizable; as the procedure cannot be repeated too often, the mucosa can only be visualized at a specific point in time; since the definition of type and degree of damage has not been standardized and the degree of inter- and intra-observer variability has not been assessed, comparisons between trials are difficult.

Finally, one should consider the fact that the short-term endoscopic studies have been carried out on the hypothesis that analysis of the results of acute NSAID administration in normal volunteers should allow the identification of the propensity of any NSAID to damage the gastrointestinal mucosa when administered to arthritic patients in daily practice. The underlying assumption of this approach is that there is a relationship between acute mucosal injury and major upper gastrointestinal tract adverse events associated with chronic use of these drugs. Unfortunately, such an assumption is far from having been demonstrated to be true. Therefore, short-term studies in normal volunteers and even in arthritic patients are of uncertain value for predicting whether chronic administration of a drug will cause gastroduodenal injury and/or major complications.

Microbleeding studies

The measurement of faecal blood loss by the ^{51}Cr-labelled red blood cells technique was employed in 53% of the studies. The main advantage of this method is that it allows the entity of bleeding from any site in the gastrointestinal tract to be measured for the entire duration of the study. If well standardized it is, in our experience [11], a reproducible technique, but many drawbacks have to be considered. It is not helpful in identifying non-haemorrhagic lesions nor in determining the site of bleeding; false positive results can occur in the case of epistaxis, gingival bleeding and contamination of faeces with menstrual blood or bleeding haemorrhoids; data may be misinterpreted in case of stypsis or incomplete stool collection; it exposes the subject to radiation and, last but not least, it is an unpleasant and time-consuming technique for both investigator and volunteer. Unfortunately there is no alternative method for accurately quantifying blood loss due to NSAID GI toxicity.

Other techniques

The various studies used a number of methods to improve or make the evaluation of gastrotoxicity by NSAIDs more complete. Histology, measurement of gastric pH or acid secretion have been rarely employed (12%, 5% and 12% of studies, respectively) and in our experience have been found useless. Gastric mucosal potential difference (GPD) measurement permits the anatomo-functional integrity of the gastric barrier to be evaluated *in vivo,* and agents such as ethanol, hypertonic solutions and biliary acids, which damage the gastric mucosa directly, are able to produce a significant drop in the GPD. However, the clinical significance of a drop in GPD is unknown and there is no standardized registration technique, making this technique suitable only for research proposals. ^{51}Cr-EDTA has been used to measure gastrointestinal permeability which is enhanced by NSAID administration but experience is very limited and its clinical significance unknown. Determination of prostanoids in the gastric mucosa and DNA recovery in the gastric juice represent techniques still restricted to research laboratories.

Symptoms

Symptoms were evaluated in 25/28 (89%) of the studies: 19/25 (76%) by simple questions and 6/25 (24%) by a specific questionnaire. All the studies reported the number of drop-outs. The evaluation of symptoms is easy, costs little, and should be included in all studies, but it is neither sensitive nor specific.

Combining different methods

Due to the many drawbacks and problems associated with any single method, there is still no ideal investigative modality for evaluating the gastro-irritancy of NSAIDs. In consequence, different methods should be used in combination in an effort to increase the reliability of assessments of gastroirritancy. However only 33% of the studies employed combinations of 2 or more gastrotoxicity evaluation techniques and attempts to correlate the results of these studies disclosed contrasting data. For example, faecal blood loss, as measured by radiochromium labelled RBC correlated well with the extent and severity of gastroscopic findings in the stomach in one study [12], but other studies [13–15] failed to reveal any such correlations, and this is also our experience [16]. Most studies found no correlation between symptoms and endoscopy, but one reported a positive correlation between symptoms and faecal blood loss [17]. Our experience is that gastric potential difference measurements and endoscopic scores do not correlate either [18]. The reasons for the lack of correlation found in most studies are not clear, but can probably be explained by the fact that the various methods explore different aspects of NSAID-induced gastrointestinal injury. A wider use of combined methods in evaluating gastrotoxicity in phase I trials is therefore warranted.

CONCLUSIONS

Review of the phase I clinical studies on NSAID gastrotoxicity published in the last 10 years indicates that the quality of trials on new NSAIDs could and should be improved, so as to provide earlier and more reliable data on the comparative benefit/risk profile of these drugs. The main defects are the small size of population studied, the lack of a placebo-treated group, the choice of a bad comparator, the lack of the compliance evaluation, the use of cross-over design and the utilization of only one method to evaluate NSAID-induced gastrotoxicity. Furthermore the available techniques have not been appropriately evaluated as far as their sensitivity, specificity and reliability are concerned.

Despite the large experience accumulated with these studies a number of questions remain unanswered. The critical question that emerges from the analysis of information derived from short-term endoscopic and microbleeding studies is: how relevant is the information to the chronic daily use of NSAID in the rheumatic population? Probably the result of the studies should be considered as doing no more than generating hypotheses that need confirmation from appropriate epidemiological studies. However, if a new compound is shown to be more gastrotoxic than the comparator or equally gastrotoxic to ASA it is probably wise to consider the withdrawal of the compound from further studies. In conclusion, we should like to propose a consensus for planning the phase I clinical trial for the evaluation of NSAID gastrotoxicity in order to generate more reliable and more comparable data:

STUDY DESIGN: randomized, parallel groups, double-blind, placebo-controlled, with at least 10 subjects for each group and with the assessment of compliance. The length of treatment must be adequate for the drug half-life.

METHODS FOR ASSESSING GASTROTOXICITY: combined endoscopy, with a standardized descriptive score, and faecal blood loss measurement with ^{51}Cr-labelled red blood cells must be employed in combination, along with the evaluation of symptoms.

REFERENCES

1. Del Favero A. Anti-inflammatory analgesics and drugs used in rheumatoid arthritis and gout. In: Dukes MNG and Beeley, eds. Side effects of drugs annual 14. Amsterdam: Elsevier; 1990:79–100.
2. Langman MJS. Epidemiologic evidence on the association between peptic ulceration and antiinflammatory drugs. Gastroenterology. 1989;96:640–644.
3. Graham DY, Smith JL. Gastroduodenal complications of chronic NSAID therapy. Am J Gastroenterol. 1988;83:1081–1085.
4. Roth SH. Nonsteroidal anti-inflammatory drugs: gastropathy, deaths and medical practice. Ann Intern Med. 1988;109:353–354.
5. Roth SH, Bennett RE. Nonsteroidal antiinflammatory drug gastropathy. Arch Intern Med. 1987;147:2093–2096.
6. Graham DY, Smith LJ, Spjut HJ, Torres E. Gastric adaptation. Gastroenterology. 1988;95:327–333.
7. Muller P, Dammann HG, Leucht U, Simon B. Comparison of the gastroduodenal tolerance of tenoxicam and diclofenac Na. Eur J Pharmacol. 1989;36:419–421.
8. Santucci L, Patoia L, Fiorucci S, Farroni F, Del Favero A, Morelli A. Esophageal lesions during treatment with piroxicam. Br Med J. 1990;300:1018.
9. Lanza FL, Royer GL, Nelson RS, Chen TT, Seckman CE, Rack MF. The effects of ibuprofen, indomethacin, aspirin, naproxen and placebo on the gastric mucosa of normal volunteers. A gastroscopic and photographic study. Dig Dis Sci. 1979;24:823–828.

10. Aabakken L, Larsen S, Osnes M. Visual analogue scales for endoscopic evaluation of nonsteroidal anti-inflammatory drug-induced mucosal damage in the stomach and duodenum. Scand J Gastroenterol. 1990;25:443–448.

11. Patoia L, Clausi G, Farroni F, Alberti P, Fugiani P, Bufalino L. Comparison of faecal blood loss, upper gastrointestinal mucosal integrity and symptoms after piroxicam beta-cyclodextrin, piroxicam and placebo administration. Eur J Clin Pharmacol. 1989;36:599–604.

12. Aabakken L, Dybdahal JH, Larsen S, Mowinckel P, Osnes M, Quiding H. A double-blind comparison of gastrointestinal effects of ibuprofen standard and ibuprofen sustained release assessed by means of endoscopy and ^{51}Cr-labelled erythrocytes. Scand J Rheumatol. 1989;18:307–313.

13. Hedenbro JL, Wetterberg P, Vallgren S, Bergqvist L. Lack of correlation between fecal blood loss and drug-induced gastric mucosal lesions. Gastrointest Endosc. 1988;34:247–251.

14. Aabakken L, Dybdahal JH, Eidsaunet W, Haaland A, Larsen S, Osnes M. Optimal assessment of gastrointestinal side effects induced by non-steroidal anti-inflammatory drugs. Scand J Gastroenterol. 1989;24:1007–1013.

15. Giilber R, Korsan-Bengtsen K, Magnusson B, Nyberg G. Gastrointestinal blood loss, gastroscopy and coagulation factors in normal volunteers during administration of acetylsalicylic acid and fluproquazone. Scand J Rheumatol. 1981;10:342–346.

16. Del Favero A, Patoia L. Non steroidal anti-inflammatory drugs: seven year's experience in preparing an annual review. Clin Exp Rheumatol. 1989;7:171–175.

17. Aabakken L, Dybdahal JH, Eidsaunet W, Haaland A, Larsen S, Osnes M. Optimal assessment of gastrointestinal side effects induced by non-steroidal anti-inflammatory drugs. Scand J Gastroenterol. 1989;24:1007–1013.

18. Santucci L, Fiorucci S, Patoia L, Farroni F, Sicilia A, Chiucchiu S, Bufalino L, Morelli A. Gastric tolerance of piroxicam-β-cyclodextrin compared with placebo and with other NSAIDs. An endoscopic and functional study by evaluation of transmucosal potential difference. Drug Invest. 1990;2(Suppl.4):56–60.

8

The ulcerogenic and anti-haemostatic effects of NSAIDs in the gut

C.J. Hawkey

Department of Therapeutics, University Hospital, Nottingham,
NG7 2UH, United Kingdom

'The desire to take medicine is one feature which distinguishes man from other animals. It is one of the most serious problems which we have to deal with.' *Osler 1894*

INTRODUCTION

When patients on NSAIDs present with haematemesis and melaena this may occur because the drugs promote ulceration by their gastric mucosal toxicity or provoke bleeding because of their anti-haemostatic activity [1]. Observations in favour of the latter proposition are that NSAIDs increase the incidence of bleeding but not uncomplicated duodenal ulcer and probably of non-ulcer bleeding; NSAID bleeding often occurs early or with sporadic consumption.

For some time we and others have used microbleeding as a method of investigating the short-term gastric mucosal toxicity of aspirin and other NSAIDs, on the assumption that this reflected mucosal injury [2,3]. Recently, we have investigated whether this is so and have shown that erosions and bleeding can be separated.

GENERAL METHODOLOGY

Figure 1 shows the general methodology used in our studies. Volunteers are endoscoped after a period of 2–28 days drug consumption. Ninety minutes after the final dose an orogastric tube is swallowed, resting juice from the stomach washed out and three timed collections of gastric washings measured for blood using the *ortho*-tolidine reaction [2–4]. Subjects then undergo unsedated endoscopy. Lesions in the oesophagus, body, antrum and duodenum are classified and counted. Four biopsy

Side-effects of Anti-inflammatory Drugs 3. Rainsford KD, Velo GP (eds), Inflammation and Drug Therapy Series, Volume V.

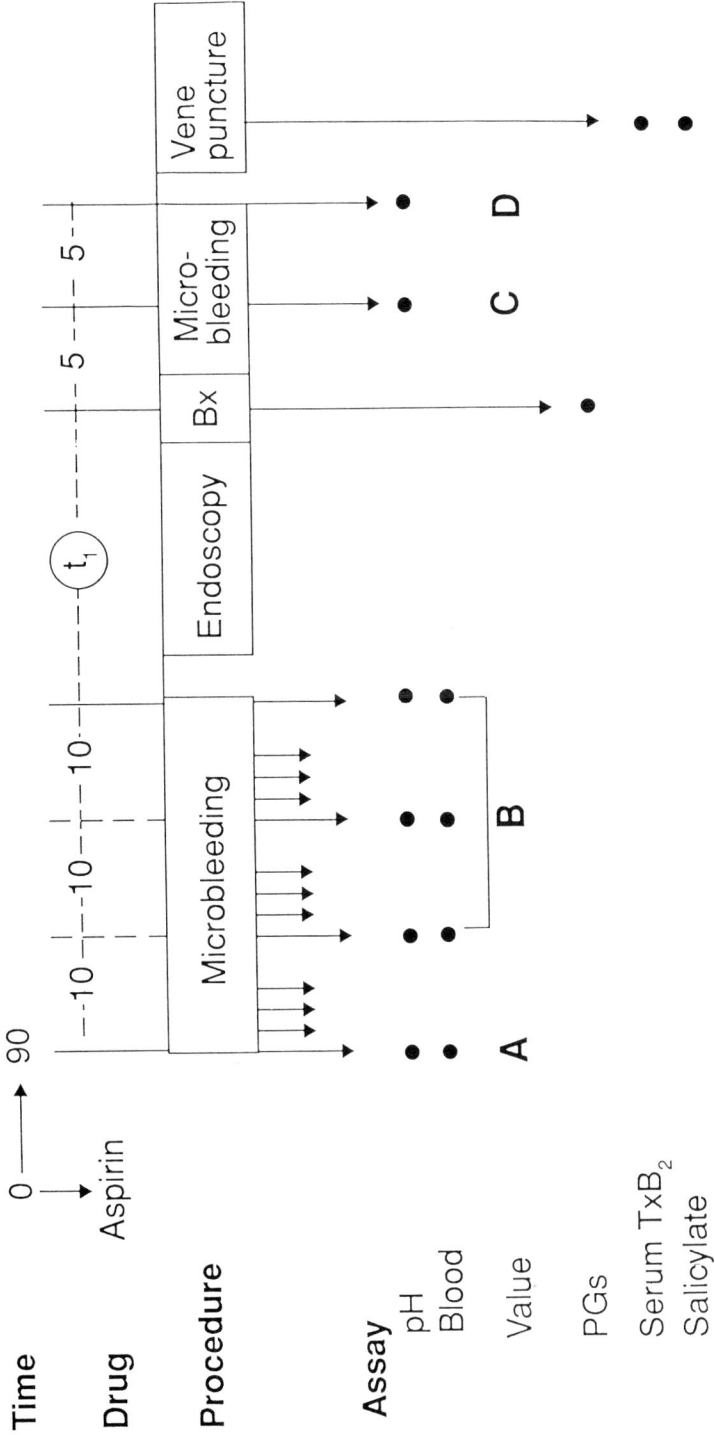

Figure 1. General protocol of volunteer experiments

specimens are then taken over ninety seconds from the greater curve. The endoscope is removed. A further orogastric tube is swallowed and biopsy-induced bleeding measured at five minute intervals for up to twenty-five minutes. Crude biopsy-induced bleeding is corrected for background spontaneous bleeding.

Validation

Three types of lesions occur after consumption of aspirin: haemorrhagic erosions, non-haemorrhagic erosions and intramucosal petechiae. Inter-observer variability studies show that haemorrhagic and non-haemor-rhagic erosions can be distinguished reliably [5]. Observers found difficulty in agreeing about the number of intramucosal petechiae. In patient studies, where additional end points of superficial and deep ulceration were offered, confusion between non-haemorrhagic erosions and superficial ulcers tended to occur (unpublished data).

We also found that using simple counts of lesions was more sensitive than converting them into grades. A comparison of aspirin 300 mg daily with aspirin 1.8–2.4 g daily showed no significant difference in the distribution of Lanza grades but a significant increase from 55 to 105 in the median number of lesions in the stomach as a whole [6].

DEVELOPMENT AND REGRESSION OF INJURY WITH ASPIRIN

A series of volunteers were given aspirin 300 mg or 2.4 g daily for five days. Aspirin 300 mg daily inhibited *ex vivo* PGE_2 synthesis by 57% and was associated with rapid onset of gastric mucosal erosions. PGE_2 inhibition by aspirin 2.4 g daily was significantly greater [7]. Both doses caused maximal reductions in serum thromboxane, and this was associated with enhanced spontaneous bleeding [6,7]. There was some evidence that a break in the mucosa and inhibition of thromboxane were required for this to occur. Thus, erosions occurring during screening endoscopy or consumption of placebo were associated with no increase in mucosal bleeding. A number of patients receiving aspirin (enteric-coated) had no erosions and, despite inhibition of thromboxane, bleeding remained at placebo levels. Thus it appears that the presence of erosions or other breaches in the mucosa and inhibition of thromboxane are required for the bleeding associated with aspirin to occur. Both of these events normally happen rapidly, so that bleeding is evident on the first day of consumption.

PIROXICAM

A completely different pattern is seen with piroxicam [8]. Piroxicam has a long half-life, and prolonged consumption is required for plateau levels of circulating piroxicam to be reached. We conducted the study in volunteers where piroxicam 10 mg bd was given for 21 days. Ten hours after the first dose of piroxicam maximal mucosal injury was seen, consisting of haemorrhagic and non-haemorrhagic erosions in both the body and antrum of the stomach. Over the next 21 days this level of injury neither progressed nor regressed, nor was there a shift in the number of erosions appearing haemorrhagic or non-haemorrhagic. In contrast to aspirin, there was no increase in the rate of spontaneous bleeding, until 21 days of piroxicam consumption, when plasma levels were similar to those previously reported to affect platelet function. Serum thromboxane was not measured in our studies. However, there was a significant correlation between the rate of spontaneous microbleeding and the plasma level of piroxicam, whereas no relationship was seen between the piroxicam levels and mucosal injury. The most likely interpretation for these data is that mucosal injury occurs early with piroxicam as a result of topical injury. Whilst some of these lesions appear to have blood in the base, this is coagulated and increases in active microbleeding do not occur until piroxicam reaches levels capable of inhibiting platelet function [9].

These studies with both aspirin and piroxicam support the notion that a broken mucosa, along with inhibition of platelet function, are required before aspirin and NSAID-associated bleeding increases.

BIOPSY-INDUCED BLEEDING

Taking a biopsy effectively creates a breach in the mucosa and can be used to measure intragastric bleeding in a way that is analogous to the skin bleeding time. Compared to basal levels of bleeding, blood rises by about ten fold [7]. Aspirin 300 mg or 2.4 g daily is associated with an approximate doubling of biopsy-induced bleeding [7].

MUCOSAL PROTECTION

The effect of two strategies of mucosal protection – enteric-coating and co-administration of an acid inhibitor – on injury and bleeding have been investigated. Enteric-coated aspirin results both in a reduced number of mucosal erosions and in a reduced rate of spontaneous bleeding compared to non-enteric-coated tablets [5,6]. The former accounts entirely for the latter and there is no effect on the rate of bleeding per erosion.

H₂ RECEPTOR ANTAGONISTS

By contrast, the phenomena of mucosal injury and haemostasis become separated when intragastric pHs change. Doses of ranitidine which have relatively little effect on the number of mucosal erosions are associated with substantial reductions in spontaneous microbleeding, and in the derived variable bleeding per erosion [10]. This is not surprising since platelet aggregation, plasma coagulation and fibrinolysis are exquisitely sensitive to pH [11]. Thus, platelet aggregation is halved at pH 6.8 and abolished at pH 5.4, whilst, at lower pH, active disaggregation occurs whilst fibrinolysis is enhanced.

SYNOPSIS

These studies suggest that the erosive and anti-haemostatic effect of aspirin can be discriminated in model systems. The implication of the studies is that some strategies such as raising intragastric pH could prevent clinically significant events such as haematemesis and melaena, without necessarily preventing NSAID-associated mucosal injury.

REFERENCES

1. Hawkey CJ. NSAIDs and ulcers: Facts and figures multiply, but do they add up? Br J Med. 1990;300:278–284.
2. Hawkey CJ, Simpson G, Somerville KW. Reduction by enprostil of aspirin-induced blood loss from human gastric mucosa. Am J Med. 1986;81(2A):50–54.
3. Pritchard PJ, Kitchingman GK, Walt RP, Daneshmend TK, Hawkey CJ. Human gastric mucosal bleeding induced by low dose aspirin, but not warfarin. Br Med J. 1989;298:493–496.
4. Fisher MA, Hunt JN. A sensitive method for measuring haemoglobin in gastric contents. Digestion. 1976;14:409–419.
5. Hawthorne AB, Hurst SM, Mahida YR, Cole AT, Hawkey CJ. Aspirin-induced gastric mucosal damage: prevention by enteric-coating of aspirin and relation to prostaglandin synthesis. Br J Clin Pharmacol. 1990;30:187–194.
6. Hawkey CJ, Hawthorne AB, Hudson N, Cole AT, Mahida YR, Daneshmend TK. Separation of aspirin's impairment of haemostasis from mucosal injury in the human stomach. Clin Sci. (in press).
7. Hawkey CJ, Sharma HK, Bhaskar NK, Didcote SM, Hawthorne AB, Daneshmend TK. High and low dose aspirin: equal gastric damage but impaired haemostasis at high dose. Gut. 1989;30:A1442.
8. Fellows IW, Bhaskar NK, Hawkey CJ. The nature and time course of piroxicam-induced injury to human gastric mucosa. Aliment Pharmacol Ther. 1989;3:481–488.
9. McQueen EG. Non-steroidal, anti-inflammatory drugs and platelet function. N Z Med J. 1986;99:358–360.
10. Cole AT, Brundell S, Hudson N, Hawthorne AB, Hawkey CJ. High dose ranitidine prophylaxis of gastric haemorrhagic lesions. Gut. 1990;31:A1187.
11. Green FW, Kaplan MM, Curtis LE, Levine PH. Effect of acid and pepsin on blood coagulation and platelet aggregation. Gastroenterology. 1978;74:38–43.

9

What role does *Helicobacter pylori* infection play in NSAID-associated gastric inflammation?

J.S.A. Collins

Royal Victoria Hospital, Grosvenor Road, Belfast, Northern Ireland,
BT12 6BA, United Kingdom

INTRODUCTION

Since the rediscovery of *Helicobacter pylori* [1] and its isolation in culture [2]; a new pathogenic factor in chronic gastritis [3] and duodenal ulcer disease [4] has been proposed. Although the organism only colonizes the epithelial cells of the gastric mucosa, it has been found in ectopic gastric mucosa and more importantly in areas of gastric metaplasia in the duodenal bulb [4], a vital link in the explanation of its role in duodenal mucosal damage. The particular form of chronic gastritis associated with *H. pylori* infection has been classified by Wyatt and Dixon [5] as Type B gastritis, characterized by polymorph infiltration in gastric pits, infiltration of the lamina propria by mononuclear cells and lymphoid hyperplasia. The form of gastritis associated with NSAID ingestion has been named Type C gastritis by the same authors and, in contrast to Type B, is associated with mucosal oedema, paucity of inflammatory cells, foveolar hyperplasia and vasodilatation. It would be reasonable to postulate that NSAID ingestion might be associated with a greater risk of gastric mucosal inflammation in *H. pylori* infected patients with or without peptic ulcer disease. The following article reviews the current literature in this field.

H. pylori AND NSAIDs – THE UNANSWERED QUESTIONS

It is logical to postulate that *H. pylori*-infected mucosa which is exposed to NSAIDs could be at higher risk of mucosal damage. However, *H. pylori* are dependent on an intact mucous layer for survival and prostaglandin inhibition may damage their habitat. This factor could lead to a paucity or eradication of the organsims or a 'mixed' form of Type B and C gastritis.

Side-effects of Anti-inflammatory Drugs 3. Rainsford KD, Velo GP (eds),
Inflammation and Drug Therapy Series, Volume V.

Studies to date have addressed the following aspects of the *H. pylori* and NSAID relationship.

1. *H. pylori* and NSAID-associated dyspepsia.
2. Prevalence of *H. pylori* in NSAID users.
3. The morphologically dominant type of gastritis in NSAID users.
4. Relationships between NSAIDs, *H. pylori* and endoscopic gastric changes.
5. Relative frequency of duodenal ulcer in *H. pylori*-positive and negative NSAID users.

H. pylori and NSAID-associated dyspepsia

The reasons for NSAID-associated dyspepsia are unclear and the tools for quantification of dyspeptic symtoms are crude [6]. Although *H. pylori*-associated gastritis is found in a significant proportion of patients with non-ulcer dyspepsia, its role is unclear and it does not have a clear correlation with dyspeptic symptoms [3,7]. Upadhyay et al. [8], compared dyspeptic symptoms in 14 patients referred for endoscopy and 38 volunteers all of whom were taking regular NSAIDs. They noted a significant correlation between the presence of *H. pylori* and severity of dyspeptic symptoms. A weakness of their study was a lack of description of symptom data. Shallcross and colleagues used a structured symptom questionnaire to record dyspepsia in a group of patients attending a rheumatology clinic. A past history of dyspepsia was more common in patients serologically positive for *H. pylori* than negative subjects. Dyspepsia was also more frequent in subgroups taking NSAIDs, but it was not significant [7].

Prevalence of *H. pylori* in NSAID-users

Both serological and endoscopic studies have assessed the prevalence of *H. pylori* infection in NSAID users and controls. Shallcross et al. have reported preliminary results of an ongoing study which measured serum antibodies to *H. pylori* in dyspeptic regular NSAID users compared to blood donor serum from the same geographical area [7]. The age-related frequency of *H. pylori* antibodies was not significantly higher in the NSAID group. Jones et al. serologically tested 100 patients who had received NSAIDs for at least 3 months and who had no dyspepsia [9]. A similar group, matched for age, sex, and smoking habits on no therapy were compared. Again, no significant difference in frequency of *H. pylori* antibodies was detected (63% NSAID group *H. pylori*-positive; 51% of control group).

An endoscopic study comparing antral biopsies from 66 patients with rheumatoid arthritis (52 were taking NSAIDs) with 122 unselected dyspeptic patients showed no significant difference in qualitative histological grade between the groups, but suggested a trend towards lower *H. pylori* prevalence in the patients on NSAIDs [10].

Type of gastritis in NSAID-users

The possible role of NSAID use in the aetiology of gastritis was reported in a large review of gastric biopsies from 444 patients undergoing gastroscopy following presentation with dyspepsia [11]. Of the patients, 261 (59%) were *H. pylori*-positive histologically and all but two had gastritis. Only 10% of the *H. pylori*-negative patients had gastritis in contrast. NSAIDs had been taken by 23% prior to endoscopy and of these 69% were *H. pylori*-positive. In the *H. pylori*-negative patients there was no significant difference in frequency of gastritis between those who had a history of NSAID ingestion and those who had not taken NSAIDs. The authors concluded that Type B chronic gastritis in NSAID users is related closely to *H. pylori* infection rather than the drug and that NSAIDs did not alter the frequency of *H. pylori* infection.

Relationships between NSAIDs, *H. pylori* and endoscopic gastric changes

One of the few studies which has examined the direct effects of NSAID ingestion on the gastric mucosa has been reported by Goggin et al. [12]. After a one week washout period, 43 patients with rheumatoid arthritis were started on NSAID treatment for 4 weeks. Endoscopy with macroscopic grading of the mucosa (LANZA score) was performed at the onset and at 4 weeks. After the washout period, the initial score was significantly higher in *H. pylori*-positive patients. After 4 weeks on NSAID treatment, there was a significant increase in score for both the *H. pylori*-positive and negative patients. However, the mean increase in grade was not significantly greater in the *H. pylori*-positive group. Unfortunately, the authors did not report histological grading before or after treatment.

Pazzi et al. have reported their findings in 51 patients who were NSAID users [13]. All patients were interviewed using a standard questionnaire for dyspepsia, endoscoped and biopsies taken from the gastric antrum. All were then randomized to treatment with 'De-Nol' + NSAID or placebo + NSAID for 4 weeks. They concluded that dyspepsia was initially more common in *H. pylori*-positive NSAID users, and not unexpectedly, at the end of 4 weeks *H. pylori* eradication was associated with 'De-Nol' treatment and improvement in gastric inflammation. Recent

61

studies would suggest that their eradication rate (12/14) at 4 weeks may be an over-estimate and that re-endoscopy should have been performed at least 4 weeks after cessation of therapy [14].

Relative frequency of duodenal ulcer in *H. pylori*-positive and negative NSAID users

To date, only one recently reported study from Taha et al. [15] has examined the link between Type C gastritis, *H. pylori*-associated or Type B gastritis and the occurrence of duodenal ulcer in NSAID users. Of 218 patients, 174 took NSAIDs and 44 did not. C gastritis was found in 46 NSAID users (26%) and in 3 (7%) not on the drugs. Duodenal ulcers were found in 22% patients without any gastritis, 48% with *H. pylori* gastritis ($p < 0.01$) and 54% with C gastritis ($p < 0.001$). The authors conclude that peptic ulcers occur more commonly in NSAID users who have concomitant *H. pylori* infection.

CONCLUSION

The implication that the combination of *H. pylori* and NSAID use could have an adverse effect on dyspepsia, gastritis and peptic ulcer disease given the wide prevalence of *H. pylori* infection and usage of these drugs is an important one. However, the literature to date is lacking large studies on this topic. It can be concluded that serological studies suggest that NSAID use is not associated with a higher prevalence of *H. pylori* infection but the controversial role of both NSAIDs and *H. pylori* in the aetiology of dyspeptic symptoms is not clarified by any study to date. The lack of an adequate, reproducible measure of the multitude of symptoms which constitute the term dyspepsia is the most important factor preventing a valid conclusion in this field. The role of *H. pylori* plus NSAID ingestion in the pathogenesis of a particular type of gastritis does not seem to have emerged clearly either. It appears that the predominant type of gastritis seen in NSAID users is that of *H. pylori* rather than NSAID-related and although *H. pylori* plus NSAIDs may produce a marked macroscopic gastric mucosal change, a clear quantitative or morphometric study on gastric biopsies before and after NSAID treatment in *H. pylori*-positive and negative groups is required.

Future work in this field should concentrate on large randomized controlled studies using reproducible quantitative histological methods. In addition, *H. pylori* eradication studies with before and after histological sampling would be helpful. Finally, a long-term follow-up of the gastritis in *H. pylori*-infected NSAID users should be carried out to assess long-term peptic ulcer risk compared to non-infected subjects.

REFERENCES

1. Warren JB, Marshall B. Unidentified curved bacilli on gastric epithelium in active, chronic gastritis. Lancet. 1983;1:1273–1275.
2. Marshal B, Warren JR. Unidentified curved bacilli in the stomach of patients with gastritis and peptic ulceration. Lancet. 1984;1:1311–1314.
3. Collins JSA, Hamilton PW, Watt PCH, Sloan JM, Love AHG. Superficial gastritis and Campylobacter pylori in dyspeptic patients – a quantitative study using computer-linked image analysis. J Pathol. 1989;158:303–310.
4. Wyatt JI, Rathbone BJ, Dixon MF et al.. Campylobacter pyloridis and acid-induced gastric metaplasia in the pathogenesis of duodenitis. J Clin Pathol. 1987;40:841–848.
5. Wyatt JI, Dixon MF. Chronic gastritis – a pathogenetic approach. J Pathol. 1988;154:113–124.
6. Larkai EN, Lacey-Smith J, Lidsky MD, Graham DY. Gastroduodenal mucosa and dyspeptic symptoms in arthritic patients during chronic non-steroidal anti-inflammatory drug use. Am J Gastroenterol. 1987;82:1153–1158.
7. Shallcross TM, Rathbone BJ, Heatley RV. Campylobacter pylori and non-ulcer dyspepsia. In: Rathbone BJ, Heatley RV, eds. Campylobacter pylori and gastroduodenal disease. Oxford:Blackwell:1989:155–166.
8. Upadhyay R, Howatson A, McKinlay A, Danesh BJZ, Sturrock RD, Russell R. Campylobacter pylori associated gastritis in patients with rheumatoid arthritis taking non-steroidal anti-inflammatory drugs. Br J Rheumatol. 1988;27:113–116.
9. Jones DM, Eldridge J, Whorwell PJ, Srivastava ED, Maxton DG. Campylobacter pylori colonisation and non-steroidal anti-inflammatory drugs. Klin Wochenschr. 1989;GI Suppl XVII:33(Abstract).
10. Pazzi P, Trevisani L, Sartori S et al. May NSAIDs have a protective role againsst Campylobacter pylori infection? Klin Wochenschr. 1989;67(Suppl XVIII):53(Abstract).
11. Shallcross TM, Rathbone BJ, Wyatt JI, Heatley RV. C. pylori is the cause of 'Non-Steroidal Gastritis'. Klin Wochenschr. 1989;67(Suppl XVIII):63(Abstract).
12. Goggin PM, Collins DA, Marrero JM, Corbishly CM, Bourke BE, Northfield TC. Does H. pylori potentiate the damaging effect of non-steroidal anti-inflammatory drugs (NSAIDs)? Rev Esp Enf Digest.1990;78(Suppl I):79(Abstract).
13. Pazzi P, La Corte R, Trevisani L, Sighinolfi D, Sartori S, Scagliarini R. Non-steroidal anti-inflammatory drug (NSAID) – induced dyspepsia: is Helicobacter pylori (HP) implicated. Rev Esp Enf Digest. 1990;78(Suppl I):69(Abstract).
14. Rauws EAJ, Tytgat GN. Campylobacter: treatment of gastritis. In: Rathbone BJ, Heatley RV, eds. Capmylobacter pylori and gastroduodenal disease. Oxford:Blackwell;1989:225–231.
15. Taha SD, Nakshabendi I, Boothman P et al. Chemical gastritis and Helicobacter pylori in patients receiving non-steroidal anti-inflammatory drugs – correlation with peptic ulcer. Gut. 1991;(Abstract in press).

10
Endoscopic evaluation of NSAID ulceration

Frank L. Lanza

Clinical Professor of Medicine, Section of Gastroenterology,
Baylor College of Medicine, Houston, Texas, USA

INTRODUCTION

The first endoscopic observation of gastric mucosal injury due to aspirin occurred in 1938 [1]. Subsequently, numerous anecdotal observations of similar injury were reported in the medical literature. The advent of fibreoptic endoscopy and photography in the 1960s made it much easier to evaluate the effects of aspirin and other non-steroidal anti-inflammatory agents (NSAIDs) on the gastric and duodenal mucosa. In 1975 we reported the first double-blind controlled endoscopic study of mucosal injury due to these agents [2]. In that study, we developed a 0 to 4 grading system which primarily dealt with mucosal haemorrhages and ulcer. In recent years, improved fibreoptic bundles and more sophisticated photographic and video-endoscopic techniques have led us to appreciate the incidence and significance of erosions as well as haemorrhages and ulcers. At the present time, there is a huge body of well-controlled endoscopic studies in the literature evaluating this injury both in normal volunteers and patients [3]. Most of these studies utilize the 0 to 4 rating scale, however, many other scoring systems have also been employed. At the present time, it is generally felt that erythema and mucosal haemorrhages are of no clinical significance. The significance of erosions depends upon their numbers and depth and whether or not they ultimately develop into ulcers. Ulcers are always highly clinically significant, since, without the ulcer lesion, the complications of haemorrhage and perforation, and the therapy-limiting occurrence of intractable pain cannot occur.

PATHOPHYSIOLOGY AND LESION DEVELOPMENT

The pathophysiological sequence of events and the relationship between these lesions is not well known. Time sequence studies after aspirin administration have shown that haemorrhages occur first, usually within

Side-effects of Anti-inflammatory Drugs 3. Rainsford KD, Velo GP (eds),
Inflammation and Drug Therapy Series, Volume V.

the first hour after administration. After about twenty-four hours erosions begin to occur. Haemorrhagic areas and erosions both tend to maximize in three to seven days [4,5]. In a small percentage of cases, a well-developed ulcer can be seen at the end of a week [3]. With the passage of time, cytoadaptation occurs and both haemorrhages and erosions begin to disappear in a majority of subjects [6]. In some subjects, however, these lesions can persist and in others frank ulceration occurs. Similar studies have not been done with the other NSAIDs. Some short-term studies with ibuprofen have shown that haemorrhages and erosions, and, indeed also some ulcers can be seen in as little as three days [7,8].

SCORING SYSTEM

With the above in mind, we have developed a scoring system which takes into account the relative importance of the lesion seen (Table 1). This system lends much greater weight to erosions and ulcers than to haemorrhages. Studies have shown that systems which give equal weight to haemorrhages and erosions tend to be very inaccurate and misleading [9,10]. In this system, scores of 0 and 1 are of no clinical significance; two is of doubtful significance; and 3 and 4 are clinically significant; therefore, it should not be possible to obtain a score of 3 or 4 unless erosions and/or ulcer are present.

We feel strongly now that haemorrhages are trivial lesions. They can occur in a significant number of normal people on no medications. There is also evidence that they arise by an entirely different mechanism than erosion or ulcers [10]. They are found more often in the upper stomach, whereas erosions and ulcers are usually confined to the lower stomach in subjects and patients taking NSAIDs. Whether some erosions ultimately become ulcers has not been determined. However, they occur in the same area and often exist side by side. At the present time the evidence points to the fact that the vast majority of erosions ultimately disappear via cytoadaptation, however, some must ultimately develop into frank ulceration. The evidence for their clinical significance, therefore, is based on this hypothesis.

Table 1. Mucosal injury scoring system

Grade	Description
0	No visible injury
1	Less than 10 haemorrhages with no erosions
2	10–25 haemorrhages and/or 1–5 erosions
3	More than 25 haemorrhages and/or 6–10 erosions
4	More than 10 erosions and/or ulcer

Unfortunately, a large majority of ulcers in both patients and volunteers are asymptomatic. In studies on both osteoarthritic as well as rheumatoid patients taking NSAIDs, a fifteen to twenty percent incidence of ulcer is seen [11,12]. Obviously, all of these patients do not bleed or perforate, or, for that matter, have significant symptomatology, but on the other hand, for these complications to occur, an ulcer must be present. The next step upward then, is obviously determining which patients taking NSAIDs who do develop ulcer subsequently develop complications. There are no controlled prospective trials addressing this problem. Retrospective and prospective case controlled case studies have shown, however, that elderly patients, especially females, patients with a prior history of peptic ulcer and patients with other debilitating diseases are more prone to these complications [13–15].

SIGNIFICANT INJURY AND PROTECTION

It is important to screen out those agents which are in themselves highly toxic, and also to determine the appropriate doses of other efficacious NSAIDs so as to protect the population at risk from the complications of NSAID therapy. It is necessary, therefore, to evaluate these agents first in normal volunteers and then in patients. To do this there must be a scoring system to evaluate injury. Among the various scoring systems proposed the 0 to 4 system has proven itself to be reliable and reproducible [3]. Agents which produce significant injury (3–4 +) in normal volunteers also do so in patients. Unfortunately, the converse is not true. Some agents which produce no injury in volunteers [16] can produce significant injury in patients. Sulindac is an excellent example of this phenomenon [17]. Nevertheless, a normal volunteer model serves as an excellent positive screen and is cheaper, quicker and safer than long-term studies in the target population, i.e. elderly and debilitated patients.

The normal volunteer model has also served well in evaluating various mucosoprotective agents. The results seen in normal volunteers with misoprostol and H_2-receptor antagonists were subsequently verified in patients taking NSAIDs. These studies showed that misoprostol in antisecretory doses protected both the stomach and duodenum, while antisecretory doses of an H_2-receptor antagonist protected primarily the duodenum and not the stomach [18]. Non-antisecretory doses of misoprostol protected the stomach but not the duodenum [19]. Subsequent studies in patients yielded essentially the same results [12,20,21]. These findings in normal volunteers are based on the 0 to 4 scale with the break point for mucosal protection being 2 or less.

Longer-term studies are now in progress to evaluate the effects of these various agents on patients with musculoskeletal diseases. In many of these the success–failure breakpoint is ulcer or no ulcer. In some studies, multiple erosions are also considered as clinically significant injury. It needs to be pointed out that only with the endoscope can the presence or absence of ulcers or erosions be confirmed. This is especially true in the stomach where even with the best radiographic techniques, only 50–75% of ulcers can be detected and erosions cannot be seen at all.

In summary, we feel strongly that a 0–4 endoscopic rating system should be employed in the evaluation of gastric and duodenal mucosal injury due to NSAIDs and other noxious agents. Clinical significance should be attached only to those findings which score 3+ or 4+ on such a scale. We also feel that the normal volunteer model is an excellent positive screen for drug toxicity and for dose-ranging studies. Lastly, we recommend that this system also should be used for the evaluation of mucoso-protective agents in normal volunteers and patients taking NSAIDs.

REFERENCES

1. Douthwaite AH, Lintott GAM. Gastroscopic observation of the effect of aspirin and certain other substances on the stomach. Lancet. 1983;2:1222–1225.
2. Lanza FL, Royer GL and Nelson RS. An endoscopic evaluation of the effects of non-steroidal anti-inflammatory drugs on the gastric mucosa. Gastrointest Endosc. 1976;21(3):103–105.
3. Lanza FL. A review of gastric ulcer and gastroduodenal injury in normal volunteers receiving aspirin and other non-steroidal anti-inflammatory drugs. Scand J Gastroenterol. 1989;24(Suppl 163):36–43.
4. O'Laughlin JC, Silvoso GR, Ivey KJ. Healing of aspirin-associated peptic ulcer disease despite continued salicylate ingestion. Arch Intern Med. 1981;141:781–783.
5. Graham DY, Smith JL, Dobbs SM. Gastric adaptation occurs with aspirin administration in man. Dig Dis Sci. 1983;38:1–6.
6. Graham DY, Smith JL, Spjut HJ, Torres E. Gastric adaptation. Studies in humans during continous aspirin administration. Gastroenterology. 1988;95:327–333.
7. Lanza FL, Royer GL, Nelson RS. An endoscopic evaluation of the effects of aspirin, non-steroidal anti-inflammatory agents and alcohol, separately and in combination on gastric and duodenal mucosa. Gastroenterology. 1983;84(5):1224.
8. Lanza FL. Endoscopic studies of gastric and duodenal injury after use of ibuprofen, aspirin and other non-steroidal anti-inflammatory agents. Am J Med (Suppl). 1984;19–24.
9. Berkowitz JM, Rogenes PR, Sharp JT, Warner CW. Ranitidine protects against gastroduodenal mucosal damage associated with chronic aspirin therapy. Arch Intern Med. 1984;148:2137–2139.
10. Lanza FL, Graham DY, Davis RE, Rack MF. Endoscopic comparison of cimetidine and sucralfate for the prevention of naproxen-induced acute gastroduodenal injury: effect of scoring method. Dig Dis Sci. 1990;35(12):1494–1499.
11. Larkai EN, Smith JL, Lidsky MD, Graham DY. Gastroduodenal mucosa and dyspeptic symptoms in arthritic patients during chronic non-steroidal anti-inflammatory drug use. Am J Gastroenterol. 1987;82:1153–1158.
12. Graham DY, Agrawal N, Roth SH. Prevention of NSAID-induced gastric ulcer with the synthetic prostaglandin, misoprostol – a multicenter double-blind placebo controlled trial. Lancet. 1988;2:1277–1280.
13. Somerville K, Faulkner G, Langham M. Nonsteroidal anti-inflammatory drugs and bleeding peptic ulcer. Lancet. 1986;1:242–244.

14. Collier D St J, Pain JA. Nonsteroidal anti-inflammatory drugs and peptic ulcer perforation. Gut. 1985;26:359–363.
15. Armstrong CP, Blower AL. Nonsteroidal anti-inflammatory drugs and life-threatening complications of peptic ulceration. Gut. 1987;28:527-532.
16. Lanza FL, Nelson RS, Rack MF. A controlled endoscopic study comparing the toxic effects of sulindac, naproxen, aspirin and placebo on the gastric mucosa of healthy volunteers. J Clin Pharmacol. 1984;24:89–95.
17. Carson JL, Strom BL, Morse L, et al. The relative gastrointestinal toxicity of non-steroidal anti-inflammatory drugs. Arch Intern Med. 1987;147:1054–1059.
18. Lanza FL, Aspinall RL, Swabb EA, et al. A double-blind placebo-controlled endoscopic comparison of the cytoprotective effects of misoprostol vs cimetidine on tolmetin-induced mucosal injury to the stomach and duodenum. Gastroenterology. 1988;95(2):289–294.
19. Lanza FL, Fakouhi A, Rubin A, et al. A double-blind placebo controlled comparison of the efficacy and safety of 50 mcg, 100 mcg and 200 mcg of misoprostol q.i.d. in the prevention of ibuprofen induced gastric and duodenal mucosal lesions and symptoms. Am J Gastroenterol. 1989;84(6):633–636.
20. Robinson MG, Griffin JW, Bowers J, Kogan FJ, Kogut DG, Lanza FL, Warner CW. Effect of ranitidine gastroduodenal mucosal damage induced by non-steroidal antiinflammatory drugs. Dig Dis Sci. 1989;34(3):424–428.
21. Ehsannulah RSK, Page MC, Tildesley G, Wood JR. Prevention of gastroduodenal damage induced by non-steroidal anti-inflammatory drugs: controlled trial of ranitidine. Br Med J. 1988;297:1017–1021.

11

Food antigen absorption in rheumatoid arthritis: effect of acetylsalicylic acid

U. Fiocco, U. Fagiolo[1], R. Paganelli[2], L. Cozzi, M. Rosada, E. Cozzi[1], M. Lama[1] and S. Todesco

Division of Rheumatology, [1]Institute of Internal Medicine, University of Padua, Padua, Italy and [2]Department of Allergy and Clinical Immunology, University La Sapienza, Rome, Italy

INTRODUCTION

Adverse reactions to food antigens have been implicated in the pathogenesis of rheumatoid arthritis, even though the mechanism by which food antigens may cause or perpetuate inflammation is still uncertain. In the case of rheumatoid arthritis (RA), dietary manipulation has been shown to alter clinical manifestations [1–3].

The increased absorption in the passage of macromolecules through the intestinal barrier may be an important step in stimulating the immune system to respond to dietary antigens, which may in turn participate in the perpetuation of arthritis [1,4]. In fact, foods often evoke an immune response in humans, as evidenced by the detection of food antigens, antibodies, circulating immune complexes (CIC) and food-sensitized lymphocytes [1,5] in the blood. On the other hand, gastrointestinal lesions represent a well-known side-effect of prolonged treatment with non-steroidal anti-inflammatory drugs (NSAIDs) [6].

Abnormal gut permeability has been reported in rheumatoid arthritis, but there is uncertainty as to whether or not it may be accounted for by the disease process itself [7,12]. At the moment, evidence is lacking that would show that it is associated with RA.

In this study, β-lactoglobulin (BLG) absorption after a cow's milk challenge in patients with untreated rheumatoid arthritis was compared to data obtained from healthy subjects. Moreover, in order to study whether or not acetylsalicylic acid (ASA) modifies intestinal permeability, a group of RA patients was examined before, during and after ASA treatment.

Side-effects of Anti-inflammatory Drugs 3. Rainsford KD, Velo GP (eds), Inflammation and Drug Therapy Series, Volume V.

In order to evaluate the relationship between ASA and intestinal permeability, BLG absorption was also studied in the control groups after the administration of ASA at various doses.

Finally, the preventive effect of cytoprotective drugs against possible alterations resulting from NSAIDs was investigated in a protocol of co-administration in healthy controls and osteoarthritis patients.

MATERIALS AND METHODS

Patients

Thirteen patients affected with RA and without evidence of atopic disease were selected according to ARA criteria [8]. Mean disease duration was greater than three years. At the time of the study, nine patients had active disease according to clinical and laboratory findings. Eleven had been previously treated with NSAIDs, six with antimalarial drugs, three with steroids and two with gold salts (Table 1).

Table 1. Patients and healthy controls

Groups	Sex M/F	Mean age (years)	Age range (years)	Drugs	
Rheumatoid arthritis	1/12	52.9 ± 10.0	52–64	NSAID	13
				Steroid	3
				Gold salts	2
Control Group A	4/6	36.6 ± 9.2	25–50		
Control Group B	2/3	30.5 ± 7.3	23–40		
Osteoarthritis	1/2	59.0 ± 4.3	56–64	NSAID	3

Three patients affected by osteoarthritis were included in the study: two with primary generalized osteoarthritis and one with secondary osteoarthritis and chronic urticaria. All had been previously treated with non-steroidal anti-inflammatory drugs (Table 1).

Fifteen normal subjects were selected among hospital staff for the absence of atopic or joint disease, or any other current inflammatory or microbial disease. All acted as controls: ten of these formed Group A for BLG absorption study, and five formed Group B for the co-administration study. None were receiving therapy or self-medication at the time of the study (Table 1). All subjects had suspended any treatment at least fifteen days prior to the study.

Oral challenge

In order to evaluate intestinal permeability to BLG all patients and controls were submitted to an oral cow's milk challenge of 10 ml/Kg body weight, after overnight fasting. Blood samples were collected before and at two and four hours after drinking the milk.

BLG absorption in RA patients before and after ASA treatment

BLG absorption was examined in thirteen RA patients after a fifteen-day wash-out period and was compared to that obtained in ten healthy controls (Group A). Nine of these patients were tested again after two and four weeks of 1g ASA treatment per day, and three healthy subjects after one single administration of 1g ASA to compare the effect of ASA on intestinal permeability in rheumatoid arthritis and under normal conditions.

Co-administration protocols

Two protocols were adopted to assess the effect of the co-administration of cytoprotective drugs, given thirty minutes before ASA, on BLG absorption. The first protocol was randomly administered to a group of five controls in single doses at one-week intervals: 1) ASA (aspirin) (300 mg); 2) misoprostol (200 mg) plus ASA (300 mg); 3) ranitidine (150 mg) plus ASA (300 mg); and 4) no treatment. In the second protocol, to a group of three osteoarthritis patients, each challenged 12 hours after completing the following one-week regimens, the following were administered: 1) no treatment (baseline); 2) ASA only (300 mg bid); 3) ranitidine (150 mg bid) plus ASA; and 4) misoprostol (200 mg BID) plus ASA.

Immunological assessment

Immunological evaluations were performed on pre-challenge blood samples of RA patients including: rheumatoid factor (latex agglutination and Waaler-Rose): total serum IgE (Phadezym PRIST, Sweden); IgG anti-IgE (Elisa) [9]; and anti-BLG IgG (RIA) [10].

Immunoreactive circulating BLG was determined in both control and patient blood samples using a solid-phase RIA as reported by Paganelli et al. [11].

71

RESULTS

Antibody response in RA patients

The mean IgE serum level was 87 ± 141 IU/ml. Two patients had IgE levels above normal (393 and 426 IU/ml). IgM rheumatoid factor was present in eight patients. IgG anti-IgE were present in seven of the thirteen cases tested. Five IgE antiglobulin-positive sera were also RF positive, but none of these were found with high IgE levels. IgG anti-BLG (above 50 ng/ml equivalents of IgG) were found in three of the 13 sera tested, which also presented low values of circulating BLG (0.11 ± 0.03 ng/ml).

BLG absorption

Circulating BLG was detected both in healthy controls and in RA patients before milk challenge, at similar levels ranging between 0.02 ± 0.06 ng/ml.

After the milk challenge, the mean maximal value found in ten normal subjects was 0.24 ± 0.12 ng/ml. The mean level of maximal BLG values in RA patients (Figure 1) after challenge was 0.25 ± 0.27 ng/ml with no difference in BLG levels in controls (p = ns) (Table 2).

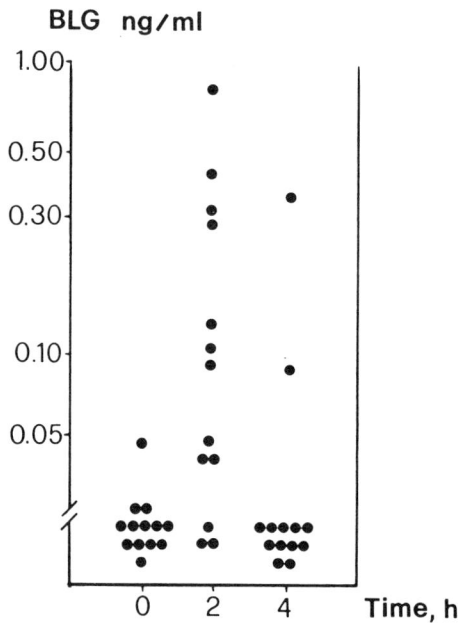

Figure 1. Concentration of BLG in RA patients' sera (n = 13) collected before, 2 and 4 h after challenge with cow's milk

Table 2. BLG absorption (ng/ml) in controls and in rheumatoid arthritis before and after ASA administration

	n	Mean ± SD		
Basal BLG level in controls	10	0.24 ± 0.12		
Basal BLG level in RA	13	0.25 ± 0.27	p:ns	(vs. controls) (Wilcoxon)
BLG level in RA after 15 days of ASA (1 g/day)	9	0.73 ± 0.79	p < 0.01	(vs. baseline) (Mann–Whitney)
BLG level in RA after 30 days of ASA (1 g/day)	9	0.54 ± 0.58	p < 0.01	(vs. baseline) (Mann–Whitney)

BLG absorption after ASA treatment

Higher circulating BLG levels were detected in nine rheumatoid arthritis patients after two and four weeks of ASA treatment (0.73 ± 79 and 0.54 ± 58 ng/ml), when compared to the basal level ($p < 0.01$ – Mann–Whitney) (Table 2). No difference was found between the two periods of ASA treatment (Figure 2). Increasied circulating BLG levels (0.82 ± 0.18 ng/ml) were also detected after the administration of 1g of ASA in three healthy subjects when compared to the basal levels (0.02 ± 0.18 ng/ml).

BLG absorption in co-administration protocol of controls

The baseline mean level of circulating BLG in five healthy subjects was 0.28 ± 0.13 ng/ml. A single test dose of 300 mg ASA induced increased BLG level: 0.78 ± 0.42 ng/ml. After ranitidine (150 mg) co-administration in three subjects, BLG was found unchanged 0.6 ± 0.53 ng/ml. After misoprostol (200 mg) co-administration in four cases, circulating BLG was reduced from a level of 0.7 ± 0.440 ng/ml to a normal level of 0.4 ± 0.22 ng/ml (Figure 3).

BLG absorption in co-administration protocol of osteoarthritis

Basal mean level of circulating BLG in three patients was 1.3 ± 3.0 ng/ml and increased to 3.47 ± 3.3 ng/ml after seven days of ASA (600 mg) treatment. Normal BLG levels were detected both after seven days of 300

BLG ng/ml

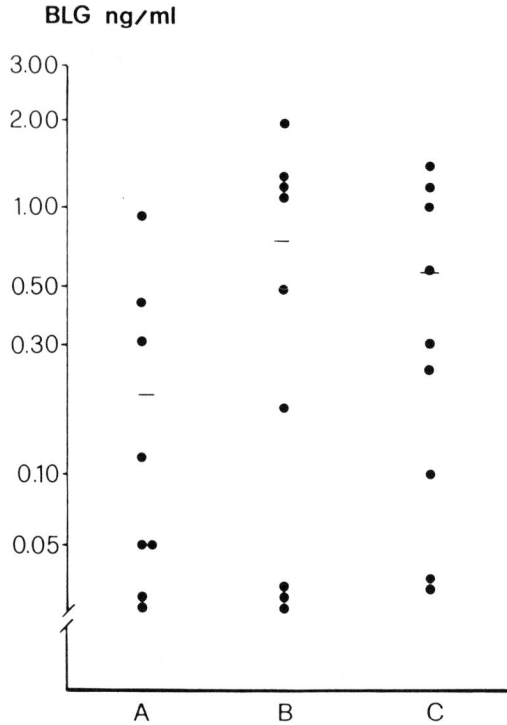

Figure 2. Serum BLG of patients with RA in three separate oral challenges with cow's milk. A: after the wash-out period; B: after 15 days ASA treatment (1 g/day); C: after 30 days ASA treatment (1 g/day)

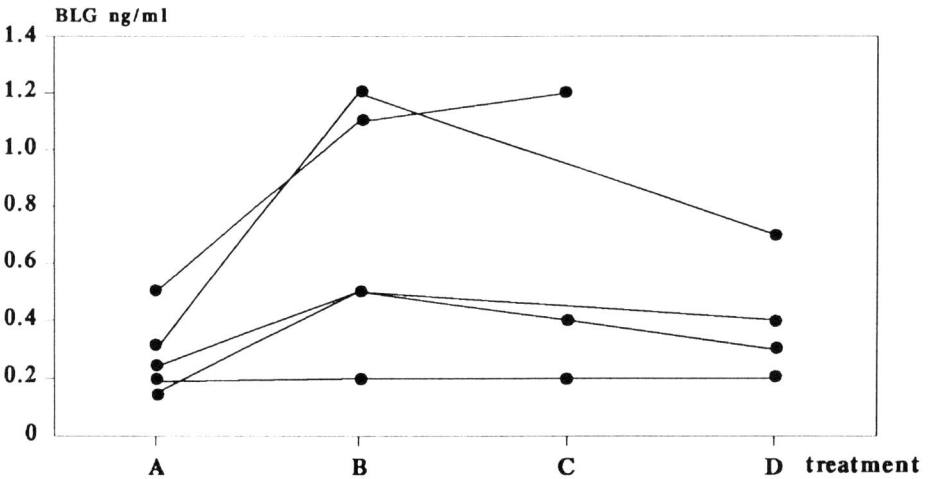

Figure 3. BLG serum before and after single test dose and milk challenge in healthy controls (A: Baseline; B: ASA; C: Ranitidine + ASA; D: Misoprostol + ASA)

mg ranitidine (300 mg) co-administration, with a mean of 0.3 ± 0.10 ng/ml and seven days of 400 mg misoprostol co-administration: 0.23 ± 0.06 ng/ml (Figure 4).

DISCUSSION

β-Lactoglobulin absorption after milk challenge in RA patients after two weeks without treatment was found to be similar to that of healthy controls. These data seem to exclude the possibility that rheumatoid arthritis is associated with changes in the intestinal barrier, at least of BLG and substances with similar molecular size.

Increased passage of BLG across the intestinal wall was detected in our patients after two weeks of ASA treatment and was still present two weeks later (Table 2, Figure 2). A similar increase in BLG immediately after milk challenge was induced by the pre-administration of 1g ASA to healthy controls, further confirming that BLG absorption is directly related to the drug. This effect, occurring after a short period of time, and from a single administration of ASA, suggests a functional and not a toxic mechanism. The results from the study of two cytoprotective molecules with distinct sites of action on the intestinal mucosa interestingly demonstrated different capacities in preventing the changes of intestinal permeability induced by ASA. Only misoprostol was found to be effective in co-administration studies both in single-dose and weekly protocols. Conflicting data

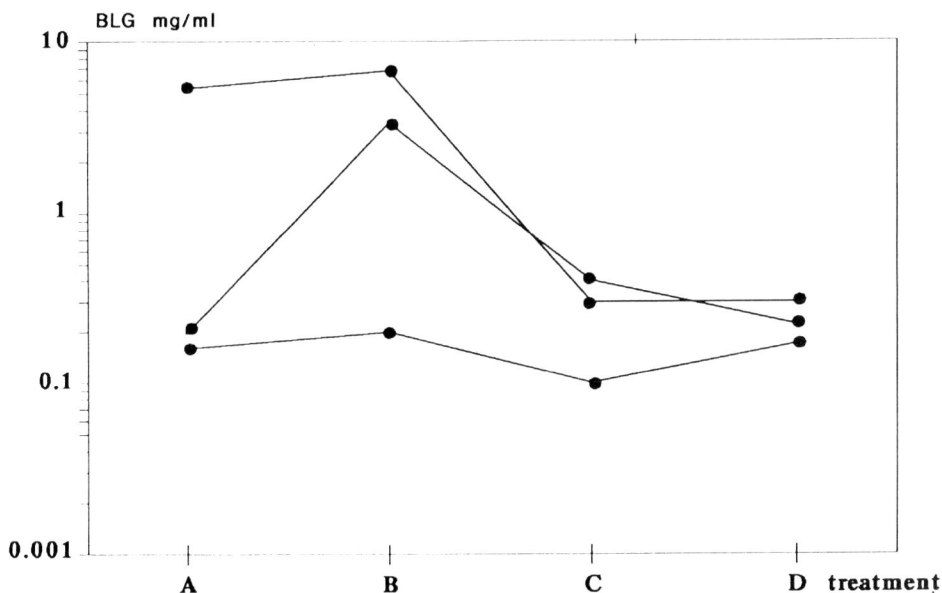

Figure 4. BLG serum level before and after weekly treatments and milk challenge in osteoarthritis (A: Baseline; B: ASA; C: Ranitidine + ASA; D: Misoprostol + ASA)

regarding intestinal permeability in rheumatoid arthritis have been reported when different probes were used [7,12,13]. The increased passage of small molecules (PEG 400) was found directly related to the disease activity [14], and in general, the probes currently used in assessing bowel permeability are smaller than dietary antigens [15]. The precise mechanism involved in the intact macromolecule uptake by the intestinal epithelium is not well understood.

Macromolecules appear to be absorbed by pinocytosis. The general mechanism involves energy-dependent endocytosis, migration to the basal lateral surface of the cell and deposition in the intercellular space [16].

We have examined the absorption of macromolecular dietary antigens in rheumatoid arthritis. Our findings agree with those of Bjarnason et al., who utilizing ^{51}Cr-EDTA, reported increased permeability both in rheumatoid arthritis and osteoarthritis patients after NSAID administration [17].

The mechanisms underlying increased intestinal permeability after NSAID treatment are still uncertain; ^{51}Cr-EDTA and BLG differ in their transport pathway across the intestinal wall, thus augmenting the difficulty in interpreting the effect of the drugs. It has been demonstrated that the uptake of small water-soluble markers does not reflect macromolecular absorption; such differences in the passage of BLG and sugar marker have been previously reported [18].

Using ^{51}Cr-EDTA it was suggested that the increase of permeability induced by the NSAIDs was proportional to the drug's efficacy in inhibiting cyclooxygenase [19]. This was not clearly confirmed in our study because single, small doses of ASA showed a marked effect on permeability (Figure 3).

Nevertheless, our data confirm the importance of local or systemic prostaglandin inhibition. The rapid increase of BLG absorption shortly after ASA intake has been evidenced, and furthermore, misoprostol, a prostaglandin analogue, has been shown to prevent increased BLG permeation induced by ASA either in a single test dose or through a weekly co-administration regimen (Figures 3, 4).

It was previously observed that endogenous and exogenous prostaglandins are also potent regulators of PEG 400 permeation, which may result via the stimulation of mucosal cAMP with inhibition of Na absorption, and therefore, a secondary influence on water flow regulation [20,21]. Prostaglandins regulate the absorption of the small molecules PEG 400 and ^{51}Cr-EDTA via changes in solvent drag and increased absorption through intercellular junctions [21]. Moreover, prostaglandins could modulate tight junctional permeability, through cAMP-mediated action, involving both the orientation of intermembranous strands [22] and contractile proteins of the terminal web [23].

Because the inhibition of cyclooxygenase can increase intestinal permeability (although through different mechanisms), this could explain the similar effect of prostaglandin inhibition on different sized molecules.

From our preliminary observations, ranitidine, an H_2 histamine receptor antagonist, was effective in preventing the ASA-induced increase of BLG absorption in osteoarthritis in a week-long treatment protocol, but showed little capacity in the single ASA dose protocol in healthy controls (Figures 3, 4). This is consistent with previous reports [24], further highlighting the role of prostaglandins in BLG absorption. Moreover, in prolonged treatment in osteoarthritis, the protective effect of ranitidine confirms the efficacy of anti-secretory agents, already reported regarding protein-losing gastropathy [25] (Figure 4).

Our approach, based on the macromolecular food protein BLG as a probe, and its detection in the sera of RA patients, may yield new insights regarding intestinal barrier function and the behavior of biologically active food proteins in rheumatoid arthritis.

Beneficial effects have been reported after diet or fasting in some cases of rheumatoid arthritis [3,12], and consequently, it has been suggested that increased food antigen absorption may be important in the perpetuation of disease [26].

Increased absorption of β-lactoglobulin in our RA patients, in whom none were found to have a history of atopic disease, was apparently unrelated to food sensitization. Nevertheless, IgG anti-IgE was detected in fifty percent of the patients, but without any correlation to the presence of RF, or other circulating immune complex formation, as we previously reported [13]. Therefore, the production of IgG anti-IgE autoantibodies might directly arise from the abnormal immune response associated with rheumatoid arthritis.

The role of IgG anti-IgE antibodies in food sensitivity reactions is controversial, even if their potential importance in basophil degranulation is well-understood [27]. Their possible role in the immune response of the RA patient to food antigens in the absence of high IgE levels, as in our patients, remains unclear.

IgG anti-BLG antibodies were found in 23 percent of our RA patients. Interestingly, these patients also presented the lowest β-lactoglobulin levels.

The production of antibodies to food antigens can lead to the formation of circulating immune complexes with either beneficial or detrimental consequences [28].

Accordingly, we have previously detected increased levels of CICs in rheumatoid arthritis patients after a milk challenge [13,29]. Up to now, it is still to be demonstrated whether IgG anti-IgE or IgG anti-BLG participate in the immunopathological mechanisms involved in the perpetuation of rheumatoid arthritis.

In conclusion, our study showed the β-lactoglobulin absorption test to be a sensitive indicator of changes in small intestine permeability and useful in monitoring cytoprotective therapy. We believe that the oral challenge for assessing food antigen absorption when combined with immunological evaluation of food sensitization may be useful in determining an early diagnosis of food intolerance and in selecting those patients who would benefit from dietary restriction.

The relationship between the absorption of food antigens in rheumatoid arthritis and their immunopathogenic consequences is open to further study.

We would like to acknowledge Rae Beno for her editing and preparation of the manuscript.

REFERENCES

1.   Panush RS. Food allergy and rheumatic diseases. Ann Allergy. 1986;56:500–503.
2.   Darlington LG. Does food intolerance have any role in the aetiology and management of rheumatoid disease? Ann Rheum Dis. 1984;44:801–804.
3.   Darlington LG, Ramsey NW, Mansfield JR. Placebo-controlled, blind study of dietary manipulation therapy in rheumatoid arthritis. Lancet. 1986;1:236–238.
4.   Panush RS. Nutritional therapy for rheumatic diseases. Ann Intern Med. 1987;106:619–621.
5.   Panush RS, Stroud RM, Webster EM. Food-induced (allergic) arthritis. Inflammatory arthritis exacerbated by milk. Arthritis Rheum. 1986;29:220–226.
6.   Fries JF, Miller SR, Spitz PW et al. Toward an epidemiology of gastropathy associated with non-steroidal antiinflammatory drug use. Gastroenterology. 1989;96:647–655.
7.   Jenkins RT, Rooney PJ, Jones DB et al. Increased intestinal permeability in patients with rheumatoid arthritis: a side effect of oral non-steroidal anti-inflammatory (NSAID) therapy? Br J Rheumatol. 1987;26:103–107.
8.   Arnett FC, Edworthy SM, Bloch DA et al. The American Rheumatism Association 1987 Revised Criteria for the classification of rheumatoid arthritis. Arthritis Rheum. 1988;31:315–324.
9.   Quinti I, Brozek C, Wood N et al. Circulating IgG autoantibodies to IgE in atopic syndromes. J Allergy Clin Immunol. 1986;77:586–594.
10. Turner MW, Paganelli R, Levinsky RJ et al. Antigen-binding radioimmunoassays for human IgG antibodies to bovine β-lactoglobulin. J Immunol Meth. 1983;56:175–183.
11. Paganelli R, Levinsky RJ. Solid phase radioimmunoassay for detection of circulating food proteins in human serum. J Immunol Meth. 1980;37:333–341.11.
12. Sundquist T, Lindstroem F, Magnusson KE et al. Influence of fasting on intestinal permeability and disease activity in patients with rheumatoid arthritis. Scand J Rheumatol. 1982;11:33–38.
13. Fagiolo U, Paganelli R, Ossi E et al. Intestinal permeability and antigen absorption in rheumatoid arthritis. Effects of acetylsalicylic acid and sodium chromoglycate. Int Arch Allergy Appl Immunol. 1989;89:98–102.
14. Smith MD, Gibson RA, Brooks PM. Abnormal bowel permeability in ankylosing spondylitis and rheumatoid arthritis. J Rheumatol. 1985;12:299–305.
15. Rooney PJ, Jenkins RT, Buchanan WW. A short review of the relationship between intestinal permeability and inflammatory joint disease. Clin Exp Rheumatol. 1990;8:75–83.
16. Walker WA, Isselbacher KJ. Uptake and transport of macromolecules by the intestine. Gastroenterology. 1974;67:531–550.

17. Bjarnason I, Williams P, So A et al. Intestinal permeability and inflammation in rheumatoid arthritis. Effects of non-steroidal anti-inflammatory drugs. Lancet. 1984;2:1171–1173.

18. Weaver LT, Coombs RRA. Does 'sugar' permeability reflect macromolecular absorption? A comparison of the gastrointestinal uptake of lactulose and β-lactoglobulin in the neonatal guinea pig. Int Arch Allergy Appl Immunol. 1988;85:133–135.

19. Bjarnason I, Williams P, Smethurst P et al. Effect of non-steroidal anti-inflammatory drugs and prostaglandins on the permeability of the human small intestine. Gut. 1986;27:1292–1297.

20. Kimberg DV, Field M, Johnson J et al. Stimulation of intestinal mucosal adenyl cyclase by cholera enterotoxin and prostaglandins. J Clin Invest. 1971;50:1218–1230.

21. Krugliak P, Hollander D, Le K et al. Regulation of polyethylene glycol 400 intestinal permeability by endogenous and exogenous prostanoids. Influence of non-steroidal anti-inflammatory drugs. Gut. 1990;31:417–421.

22. Duffey ME, Hainan B, Ho S et al. Regulation of epithelial tight junction permeability by cyclic AMP. Nature. 1981;294:451–453.

23. Madara JL. Tight junction dynamics: is paracellular transport regulated? Cell. 1988;53:497–498.

24. Bjarnason I, Smethurst P, Fenn CG et al. Misoprostol reduces indomethacin-induced changes in human small intestinal permeability. Dig Dis Sci. 1989;34:407–411.

25. Overholt BF, Jeffries GH. Hypertrophic, hypersecretory protein-losing gastropathy. Gastroenterology. 1979;58:80–86.

26. Panush RS. Food-induced (allergic) arthritis: clinical and serologic studies. J Rheumatol. 1990;17:291–294.

27. Johansson SGO. Anti-IgE antibodies in human serum. J Allergy Clin Immunol. 1986;77:555–557.

28. Paganelli R, Quinti I, D'Offizi GP et al. Immune complexes in food allergy: a critical reappraisal. Ann Allergy. 1987;59:157–161.

29. Fagiolo U, Ossi E, Paganelli R et al. Food antigen absorption and immune complex behaviour in chronic urticaria with associated joint involvement and in rheumatoid arthritis. Progr Rheumatol. 1987;3:141–146.

12

Intestinal mucosal permeability in inflammatory rheumatic diseases

H. Mielants, E.M. Veys, S. Goemaere, M. De Vos, C. Cuvelier, M. Maertens and C. Ackerman

Department of Rheumatology, Ghent University Hospital, Ghent, Belgium

INTRODUCTION

The gut must be considered an outside surface. Before material enters the body, it must traverse the mucosa either actively or passively. The gut acts as a selective barrier to the luminal material, consisting not only of nutrients, water and electrolytes but also of bacteria and antigens. Abnormalities in the gut membrane, e.g. inflammation or disturbed permeability, could lead to an enhanced uptake of antigens which can induce inflammatory responses in target organs.

Permeability implies transfer by passive diffusion. This can occur paracellularly (as determined by ^{51}Cr-EDTA, lactulose, oligosaccharides) or transcellularly (as assayed with monosaccharides, PEG 400).

Increased gut permeability has been demonstrated in ankylosing spondylitis [1,2] and in rheumatoid arthritis [1,3].

Bjarnason et al. have demonstrated that non-steroidal anti-inflammatory drugs (NSAIDs) are capable not only of increasing gut permeability [4,5] but also of inducing gut inflammation [6].

Since most patients suffering from inflammatory rheumatic diseases frequently take NSAIDs or corticosteroids, the first part of this study is concerned with the effect not only of NSAIDs but also steroids on gut permeability in inflammatory rheumatic diseases and in controls.

On the other hand some authors demonstrated that patients with ankylosing spondylitis [1,2] or rheumatoid arthritis [1,7,8] taking no NSAIDs have an increased gut permeability or ileocaecal inflammation on indium-111 (^{111}In) leucocyte scans.

We obtained ileocolonoscopic evidence of subclinical gut inflammation in the spondylarthropathies [9] which correlated with the presence of joint inflammation [10]. We were able to subdivide the gut inflammation into

Side-effects of Anti-inflammatory Drugs 3. Rainsford KD, Velo GP (eds), Inflammation and Drug Therapy Series, Volume V.

two different histologic forms (acute and chronic) [11] with not only specific histologic features but also a different genetic basis [12] and probably a different pathogenetic relation [13].

In the second part of this study we have tried to establish whether the gut inflammation found on ileocolonoscopy had any influence on gut permeability.

MATERIALS AND METHODS

Subjects

Two-hundred and twenty-six subjects were included in the study (Table 1): 129 patients suffering from inflammatory joint diseases (73 patients with spondylarthropathies, 56 patients with active rheumatoid arthritis). The male:female ratio was 66:63; mean age 48 years. Of those patients 72 were taking NSAIDs, 17 patients steroids only and 30 patients both drugs; 10 patients had never taken any anti-inflammatory medication; 97 controls (male:female ratio 38:59; mean age 42 years) including 42 patients admitted for osteoarthritis or herniated intervertebral disc. Twenty-seven patients were taking only NSAIDs, 13 patients steroids only and 2 patients both. The remaining 55 controls were healthy volunteers taking no anti-inflammatory drugs. The 30 arthritis patients and the 2 control patients taking both drugs were excluded from the present evaluation. NSAIDs used in both groups were mainly indomethacin, piroxicam and naproxen at conventional anti-inflammatory dosages. Steroids were given in dosages ranging between 5 mg and 20 mg prednisolone per day.

Eighteen patients with histologic evidence of inflammatory bowel disease (IBD) (10 males:8 females; mean age 35 years) were added. This group consisted of 14 patients with Crohn's disease and 4 patients with ulcerative colitis. The mean duration of disease was 5 years (min 0.5 year – max 20 years) and all patients had active disease at the time of gut permeability measurement. Five patients had previously undergone gut surgery. Of these patients, eight were on anti-inflammatory drug treatment (NSAID or corticosteroids).

Table 1. Investigated patients and intake of NSAID

	Total	Only NSAID	Only steroids	Both drugs	No NSAID
Controls	97	27	13	2	55
RA	56	14	14	28	0
SpA	73	58	3	2	10
Total	226	99	30	32	65
IBD	18	1	4	3	10
Total	244	100	34	35	75

Gut permeability measurement

After an overnight fast, the subjects were given 100 µCi ^{51}Cr-EDTA (Medgenix diagnostics) in 20 ml of water at 08.00 a.m., followed by approximately 300 ml of water. Normal food and fluid intake (except for alcoholic beverages) was allowed 2 hours later. Urine was collected from 0–6 hour and from 6–24 hour in order to determine the possible site of increased permeability. Urine samples were placed in polyethylene bottles and water was added to a final volume of 2 litres. Radioactivity was measured using a gamma scintillation counter (MBLE – Philips combination). For each sample 10,000 counts were made or, in cases of lower activity, counting was continued for 10 minutes (SD 1%). The minimum detectable activity was 0.01 µCi.

Ileocolonoscopy

Ileocolonoscopy was performed by an experienced ileocolonoscopist unaware of the clinical diagnosis. A type IB Olympus CF colonoscope was used and premedication consisted of diazepam IV and hyoxine butylbromide (Buscopan®). A mean of 13 biopsy specimens per ileocolonoscopy were studied. The tissue was fixed in 10% formalin or in sublimate formaldehyde for 3–4 h at room temperature. After fixation the samples were routinely processed and embedded in paraplast. Tissue sections were cut at 5 µm and stained with haematoxylin–eosin. The samples were interpreted by an experienced pathologist unaware of the clinical findings or macroscopic abnormalities. They were classified as acute or chronic lesions [11].

Ileocolonoscopy was performed in 66 of 73 patients suffering from spondylarthropathies (Table 2). In 45 patients no histologic abnormalities were seen (normal ileocolonoscopy); 6 of these patients were taking no NSAIDs. Twenty-one patients had histologic evidence of gut inflammation (in 7 patients macroscopic lesions were seen): 12 patients, of whom 2 were taking no NSAIDs, were classified as having acute lesions; 9 patients, of whom 2 were taking no NSAIDs, as having chronic lesions. ^{51}Cr-EDTA

Table 2. Results of ileocolonoscopy in the patients with SpA. Intake of NSAID is shown

	Total	Anti-inflam. drugs	No anti-inflam. drugs
Ileocolo. not done	7	7	0
Ileocolo. normal	45	39	6
Ileocolo. acute lesions	12	10	2
Ileocolo. chronic lesions	9	7	2
Total	73	63	10

excretion was determined 1 to 2 days prior to ileocolonoscopy; the pathologist, the ileocolonoscopist and the clinician were all unaware of the results of the ^{51}Cr-EDTA excretion test.

RESULTS

Since no statistically significant differences were found between the 0–6 and the 6–24 h collection in any of the investigated groups, a 24-hour urine collection was used to evaluate ^{51}Cr-EDTA.

Statistical analysis demonstrated that there was no correlation between sex or age and the results in all investigated groups. The median 24-hour urine collection of ^{51}Cr-EDTA in control subjects not taking any drug, was 1.83% (3rd percentile 0.67%, 97th percentile 3.05%) of the orally administered dose.

In the control group ^{51}Cr-EDTA urine excretion in patients on NSAIDs alone was significantly elevated as compared to the patients not taking NSAIDs. In the arthritis group gut permeability was not significantly increased in patients taking only NSAIDs as compared to patients taking no anti-inflammatory drugs. We found a significant increase in gut permeability in the control patients taking only corticosteroids. This was not the case for the arthritis group. Finally, when patients taking only steroids were compared with patients taking only NSAIDs, no significant difference in gut permeability was found.

A significant increase of gut permeability was found in the 3 investigated patient groups in comparison to the control group. No significant differences were found when the 3 investigated groups were compared among themselves.

When patients on anti-inflammatory drugs were excluded, we still found a significant increase of gut permeability in SpA patients and IBD patients in comparison to controls (Figure 1). This comparison could not be made for RA patients as these were all taking anti-inflammatory drugs. Patients suffering from IBD, and taking no anti-inflammatory medication, had a significant increase of gut permeability as compared to the SpA patients who were taking no drugs.

SpA patients with histologic gut lesions on ileocolonoscopy did not show a significant increase of gut permeability as compared with patients without gut lesions (Figure 2). However, when the type of gut inflammation was considered, it appeared that patients with chronic gut lesions had a significantly elevated ^{51}Cr-EDTA excretion as compared to patients presenting acute gut lesions.

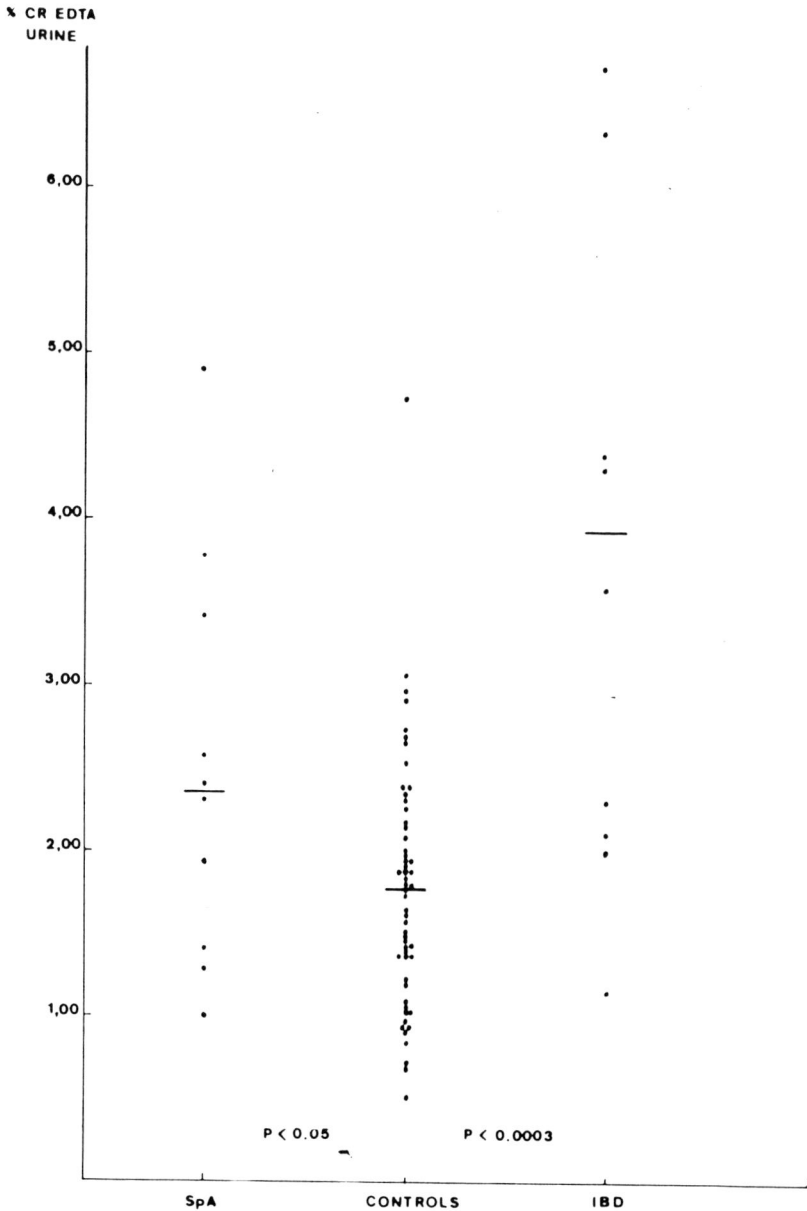

Figure 1. Urinary excretion of ^{51}Cr-EDTA (expressed as a percentage of the orally administered dose) in patients not taking anti-inflammatory medication in the different diagnostic groups. (Statistical analysis is indicated on the figure: NS denotes not significant; —— is the median)

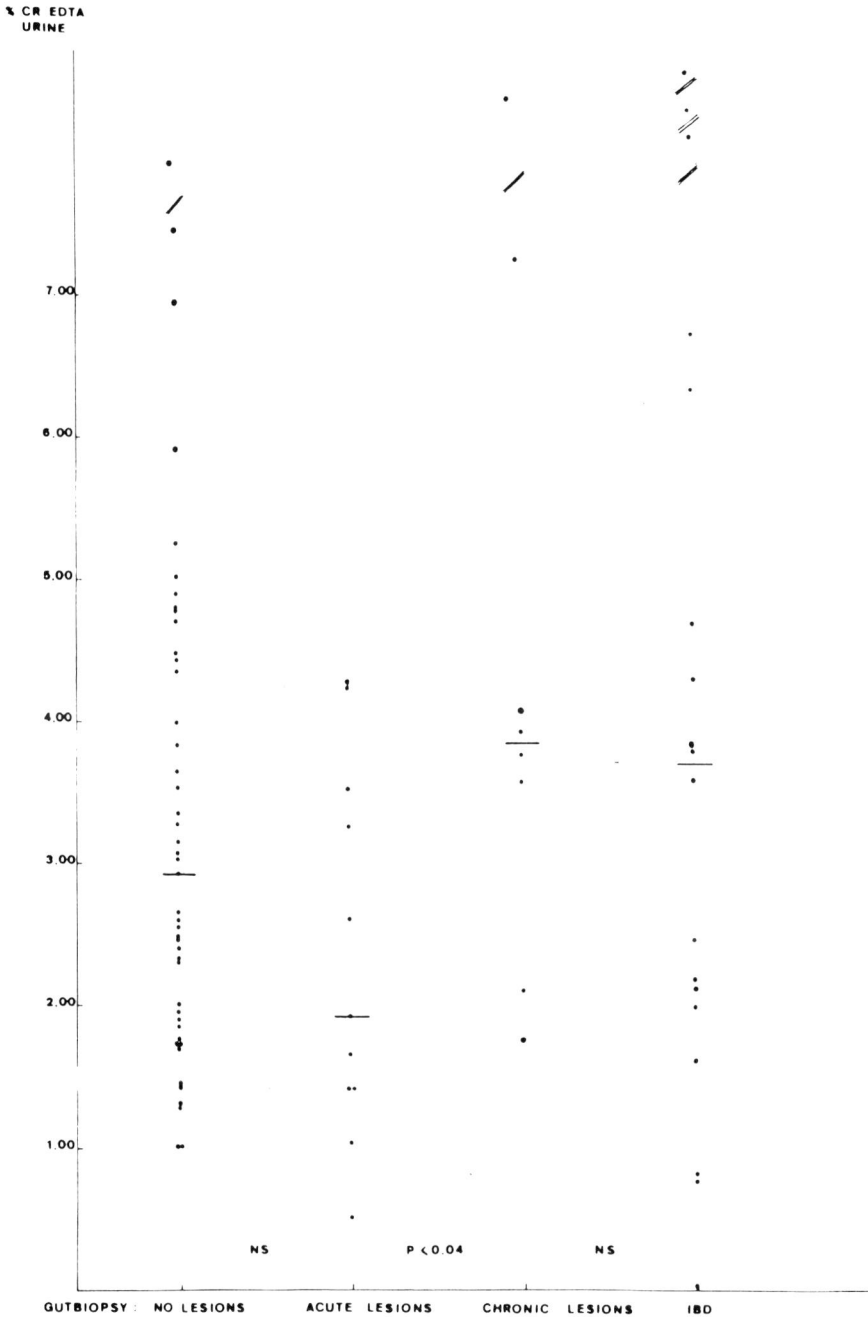

Figure 2. Urinary excretion of ^{51}Cr-EDTA (expressed as a percentage of the orally administered dose) in relation to the results of ileocolonoscopy (normal = normal histology; acute = acute lesions; chronic = chronic lesions). (Statistical analysis is indicated on the figure: NS denotes not significant; —— is the median)

DISCUSSION

The gut may play an important role in the pathogenesis of inflammatory joint diseases by permitting dietary, bacterial or viral antigens to gain access to the circulation thus provoking exaggerated immune responses causing inflammation. One of the possible mechanisms of transgression of the mucosal gut barrier is an increased gut permeability. This phenomenon has been clearly demonstrated by the development of an inflammatory polyarthritis after intestinal bypass surgery for morbid obesity [14–15].

Urinary excretion of ^{51}Cr-EDTA has proved to be a valuable method in measuring gut permeability [16]. This method specifically measures intercellular permeability [17,18].

Nonsteroidal anti-inflammatory drugs have been shown to significantly increase gut permeability in inflammatory joint diseases and in osteoarthritis [4,5].

Our study confirms the findings of Bjarnason et al. [4,5] as NSAIDs were found to play an important role in increasing gut permeability in the control groups.

Little seems to be known about the effect of corticosteroids on gut permeability. We found that in the control population steroids significantly increased gut permeability. This was not so in the arthritis group, although these patients usually take steroids for a longer time and at higher dosages. The fact that in this group there is no significant difference in gut permeability can be explained either by the restricted numbers or by the possible influence of a disease-related permeability. The NSAID-induced increase of gut permeability did not significantly differ from the steroid-induced increase.

The mechanism of NSAID-induced increased gut permeability is unknown, but a reduced synthesis of mucosal prostaglandins [19] through an inhibition of mucosal cyclooxygenase activity [20] is one of the possible explanations. In rats Whittle [20], however, did not find a temporal relationship between the inhibition of cyclooxygenase and the formation of intestinal lesions, and suggested that other enzymatic pathways including the arachidonic lipoxygenase system should be considered. The current study suggests that not only local inhibition of cyclooxygenase activity is implicated in drug-induced increased gut permeability but perhaps also other enzymatic pathways in the arachidonic cascade. Since corticosteroids act on phospholipase A2 at the beginning of the arachidonic cascade, this enzyme could play a role in maintaining gut integrity.

Increased gut permeability has been demonstrated not only in patients with inflammatory bowel diseases [21–23] but also in their clinically healthy relatives [24], indicating that this abnormality could be a primary defect and an aetiological factor. This study confirms the important disturbance of gut permeability in IBD, not influenced by anti-inflammatory drug intake. IBD is a disease belonging to the concept of spondylarthropathies.

Increased gut permeability has also been described in other forms of spondylarthropathies, such as *Yersinia* infections [25] and ankylosing spondylitis (AS) [1,2]. The finding of Wendling [2] of an increased permeability in AS patients taking no NSAIDs would suggest that a disease-related factor is involved.

The present study confirms these findings not only with respect to an increased gut permeability in the total group of SpA patients in comparison to controls, but also in untreated SpA patients.

By performing ileocolonoscopies we have demonstrated the presence of subclinical gut inflammation, mainly in the ileocaecal region in patients with SpA [9,26]. Repeat ileocolonoscopies have directly related the gut inflammation to the joint inflammation [10]. Since elevated urinary ^{51}Cr-EDTA excretion is directly related to the extent of gut inflammation in IBD [21], we have determined this excretion in SpA patients with inflammatory gut lesions, but found no significantly increased permeability.

Gut inflammation in SpA can be histologically subdivided into two forms [11], i.e. (a) patients with acute lesions resembling acute bacterial enteritis, and (b) patients with chronic lesions resembling the lesions of inflammatory bowel disease. These groups were not only histologically different, but also with regard to clinical expression (gastrointestinal, urogenital and rheumatological symptoms), radiological abnormalities, and genetic basis (HLA-BW62) [12].

A significant increase in gut permeability was found in patients with chronic gut lesions in comparison to patients with acute gut lesions, although the number of patients examined was relatively small (9 and 12 patients).

This finding supports the view that the chronic gut inflammation seen in SpA is fundamentally different and could have a different aetiopathogenic mechanism than the acute lesions. It also favours the hypothesis that some patients with SpA suffer from a form of subclinical Crohn's disease of which the joint inflammation is the only clinical expression [13].

REFERENCES

1. Smith MD, Gibson RA, Brooks PM. Abnormal bowel permeability in ankylosing spondylitis and rheumatoid arthritis. J Rheumatol. 1985;12:299–305.
2. Wendling G, Bidet A, Guiot M. Intestinal permeability in ankylosing spondylitis. J Rheumatol. 1990;17:114–115.
3. Jenkins RT, Rooney RT, Jones DR, Bienenstock J, Goodacre RL. Increased intestinal permeability in patients with rheumatoid arthritis: a side-effect of oral non-steroidal anti-inflammatory drug therapy? Br J Rheumatol. 1987;26:103–107.
4. Bjarnason I, Williams P, So A et al. Intestinal permeability and inflammation in rheumatoid arthritis: effects of non-steroidal anti-inflammatory drugs. Lancet. 1984;2:1171–1173.

5. Bjarnason I, Williams P, Smethurst P, Peters TJ, Levi AJ. Effect of non-steroidal anti-inflammatory drugs and prostaglandins on the permeability of the human small intestine. Gut. 1986;27:1292–1297.

6. Bjarnason I, Zanelli G, Smith T et al. Non-steroidal anti-inflammatory drug-induced intestinal inflammation in humans. Gastroenterology. 1987;93:450–459.

7. Segal AW, Isenberg DA, Hajirousou W, Tolfree S, Clarck J, Snaith MC. Preliminary evidence for gut involvement in the pathogenesis of rheumatoid arthritis? Br J Rheumatol. 1986;25:162–166.

8. Rooney PJ, Jenkins RT, Smith KM, Coates G. [111]Indium-labelled polymorphonuclear leucocyte scans in rheumatoid arthritis – an important clinical cause of false positive results. Br J Rheumatol. 1986;25:167–173.

9. Mielants H, Veys EM, Cuvelier C, De Vos M. Ileocolonoscopic findings in seronegative spondylarthropathies. Br J Rheumatol. 1988;27(Suppl II):95–105.

10. Mielants H, Veys EM, Joos R, Cuvelier C, De Vos M. Repeat ileocolonoscopy in reactive arthritis. J Rheumatol. 1987;14:456–458.

11. Cuvelier C, Barbitis C, Mielants H, De Vos M, Roels H, Veys EM. The histopathology of intestinal inflammation related to reactive arthritis. Gut. 1987;28:394–402.

12. Mielants H, Veys EM, Joos R, Noens L, Cuvelier C, De Vos M. HLA-Antigens in seronegative spondylarthropathies, reactive arthritis and arthritis in ankylosing spondylitis: relation to gut inflammation. J Rheumatol. 1987;14:466–471.

13. Mielants H, Veys EM. Editorial. The gut in the spondylarthropathies. J Rheumatol. 1990;17:7–9.

14. Wands JR, Le Mont JT, Mann E, Isselbacher KJ. Arthritis associated with intestinal bypass procedure for morbid obesity. N Engl J Med. 1976;294:121–124.

15. Clegg DO, Zone JJ, Samuelson CO Jr, Wands JR. Circulating immune complexes containing secretory IgA in jejunoileal bypass disease. Ann Rheum Dis. 1985;44:239–244.

16. Jenkins RT, Jones DB, Goodacre RL, Collins SM et al. Reversibility of increased intestinal permeability to ^{51}Cr-EDTA in patients with gastrointestinal inflammatory diseases. Am J Gastroenterol. 1987;82:1159–1164.

17. Axon ATR, Creamer B. The exsorption characteristics of various sugars. Gut, 1975;16:99–104.

18. Bjarnason I, Peters TJ, Levy AJ. Intestinal permeability: clinical correlates. Surv Dig Dis. 1986;4:83–92.

19. Miller TA, Jacobson ED. Gastrointestinal cytoprotection by prostaglandins. Gut, 1979;20:75–87.

20. Whittle BJR. Temporal relationship between cyclooxygenase inhibition as measured by prostacyclin biosynthesis and the gastrointestinal damage induced by indomethacin in the rat. Gastroenterology. 1981;80:94–98.

21. Jenkins RT, Jones DB, Goodacre RL, Collins SM et al. Reversibility of increased intestinal permeability to [51]CR-EDTA in patients with gastrointestinal inflammatory diseases. Am J Gastroenterol. 1987;82:1159–1164.

22. Bjarnason I, O'Morain C, Levi J, Peters TJ. Absorption of [51]Chromium-labeled ethylenediamine-tetracetate in inflammatory bowel disease. Gastroenterology. 1983;85:318–322.

23. Olaison G, Leandersson P, Sjödahl R, Tagesson C. Intestinal permeability to polyethyleneglycol 600 in Crohn's disease. Peroperative determination in a defined segment of the small intestine. Gut. 1988;29:196–199.

24. Hollander D, Vadheim C, Brettholz E et al. Increased intestinal permeability in patients with Crohn's disease and their relatives. Ann Intern Med. 1986;105:883–885.

25. Serrander R, Magnusson KE, Kihlstrom E. Acute Yersinia infections in man increase intestinal permeability for low molecular polyethylene glycols. Scand J Infect Dis. 1986;18:409–413.

26. Mielants H, Veys EM, Cuvelier C, De Vos M, Botelberghe L. HLA-B27 related arthritis and bowel inflammation. Part 2: Ileocolonoscopy and bowel histology in patients with HLA-B27 related arthritis. J Rheumatol. 1985;12:244–248.

13

Comparison of effects on gastrointestinal blood loss and gastric mucosal appearance of piroxicam-β-cyclodextrin, piroxicam and placebo

S. Warrington, N. Debbas, M. Farthing[1], M. Horton[1], A. Thillainayagam[1] and A. Umile[2]

Charterhouse Clinical Research Unit Ltd, London, UK;
[1]St Bartholomew's Hospital, London, UK;
and [2]Medical Department, Chiesi Farmaceutici SpA, Parma, Italy

INTRODUCTION

Piroxicam-β-cyclodextrin is a form of physical pro-drug for the widely-used NSAID piroxicam. It is a complex of piroxicam and the cyclic oligosaccharide β-cyclodextrin; the latter forms an inclusion compound, thus increasing hydrosolubility and bioavailability of piroxicam [1]. The complex dissociates in the gastrointestinal tract, releasing piroxicam dissolved in the gastrointestinal fluid so that the drug can be absorbed more readily, and β-cyclodextrin, which is transformed into linear chain derivatives and finally to glucose monomers that enter the usual metabolic pathway of sugars. The mean plasma piroxicam concentrations at 15 and 30 minutes after administration of piroxicam-β-cyclodextrin were 10 and 3 times greater, respectively, than those after administration of plain piroxicam [2], thus allowing a more rapid onset of analgesia [3].

Increasing the rate of absorption of piroxicam by incorporation in β-cyclodextrin should shorten the contact time between drug and gastrointestinal mucosa. Furthermore, rapid absorption should lead to reduction in exposure of distal small intestinal mucosa to the drug, thus reducing the likelihood of a piroxicam-induced enteropathy. Two previous studies [4,5] have suggested that piroxicam-β-cyclodextrin may indeed cause less injury to the gastrointestinal tract, as measured by upper gastrointestinal endoscopy, gastric transmucosal potential difference, and faecal erythrocyte excretion.

Side-effects of Anti-inflammatory Drugs 3. Rainsford KD, Velo GP (eds), Inflammation and Drug Therapy Series, Volume V.

The available data justified the undertaking of a further study, comparing piroxicam-β-cyclodextrin or piroxicam with placebo treatment in volunteers, of protracted (28-day) administration, with daily collection of faeces for blood-loss analysis and 'before and after' endoscopy.

The results of this study are also published elsewhere [14].

SUBJECTS AND METHODS

The protocol was approved by the District Ethics Committee of St. Bartholomew's Hospital. Written informed consent was obtained. The study was carried out in double-blind conditions, using the double-dummy technique to avoid difficulties due to different formulations of the two drugs.

The subjects were enrolled in the study, after clinical examination, if they satisfied the inclusion criteria: male sex, normal clinical history, physical examination, ECG and routine haematological, biochemical and urinalysis, normal endoscopic findings, regular bowel habit, negative evidence of past or present gastrointestinal disease.

Thirty-six healthy men aged 19–31 years, weight 57–90 kg, were randomized in blocks of 12 subjects/treatment, to the three treatment groups.

Between 1 and 3 days before Study Day 0, subjects underwent upper gastrointestinal endoscopy. All examinations were performed in the afternoon, with the subjects having fasted after a light early breakfast. Pre-medication was limited to 3–5 sprays of the pharynx with lignocaine hydrochloride (xylocaine). The endoscope was passed via the mouth to the duodenum; duodenal and gastric mucosa was examined both on entry and on withdrawal, and the appearance scored as described by Lanza et al. [6]

Grade 0 = normal

Grade 1 = one submucosal haemorrhage or superficial ulceration

Grade 2 = more than one submucosal haemorrhage or superficial ulceration but not numerous or widespread

Grade 3 = numerous areas of submucosal haemorrhage or superficial ulceration

Grade 4 = widespread involvement of the stomach with submucosal haemorrhage or superficial ulceration. Invasive ulcer of any size. (Invasive ulcer was defined as a lesion which produces an actual crater: i.e. a depression below the normal plane of the mucosal surface)

On Study Day 0, 10 ml venous blood was taken from the subject, labelled with a maximum of 200 µCi ^{51}Cr using standard methods [7] and reinfused. The amount of radioactivity administered was about 50 µCi. Six days were allowed for the reinfused red cells to appear into the faeces. Complete faecal collections were then made from day 6–12.

From day 13–40 (28 consecutive days) subjects received one of the three study treatments: piroxicam-β-cyclodextrin (20 mg/day); piroxicam (20 mg/day); matching placebo daily.

The subjects were asked to take the medicine with their evening meals, and to avoid taking breakfast cereals, any alcoholic drinks and any other medicines (including over-the-counter medications) during the entire study period.

Complete daily faecal collections were made for the entire 4 weeks' treatment. Venous blood samples (10 ml) for determination of ^{51}Cr specific activity were taken on Days 6, 13, 20, 27 and 34. Blood was taken into lithium heparinized tubes. The specific activity of the red cells, the haematocrit and the activity of the faecal collection were determined and the whole blood content of each faecal specimen was calculated. Counting was done with a Packard Tricarb scintillation spectrometer model 3002. A high precision standard clinical method was used, recording the number of counts in 3 minutes from the faecal samples; for blood samples the time taken for 10,000 counts to be made was recorded. Faecal blood loss for each subject was calculated as mls whole blood lost during each day of the 7-day collection periods.

On Days 20, 27 and 34, a further 10 ml venous blood sample was taken into lithium heparinized tubes for piroxicam assay as verification of subjects' compliance with treatment.

Tolerability assessments were made on Day 20. Adverse events were recorded, including subjects' response to the question "how have you been feeling during the last week?".

Upper gastrointestinal endoscopy was repeated on the afternoon of Day 41, 16–20 h after the last dose of medication. The appearance was graded in the same way as the initial examination.

Primary efficacy was dependent on the faecal blood loss findings; of secondary importance were the endoscopic findings. Differences between treatments were tested using the Kruskall–Wallis test. If the Kruskall–Wallis test was significant then pairwise comparisons were made using the Wilcoxon 2 samples test.

RESULTS

The main measures of outcome in this study were endoscopic appearance, and faecal blood loss.

Endoscopic appearance was within normal limits before and after treatment in the great majority of subjects. The appearance showed no change in any subject receiving placebo, whereas 3 subjects in each of the treatment groups showed changes; but no grade worse than 2, which was considered as acceptable for inclusion in the study, was found after treatment (Table 1).

Table 1. Endoscopy scores before and after treatment with placebo, piroxicam-β-cyclodextrin and piroxicam

	Placebo (n=12)		Piroxicam-β-CD (n=11)		Piroxicam (n=12)	
	Before	After	Before	After	Before	After
	2	2	0	2	0	1
			0	2	0	2
			0	2	0	2
Total scores	2	2	0	6	0	5

Results from subjects with zero scores throughout have been excluded

With regard to faecal blood loss, there were clear-cut differences between placebo on the one hand and the active treatments on the other, while there were no significant differences between piroxicam-β-cyclodextrin and piroxicam (Tables 2 and 3). Before any treatment began, median blood losses in all treatment groups were similar and within the range to be expected in normal subjects. Both piroxicam-β-cyclodextrin and piroxicam caused significant increases in median total blood loss compared with placebo, but the effects of piroxicam-β-cyclodextrin did not differ significantly from those of piroxicam.

Figure 1 shows the cumulative mean blood loss for each treatment. The trend for cumulative blood loss for piroxicam to be higher than the other treatments in the last 10 days of dosing was mainly due to exceptionally high losses in 3 subjects receiving piroxicam.

Two subjects were withdrawn from treatment because of abdominal pain: one subject was withdrawn after 10 days' piroxicam-β-cyclodextrin treatment and the other subject after 26 days' piroxicam treatment. Neither subject was replaced. Overall, 12 of the 36 subjects experienced adverse events during treatment: 5 receiving placebo, 2 piroxicam and 5 piroxicam-β-cyclodextrin. Of these subjects, 4 receiving placebo, 2 piroxicam and 4 piroxicam-β-cyclodextrin had gastrointestinal symptoms; the other adverse events were minor and probably unrelated to treatment.

Table 2. Median total blood loss for collection periods before and during treatments (ml)

	Pre-treatment (days 6–12)	During treatment (days 13–41)
Placebo	1.48	12.94
Piroxicam-β-cyclodextrin	1.91	21.50
Piroxicam	1.44	23.84
p values for differences between treatments (Kruskall–Wallis test)	0.6203	0.0034

Table 3. Results of Wilcoxon 2 samples test for piroxicam-β-cyclodextrin versus piroxicam and placebo, and piroxicam versus placebo (median total blood loss for days 13–41)

	Piroxicam-β-CD versus Placebo	Piroxicam-β-CD versus Piroxicam	Piroxicam versus Placebo
p values (Wilcoxon 2 samples test)	0.001	0.4755	0.0033

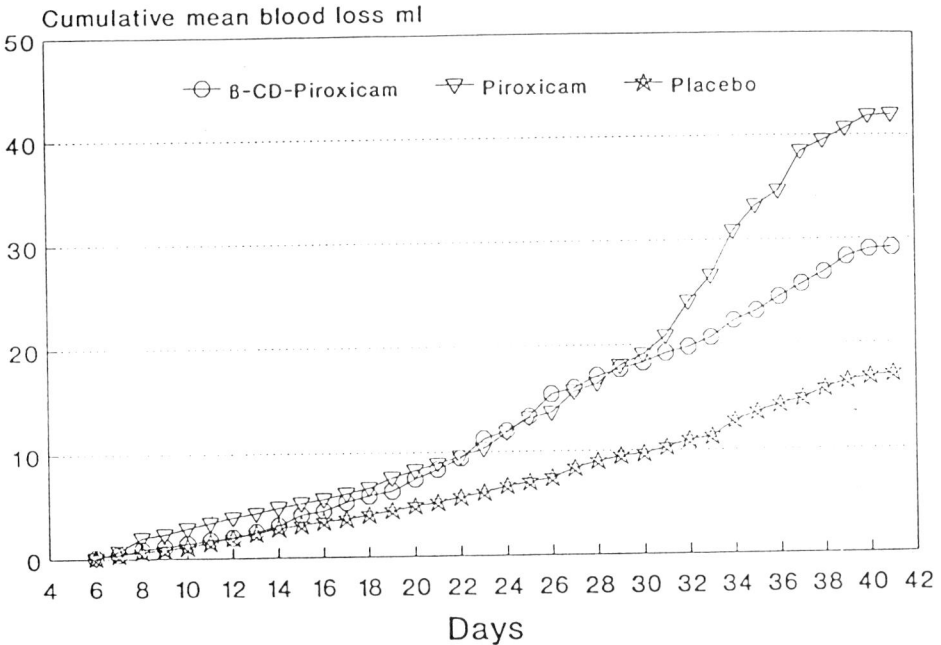

Figure 1. Cumulative total blood loss for each treatment, divided by number of subjects in each group ($n = 11$ for piroxicam-β-cyclodextrin; $n = 12$ for piroxicam and placebo). Treatment period: days 13–40

93

DISCUSSION

In this study, piroxicam-β-cyclodextrin and piroxicam had only mild effects on the appearances of gastric and duodenal mucosa. This is consistent with the findings of Bianchine et al. [8] with piroxicam alone, but in that study the medication was given for only 4 days. Patoia et al. [4] studied healthy volunteers receiving piroxicam or piroxicam-β-cyclodextrin for 28 days, and found only minor effects of the complex on endoscopic appearances; in contrast with our experience, however, piroxicam itself was associated with Grade 4 mucosal lesions in 4 out of 7 subjects. The study population included women, which might account for some of the differences between their findings and ours; furthermore, only 7 subjects received each treatment so the study sample was a small one. Santucci et al. [5] also compared piroxicam with piroxicam-β-cyclodextrin complex (14 days' treatment, 8 subjects per treatment group), and found that endoscopic appearances deteriorated significantly on both treatments but only piroxicam differed significantly from placebo. We found that neither piroxicam nor its complex with β-cyclodextrin frequently caused important mucosal injury after 28 days' treatment, whereas the findings of Patoia et al. [4] and Santucci et al. [5] suggest that the complex may be less irritant to gastric and duodenal mucosa than is piroxicam itself. Overall, it seems safe to conclude that increasing the dissolution rate of piroxicam by incorporating the molecule in β-cyclodextrin has certainly not increased the local irritant effect of the drug, and it is possible that it has actually reduced it.

Although only minor effects on gastric and duodenal mucosa were observed in our study, both piroxicam and its complex with β-cyclodextrin caused similar, significant increases in median daily faecal blood loss. Our findings for piroxicam are consistent with 3 previous reports [9–11]; the failure of Bianchine et al. [8] to show any effects of piroxicam on gastrointestinal blood loss was probably due to the administration of the study drug for only 4 days.

For the piroxicam-β-cyclodextrin complex, our results broadly confirm those of Patoia et al. [4]; these workers were not able to obtain comparable data for piroxicam-induced faecal blood loss because of poor tolerability of the drug in their study population.

Cumulative mean blood loss increased quite strikingly in the piroxicam group compared with piroxicam-β-cyclodextrin during the last 12 days of treatment. This phenomenon was due to exceptionally high losses in three piroxicam-treated subjects, whereas no subject receiving piroxicam-β-cyclodextrin was similarly affected.

There is evidence that piroxicam-induced injury to the gastrointestinal mucosa occurs in part as a result of a systemic action via the inhibition of cyclo-oxygenase and partly due to a direct irritant effect of the agent on the gastrointestinal wall [12]. It is tempting to speculate that the incorporation of piroxicam in a complex with β-cyclodextrin could actually decrease the propensity of the active moiety to cause gastrointestinal bleeding. This difference could be reasonably attributed to the faster absorption of piroxicam from piroxicam-β-cyclodextrin and the consequently shorter time the drug is in contact with the gastrointestinal mucosa.

There is some clinical evidence that the complex may be better tolerated than native piroxicam [4,13]. Our results indicate that piroxicam-β-cyclodextrin and piroxicam in equivalent dosage for 4 weeks in healthy volunteers cause similar effects on endoscopic appearance and faecal blood loss but with a trend for cumulative blood loss to increase towards the end of treatment with piroxicam.

Further clinical studies are needed to show whether piroxicam-β-cyclodextrin is less likely than piroxicam to injure the gastrointestinal tract in patients with rheumatic disease.

ACKNOWLEDGEMENTS

We thank Dr A.J. Jouhar, of Information Transfer International, for his help in setting up and conducting this project.

REFERENCES

1. Acerbi D, Bonati C, Boscarino G, Bufalino L, Cesari F et al. Pharmacokinetic study on piroxicam at the steady-state in elderly subjects and younger adults after administration of piroxicam-β-cyclodextrin. Int J Clin Pharmacol Res. 1988;8:175–180.
2. Acerbi D, Lebacq Jr E, Rondelli I, Stockis A, Ventura P. Rapid oral absorption profile of piroxicam from its beta-cyclodextrin complex. Drug Invest. 1990;2(Suppl 4):50–55.
3. Tiengo M. Review of the analgesic activity effects of piroxicam-β-cyclodextrin. Drug Invest. 1990;2(Suppl 4):61–66.
4. Patoia L, Clausi G, Farroni F, Alberti P, Fugiani P, Bufalino L. Comparison of faecal blood loss, upper gastrointestinal mucosal integrity and symptoms after piroxicam-β-cyclodextrin, piroxicam and placebo administration. Eur J Clin Pharmacol. 1989;36:599–604.
5. Santucci L, Fiorucci S, Patoia L, Farroni F, Sicilia A, Chiucchiu S, Bufalino L, Morelli A. Gastric tolerance of piroxicam-beta-cyclodextrin compared with placebo and with other NSAIDs: An endoscopic and functional study by evaluation of transmucosal potential differences. Drug Invest. 1990;2(Suppl 4):56–60.
6. Lanza FL, Panagides T, Salom I. Etodolac compared with aspirin: an endoscopic study of the gastrointestinal tracts of normal volunteers. J Rheumatol. 1986;13:299–303.
7. Dacie JV, Lewis SM. Practical haematology. 6th ed. Edinburgh: Churchill Livingstone; 1984.
8. Bianchine JR, Proctor RR, Thomas FB. Piroxicam, aspirin and gastrointestinal blood loss. Clin Pharmacol Ther. 1982;32:247–252.
9. Bird HA, Hill J, Ardley RG, McEvoy M, Wright V. A comparison of faecal blood loss caused by two prolonged-release formulations of indomethacin (Flexin Continus and Indocid R) in normal healthy male volunteers. Curr Med Res Opin. 1988;11:4–9.
10. Hooper JW, Anslow JA, Martin WS, Araujo P, Darke A. Faecal blood loss during isoxicam and piroxicam administration for 28 days. Clin Pharmacol Ther. 1985;38:533–537.
11. Jallad NS, Sanda M, Salom I et al. Gastrointestinal blood loss in arthritic patients receiving chronic dosing with etodolac and piroxicam. Am J Med Sci. 1986;292:272–276.

12. Schiantarelli P, Cadel S. Piroxicam pharmacological activity and gastrointestinal damage by oral and rectal routes. Comparison with oral indomethacin and phenylbutazone. Arzneim Forsch. 1981;31:87–92.
13. Ambanelli U, Nervetti A, Colombo B et al. Piroxicam-β-cyclodextrin in the treatment of rheumatic diseases: a prospective study. Curr Ther Res. 1990;48:58–68.
14. Warrington S, Debbas N, Farthing M, Horton M, Thillainayagam A, Umile A. Comparison of effects on gastrointestinal blood loss and gastric mucosal appearance of piroxicam-β-cyclodextrin, piroxicam and placebo. Int J Tissue React. [in press]

14

Mechanisms of gastrointestinal ulceration from non-steroidal anti-inflammatory drugs: a basis for use and development of protective agents

K.D. Rainsford

Departments of Biomedical Sciences and Pathology,
McMaster University Faculty of Health Sciences, Hamilton,
Ontario, L8N 3Z5, Canada

INTRODUCTION

The past decade or so has seen an upsurge in interest on the clinical importance of gastrointestinal (GI) ulceration as a major side-effect of the non-steroidal anti-inflammatory drugs (NSAIDs) and with this research on the mechanisms thereof has also increased. A number of reviews on the clinical importance of GI side-effects from NSAIDs have been published [1-6]. The epidemiological evidence suggests that there is an appreciable risk of NSAID gastropathy in rheumatic patients [3,4], the risk being much greater in the elderly female patient [5].

THE CASE FOR PROTECTION AGAINST NSAID ULCERATION:

The clinical problem of treating patients with peptic ulcer diseases (PUD) with NSAIDs has been debated [1,2] and the problem so difficult that no clear concensus has been reached. This makes it important to search for approaches/therapies to reduce the risk in rheumatic patients in whom endoscopically-observed gastroduodenal lesions and ulcers are of high frequency when receiving NSAIDs [1,2].

While much emphasis has been placed on the risk of ulceration and bleeding in the stomach (so-called 'NSAID gastropathy') and duodenum in patients with rheumatic conditions receiving these drugs for long periods, recent studies by Bjarnason et al [7] and other groups (e.g. ref. 8) have recognized that 'deeper' regions of the intestinal tract somewhat inaccessible to routine endoscopy may show permeability changes and

Side-effects of Anti-inflammatory Drugs 3. Rainsford KD, Velo GP (eds),
Inflammation and Drug Therapy Series, Volume V.

signs of inflammation in these subjects. Thus NSAIDs may not only produce iatrogenic ulceration in the upper GI tract but also the intestine, especially the colon [8].

The case for use and development of procedures to reduce or even eliminate GI ulceration and bleeding therefore rests on recognizing the nature of the mechanisms of mucosal injury in these different regions of the GI tract. Evidence suggests that these differ considerably depending on the type of drug, physiological, dietary and environmental factors, and mucosal region affected [9].

The main practical developments in recent years to reduce NSAID ulceration have been to employ anti-ulcer agents, usually in subjects at risk (the elderly, those with PUD). No attempt is made here to review the efficacy and effects of established anti-ulcer agents (prostaglandins such as misoprostol, H_2 receptor antagonists, H-pump blockers, and sucralfate) for preventing NSAID ulceration since these are reveiwed at length elsewhere in this volume. However, the conclusions from these and other recent literature suggest that misoprostol is probably more likely to prevent NSAID ulceration in the entire GI tract than H_2 blockers. The use of misoprostol is limited because of the occurrence of diarrhoea (though this appears to only occur for a few days and when the drug is taken before meals), and the inevitable extra cost (though offset by reduction in treatment from morbidity and mortality from serious GI ulceration and haemorrhage). H_2-receptor antagonists and, to a greater extent, H-pump blockers may find utility where symptoms of hyperacidity (notably epigastric distress), or an acid related factor is implicated such as PUD or simply duodenal injury for the individual. The choice is clearly dependent on patient related factors (see elsewhere in this volume). Albeit, the clinical studies on the use of anti-ulcer agents show that ulceration from NSAIDs is not eliminated entirely in the long term. The case for devising novel procedures or NSAIDs with even lower ulcerogenicity than drugs such as indomethacin or aspirin is obviously of much importance.

The scope of the present paper is, therefore, to discuss (a) the current concepts of GI mucosal injury of NSAIDs as they are relevant to the problem of instituting therapies or procedures to prevent the occurrence of GI ulceration and haemorrhage, and (b) based on these concepts some of our recent studies exploring some novel approaches for reducing GI injury by NSAIDs as well as results of studies on misoprostol indicating novel actions which may be exploited in the future. The potential use of vasoactive and growth regulatory peptides, nitric oxide generators and other vascular agents is not considered since these are discussed elsewhere by others in this volume.

CONCEPTS OF THE PATHOGENESIS OF GI MUCOSAL INJURY

Several recent reviews summarize the current information of gastric and intestinal ulceration from NSAIDs [9-18]. Table 1 shows a summary of the current concepts. As a principle, NSAIDs exhibit mutiple attack on some or all of the mucosal defences; the diagrammatic representation of these defences is shown in Figures 1-3. Some effects of these drugs predominate in their consequences on the integrity of mucosal cells. For example, we consider that vascular injury is among the important early events involved in the initiation of gastric, and possibly intestinal mucosal damage (Figure 4). It is clear that in addition to the inhibition of vasodilatatory prostaglandins (PGs), diversion of arachidonic acid through the lipoxygenase (LO) pathway to produce an excess of vasoconstrictor peptido-leukotrienes and H(P)ETEs, combined with release of histamine from mast cells are among the important inflammatory mediators produced in response to NSAIDs and cause vascular changes (Figures 4 and 5) [19-22].

It is important, also, to recognize that some NSAIDs have more potent or profound actions on mucosal defensive processes than others. Thus it is not possible to generalize about the actions of NSAIDs collectively. To reiterate, it is also important to recognize that some NSAIDs have greater gastro-ulcerogenicity while being more injurious to the intestinal mucosa than others and vice versa.

Strategies to reduce mucosal injury from existing NSAIDs take essentially one of two approaches: (a) add an anti-ulcer agent, or (b) modify the chemical properties of the NSAID (e.g. form a pro-drug). For (a) the anti-ulcer agent must essentially overcome the mucosal defences which have been affected by the NSAID. In many respects the current range of agents would not be expected to completely overcome the impaired mucosal defences produced by NSAIDs. It is, indeed, remarkable that they are so effective at all. However, the results with standard anti-ulcer agents give clues that some of the processes which they affect clearly are partially important in the pathogenesis of mucosal injury by NSAIDs.

CHEMICAL MODIFICATION TO REDUCE ULCEROGENICITY

The development of pro-drugs underlying the second strategy has been explored extensively [9, 23-26] and there is still some interest in this approach today. Of the pro-drugs developed only fenbufen, nabumetone, proquazone and salsalate have shown any measurable reduction in gastric injury in humans in the long-term studies in the clinic [25,26], but there has been no elimination of the GI ulcerogenicity with these drugs. This strategy shows at least that some success is possible by developing pro-drugs, especially if they are non-carboxylates. The lack of success of sulindac in

Table 1: Summary of physiopathological and biochemical changes involved in the pathogenesis of GI mucosal injury by NSAIDs

Factor	Principal consequences
Immediate (Primary Actions):	
Acidity of drug (organic acid)	Loss of membrane integrity
Sloughing of surface mucus, decreased HCO_3^-, and altered phospholipid hydrophobicity	Impaired surface mucus and surface membrane protection
Back diffusion of acid from acidic drugs	Local decrease in cell pH (promotes drug uptake and local cellular autolysis)
Inhibition of cyclo-oxygenase leading to (a) decreased PGI_2 and PGE_2 synthesis, and (b) ? diversion of arachidonate to lipoxygenase products	Altered blood flow → anoxia. Platelet-vessel adhesion promotes microvascular injury. Reduced 'cyto'-protection by: decreased mucus production, decreased HCO_3^- secretion (probably PGE/I effect only). Promotion of leucocyte accumulation, adhesion (? from increased LTB_4 production and/or degradation chemotactic peptides from local cell injury).
Release of lysosomal hydrolases	Local cellular autolysis
Cholinergic activation	Acid/pepsin secretion enhanced in stomach
Histamine release from mast cells	Promotes acid secretion, vasodilation (stomach)
Enhanced oxyradical production	Localized tissue destruction
Reduced sulphydryls	Possible loss of reductive protection by mucosal bio-molecules against oxyradical damage and perturbed eicosanoid metabolism
Longer Time Effects:	
Enhanced motility (amplitude)	Altered GI transit ? relation to prostaglandin control of smooth muscle functions
Inhibition of ATP production	Reduced capacity to resist cell injury from mucus and other synthetic reactions.
Altered cAMP levels (? from phosphodiesterase inhibition)	Altered cell metabolism, including effects on acid and mucus secretion (stomach)
Inhibition of production of mucus layer and inhibition of mucus biosynthesis (at enzyme level)	Reduced mucus protection

It should be emphasised that some of these drug actions are rather speculative at the present state of knowledge.
Based on refs 9–27, 46, 47 and 57

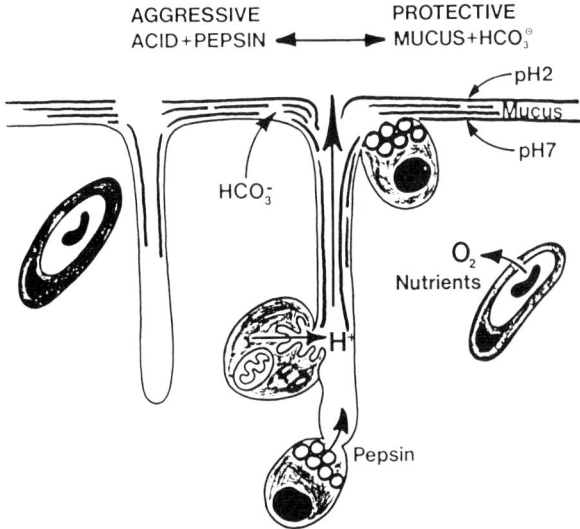

MUCOSAL DEFENCE MECHANISMS 1

Figure 1: The classical view of the role of aggressive (acid + pepsin) and preventative or protective (mucus + bicarbonate) events in the maintenance of mucosal defences in the stomach, imbalance in favour of aggressive factors favouring ulcer formation. As noted in Table 1 the mucus layer can be physically removed (sloughed) by NSAIDs (especially aspirin and other salicylic acids).

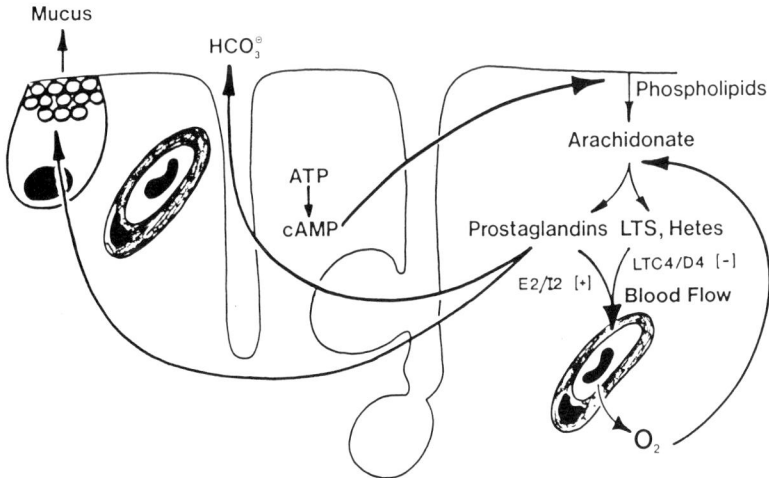

MUCOSAL DEFENCE MECHANISMS 2
— THE ROLE OF PROSTAGLANDINS

Figure 2: Role of prostaglandins E_2 and I_2 in blood flow, the dynamics of vascular smooth muscle function, consequent local cell oxygenation, and mucus-bicarbonate production. The regulation of mucus and bicarbonate production is achieved by PGE_2, cyclic 3',5'-AMP, cAMP and ATP. In turn cAMP regulates release of arachidonate. Prostaglandins also negatively regulate release of leukotrienes. [-] denotes negative effect, [+] denotes positive actions.

101

ACID + PEPSIN

PROTEINS

AMINO ACIDS

GLUCOSE

HCO$_3^-$ GLUTAMATE

Mucus

Mitochondria

ATP

O$_2$

Nutrients

ATP

cGMP cAMP Cell Regulation of
Synthesis, Secretion

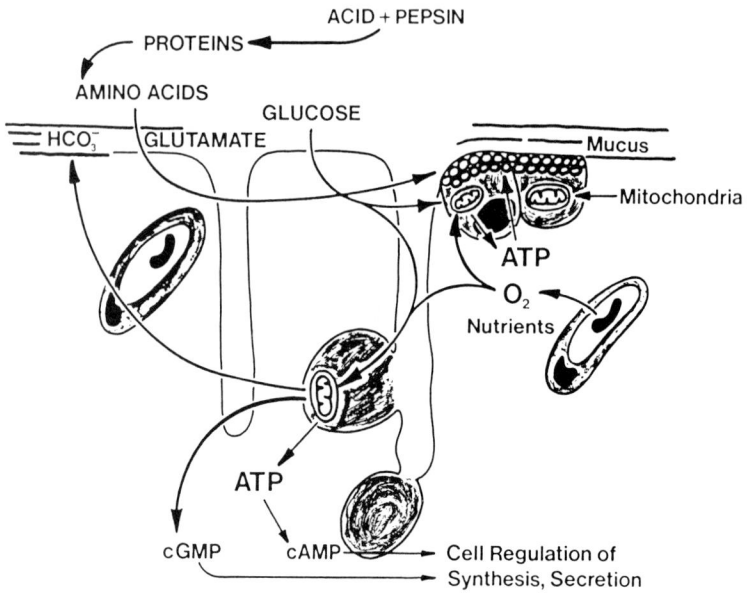

MUCOSAL DEFENCE MECHANISMS 3

Figure 3: Gastric supply of nutrients regulates mucosal metabolism promoting defensive biochemical reactions. Linked to this is the vascular status and supply of oxygen and the regulation by cyclic nucleotides via receptor activation by PGE/I (of cAMP), or cholinergic and PGF$_2$ receptors (of cGMP).

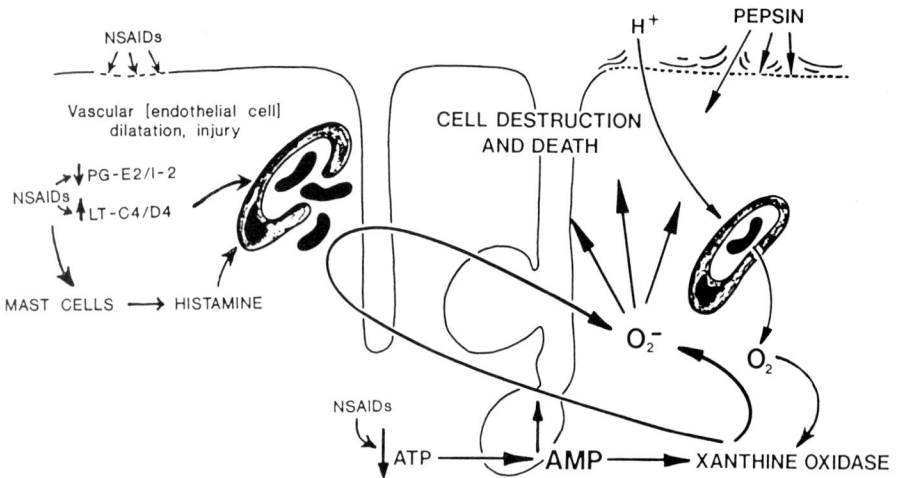

NSAIDs

H$^+$ PEPSIN

Vascular [endothelial cell]
dilatation, injury

CELL DESTRUCTION
AND DEATH

↓PG-E2/I-2

NSAIDs
↑LT-C4/D4

MAST CELLS ⟶ HISTAMINE

O$_2^-$

O$_2$

NSAIDs

↓ATP ⟶ AMP ⟶ XANTHINE OXIDASE

Figure 4: Oxygen radicals generated from (a) perturbed eicosanoid metabolism (i.e. peroxy-derived radicals), and (b) activation of xanthine oxidase in local reperfusion reactions consequent upon vascular injury by NSAIDs, and superoxide so produced, combine to potentiate cellular injury. Vascular endothelial-smooth muscle changes (in a sense "stressful") are promoted by (a) histamine released from mast cells whose membranes are made unstable by NSAIDs, (b) vasoconstrictor effects of peptido-leukotrienes, and (c) the consequent negative influence of deficiency in vasodilatatory prostaglandins E/I.

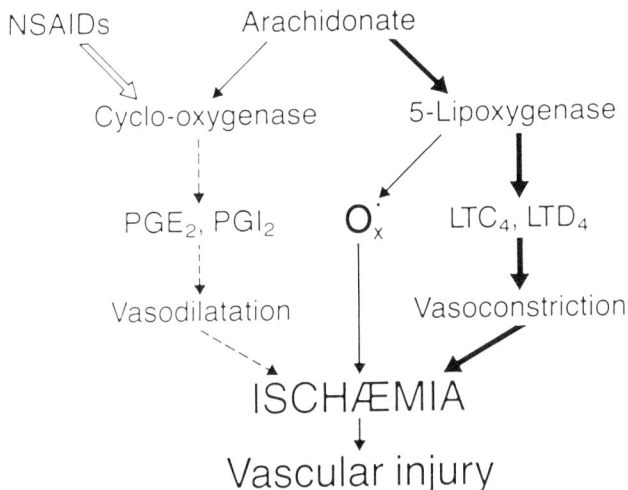

Figure 5: Diversion of arachidonate by cyclo-oxygenase inhibition caused by NSAIDs leads to enhanced peptido-leukotrienes that promote with histamine vasocontriction (see also Figure 4). The regulation of lipoxygenase activity may be influenced not only by substrate availability but also via the reduction in negative regulation by PGE/I, cyclic nucleotides and ATP (from ref 57 with permission).

reducing the GI ulcerogenicity compared with its congener, indomethacin [11,21,27-30] is probably due to its rapid conversion to the active metabolite, sulindac sulphide such that appreciable quantities are evident in the GI mucosa and produce consequent cyclo-oxygenase (CO) inhibition-dependent cellular injury therein [28-30].

Another strategy we have employed is to examine the structural features of those NSAIDs which we can identify as being of low relative ulcerogenicity compared with those of established drugs such as indomethacin and aspirin [11,21,27-31], where the case is proven for their ulcerogenic effects, so as to identify structural features underlying ulcerogenicity of NSAIDs [30,31].

Recently, it was suggested [32,33] that the low ulcerogenicity of azapropazone [11,21,27-33] might be due to the amphiprotic character conferred by the intermolecular association of the nitrogen group in the dimethyl-amino moiety with the hydroxyl group in this drug (Figure 6) [32,33]. A consequence of this amphiprotic property is that it may account for the high relative aquo-solubility of azapropazone under acidic conditions [33].

To test this hypothesis we compared the ulcerogenic effects of the des-dimethyl-amino-derivative of azapropazone (DDA) (which we prepared) with that of azapropazone (APZ) itself reasoning that if the dimethyl-amino-nitrogen association with the hydroxyl group has any significance

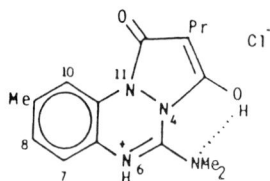

Azapropazone (HCl salt)

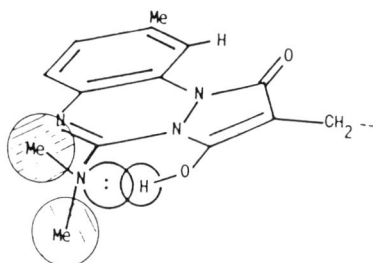

Out-of-plane view
showing N-diMe---HO-
interactions

Figure 6: Structure of azapropazone showing the hydrogen bonding of the *N*-dimethyl-amino nitrogen to the hydroxyl group, both in planar and out of plane steric view.

then DDA should be more ulcerogenic than APZ [unpublished data]. The data we obtained in cholinomimetic-stimulated mouse gastric ulcer assay showed that these two drugs were equi-ulcerogenic [unpublished data – studies in preparation]. We, therefore, conclude that the dimethyl-amino group confers little if any significant influences on the low ulcerogenicity of APZ. It is possible that the solubility properties of APZ do give it properties of slow absorption from the stomach and this may be a minor contributory factor to the low ulcerogenicity of APZ. Other features should be sought perhaps relating to the electronic character of the benzotriazine ring system which is unique among NSAIDs and this might be important in the low ulcerogenicity of this drug. Certainly, in comparison with phenylbutazone and oxyphenbutazone which are keto-enolates but without the benzotriazine ring system of APZ these two former drugs are appreciably more ulcerogenic than APZ [29-31] suggesting the benzotriazine structure of APZ is of major significance. The ring structure of other NSAIDs has been shown to be of considerable importance in ulcerogenicity especially when electron-withdrawing substituents (e.g. halogens) are added to increase anti-inflammatory potency; this coincidently leading to increased ulcerogenicity in many compounds [34].

The role of carboxylic acid moieties of NSAIDs in gastric ulcerogenesis has classically been shown by the protection against mucosal damage afforded by esters of these drugs [23,24]. Drugs such as keto-enolates with an acidic function which are not carboxylates may be less irritating because of their higher pKa compared with that of the latter [33].

While it is not possible to review at length other important physico-chemical features of NSAIDs underlying their ulcerogenicity, these and other studies underway may give insight into this aspect and help in the design of less ulcerogenic drugs.

Role of lipid mediators

Prostaglandin inhibition in gastric mucosal damage by NSAIDs

Inhibition by anti-inflammatory drugs of the synthesis of mucosal protective prostaglandins (PGs) has been much studied and recognized as a major factor in the initiation of gastric mucosal injury by NSAIDs [9,10, 14-17]. A number of mechanisms have been proposed to explain the consequences of these inhibitory effects in the stomach (e.g. reduced production of mucus and bicarbonate, damage to the microvasculature with alterations in blood flow, and alterations in the regulation of acid and pepsin secretion) (reviewed in refs. 9,16,34).

The importance of PGs in the maintenance of mucosal integrity has been demonstrated by the well-known potent effects they exhibit in preventing gastric mucosal injury by noxious irritants including NSAIDs and their clinical utility as anti-ulcer agents [35,36; see other chapters in this book]. However in NSAID-induced gastric mucosal damage there does not appear to be a specific link between inhibition of PG synthesis and development of gastric mucosal damage [9,15]. It has been shown by several authors that oral or parenteral administration of aspirin (in low doses), chloroquine, indomethacin or oxaprozin to rats can reduce mucosal concentrations of PGE_2 and/or PGI_2 (prostacyclin) in vivo without causing the appearance of gastric lesions [9,15,26,27,37-39].

These apparent negative observations contrast, however, with evidence that the inhibitory effects of NSAIDs on PG synthesis in isolated microsomes and other in vitro systems correlates with the gastric ulcerogenic potency of these drugs in various rat models [15]. There is, however, one reported exception to this where piroxicam was found to be a relatively weak inhibitor of PG synthesis in human microsomes and scrapings in vitro [40] even though this drug is of high ulcerogenicity in sensitive models of NSAID gastric irritancy in rats [28], mice [30], pigs [21] and is well-known to be associated with gastric ulcers in man [29]. Piroxicam is, however, a reversible inhibitor of cyclo-oxygenase (CO) with respect to its substrate arachidonate [41]. Since release of arachidonate

105

occurs during incubation with the drug *in vitro* this substrate might well over-ride the CO inhibitory effects of the drug. In contrast to these *in vitro* results, it has been found that gastric mucosal concentrations of PGE_2 are reduced *in vivo* 1 hour following oral administration of piroxicam to rats [9]. The difference in the results from *in vitro* experiments might be explained by arachidonate reversing the drug induced inhibition of CO. Given the important role of the kinetics of drug uptake into the gastric mucosa in determining inhibitory effects on PG production [26,27] the correlation between inhibitory potency of NSAIDs on CO and their gastric ulcerogenicity still requires reconciling with the lack of a strict linkage of CO-inhibitory effects of NSAIDs to the time-sequence of the appearance of mucosal damage [15]. It seems, therefore, reasonable to look for additional consequences of cyclo-oxygenase (CO) related effects which could be important in the pathogenesis of NSAID gastric ulceration.

Activation of the lipoxygenase pathway

A number of studies indicate that some NSAIDs could, by inhibiting CO activity, cause diversion of arachidonate through the lipoxygenase pathway as postulated (Figure 5) [14]. This might lead to excess vasoactive PEP-LTs and peroxy-derived cell-destructive oxyradicals (Figure 4). Evidence in support of this hypothesis comes from observations that (a) administration of 5-lipoxygenase inhibitors or leukotriene antagonists reduces the development of NSAID-induced gastric mucosal lesions in rodents [22], and (b) some NSAIDs which are of low ulcerogenicity (e.g. azapropazone, benoxaprofen) have some modest effects in inhibiting 5-LO activity [20,27]. The implications from these studies are that NSAIDs may somehow cause an imbalance of eicosanoid metabolism by their CO-inhibitory effects. It is possible that dual CO-LO inhibitors (e.g. BW755C) are less ulcerogenic because they do not induce such perturbations [31] though it should be appreciated that many of these drugs have antioxidant activity and other actions which contribute to their low ulcerogenicity.

The lipoxygenase pathway could be implicated in the development of gastric mucosal damage by its products inducing damage to vascular and other mucosal cells [14,16,42]. These include the production of oxygen radicals and reduced sulphydryl group reactivity [14]. Oxyradicals could be produced in the conversion of peroxy- to hydroxy acids as well as being involved in these reactions other sources of oxyradicals are involved in arachidonic acid release and metabolism [14]. The reduced sulphydryl reactions could result in part, from incorporation of glutathione in the synthesis of peptido-leukotrienes. However, there could be other mechanisms where oxyradicals and thiols are important (e.g. superoxide anion generation, involvement of thiols in cell regulation). Thiols would also be expected to be oxidized by oxyradicals. The evidence for the

106

involvement of oxyradicals and thiol groups in NSAID-induced mucosal injury has been derived from experiments with agents (e.g. oxyradical scavengers, thiol-containing agents) [14,16] which are not very specific in their actions. The nature of the oxyradicals produced and of the thiols oxidized or otherwise altered has not been determined. Likewise, the apparent gastro-protective effects of the agents has not been correlated with their actions on the postulated biochemical system i.e. by way of measurements of changes in products of oxyradical attack (e.g. lipid peroxides) or specific thiols (e.g. cysteine, glutathione).

Aside from one isolated report [43] the evidence to date suggests that NSAIDs increase products of the lipoxygenase pathway. As shown in Figures 7 and 8 the two potent CO inhibitors, indomethacin and diclofenac, given to pigs under single or multiple dose regimes both cause enhancement of leukotriene production in the gastric mucosa of these animals. The gastric injury produced by these NSAIDs is associated with extravasation of blood cell components and fine structural evidence of damage to both pigs and rats [19,20,27,28]. That products of the 5-LO pathway could affect the integrity of the gastric mucosa receives support from the studies of Pendleton and Stavorski [44]. They fould that intravenous infusion of LTD_4 to anaesthetized cats resulted in (a) a

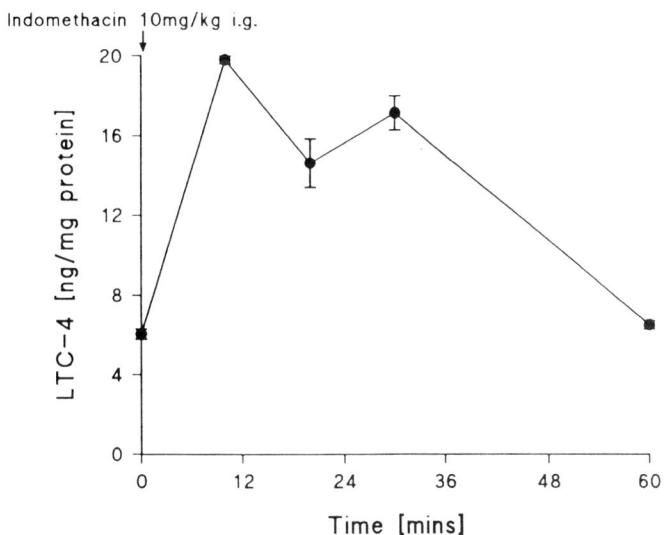

Figure 7: Effects of intragastric administration of 10 mg/kg indomethacin on the production of radio-immunoassayable leukotriene C_4 in the plasma of the efferent gastrosplenic circulation of halothane-nitrous oxide anaesthetized pigs (procedures as described in ref. 21). The same dose of the NSAID also decreases the production of PGE_2 in the gastric mucosa of pigs over the same time period; the animals being treated in the same way (except for cannulation of the blood supply) as described in ref. 21.

107

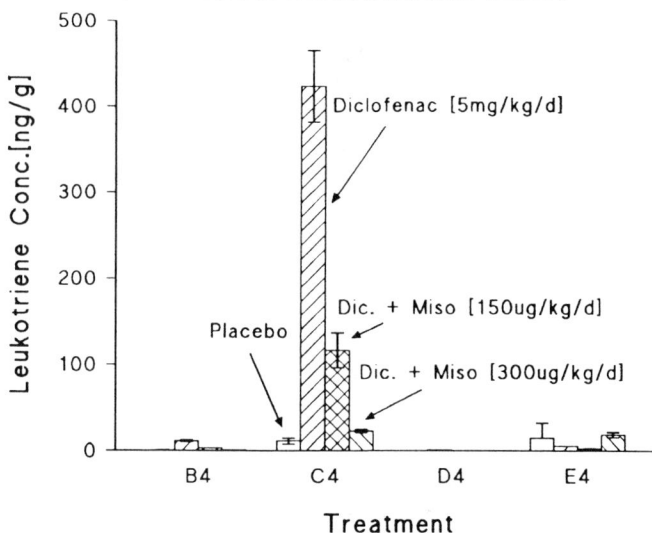

Figure 8: Effects of repeated daily administration of diclofenac (5 mg kg^{-1} day^{-1} for 10 days in divided doses) on the production of leukotrienes (LTs) B_4, C_4, D_4 and E_4 in the gastric mucosa of pigs at 2 h after the final dose, and the effects of co-administration of misoprostol (150 and 300 μg kg^{-1} day^{-1}) in reducing the production of LTs.

marked reduction in transmucosal electropotential difference reflecting breakdown of the gastric mucosal barrier, and (b) enhanced secretion of pepsin which could contribute to ulcer development by proteolysis.

Vasoconstrictor effects of LTs on the microvasculature might be one means of initiating ischaemia providing there is a reperfusion of oxygenated blood which follows so enabling superoxide to be produced [14]. One other source of vaso-active mediators derived from LO activity in the gastric micro-circulation was demonstrated by Salvati and Whittle [45]. These authors showed that infusion of various hydroperoxyeicosatetrae-noic acids (HPETEs) cause vasodilatation of the gastric blood vessels whereas the corresponding hydroxy acids (HETEs) were without effect. This suggests that vasodilatory activity is associated with the peroxy-moiety of these acids. It is clear, therefore, from these published studies that the main products of the 5-LO pathway, i.e. PEP-LTs and HPETEs do have potent effects on the vascular integrity of the gastric mucosa which could be considered important in their potential for reducing mucosal integrity.

Recently, Wallace et al. have shown that NSAID-associated mucosal injury is a neutrophil-dependent reaction [46,47]. It is possible that this reaction is due to the diversion of arachidonate following CO inhibition by NSAIDs to yield production of LTB$_4$, a lipoxygenase product which is well-known to promote accumulation and adhesion of leucocytes to blood capillaries [42].

Exogenous PGs could also prevent both the leucocyte accumulation and adhesion at sites of mucosal injury but also may modulate 5-LO activity. As shown in Figure 8 co-administration of misoprostol with diclofenac reduced the production of leukotrienes caused by the latter. The mechanism of this effect may be related to the reduction of LT production following stimulation of cyclic-AMP by the PGE analogue [48,49].

ROLE OF NUTRIENTS

We have been interested for a number of years in the effects of NSAIDs on mucosal intermediary and trace metal metabolism in the genesis of mucosal ulceration by these drugs. The effects of salicylates and other NSAIDs on the metabolism of glucose, the functions of the tricarboxylic acid (Kreb's or TCA) cycle and mitochondrial production of adenosine triphosphate (ATP) formed the initial focus of our interest since these metabolic events would seem to be important in the maintenance of mucosal protective functions which are so dependent upon ATP (Figure 9).

We originally decided to test the hypothesis that depletion of glucose and TCA metabolism caused by aspirin (or its mucosal metabolite salicylate) inhibiting enzymes involved in these pathways and the uncoupling of oxidative phophorylation in mitochondria by examining the potential protective effects of glucose and TCA cycle intermediates or

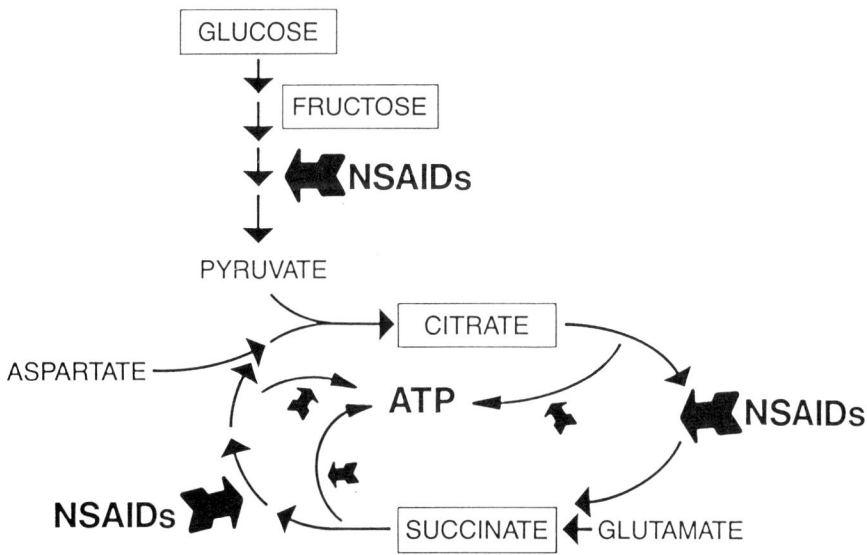

Figure 9: Sites of action of some NSAIDs on the glycolytic and tricarboxylate pathways ultimately affecting the mitochondrial and extramitochondrial production of adenosine triphosphate (ATP). Arrows show sites of inhibition of enzymes by NSAIDs.

precursors given in combination with aspirin to rats [50]. We found that substantial, but not complete, reduction in gastric mucosal injury by aspirin, and indeed other NSAIDs, was achieved by glucose or other glycolytic precursors or intermediates given with TCA cycle intermediates or precursors, but not when these were given alone or when non-metabolizable analogues of these metabolites (e.g. 2-deoxy-glucose) in a variety of different test systems in laboratory animal models [50-54]. Moreover, the reduction of gastric mucosal injury by aspirin given in combination with glucose and sodium acetate coincided with restoration of mucosal ATP levels and glucose utilization in the mucosa to near normal levels [50].

To our surprise (and despite initial disbelief that this could occur!) we were able to show in collaborative studies that reduction in GI injury could occur in human volunteers given specially formulated combinations of glucose and citrate with the drugs [52-54]. We had to work out the optimal ratios of glucose and citrate required for GI mucosal protection and at the same time retaining drug stability details of which have been reported in part elsewhere [52,54] and will be described fully later. Furthermore, it appears at least with indomethacin and azapropazone that these formulations do not lead to any reduction in bioavailability or anti-inflammatory/analgesic activity of the NSAIDs [53,54; unpublished observations]. Recently, we reported that a 1:1:1 formulation of azapropazone/glucose/sodium acid citrate caused a slight reduction in what is normally a low rate of blood loss observed with azapropazone alone and reduced the otherwise severe GI symptoms in a small group of subjects who were known to be severely intolerant in the GI tract to NSAIDs [54]. The pharmacokinetics of the drug were unaltered by the addition of the glucose-citrate combination [54]. Not surprisingly, little effect of the combination was shown in reducing endoscopically observed injury in the gastro-duodenal mucosa in subjects with rheumatoid arthritis [54], since azapropazone itself is relatively of low ulcerogenicity. More striking differences in blood loss and other observations of GI injury have been observed with the indomethacin formulation of glucose + citrate (15:15 ratio with respect to indomethacin = 1) [52; unpublished studies]. These results give encouragement to the potential of nutrient mixtures for reducing the ulcerogenicity of NSAIDs and also, quite significantly, highlight the importance of NSAID effects on mucosal metabolism in the development of mucosal ulceration in the GI tract.

Our interest in the effects of trace metals in NSAID ulcerogenesis may be linked, in part, to the effects of some of these metal ions (e.g. Cu, Zn) on thiols in biomolecules of the mucosa [16].

Recently, we have investigated the effects of a slow-release complex of zinc for its effects in protecting the gastric mucosa against NSAID ulceration. This complex, zinc monoglycerolate [ZMG; Glyzinc (TM),

110

Glyzinc Pharmaceuticals Ltd., 6 Janet Court, Highbury, South Australia, Australia] has a well-defined, pH-dependent capacity to slowly release zinc in a sustained fashion in the stomach, so avoiding rapid absorption and the profound astringency observed with zinc salts (e.g. zinc sulphate which have been previously shown to have some anti-ulcer activity). We showed in several ulcer models (e.g. arthritic rats exposed to brief chilling, cholinomimetic-treated mice, both of which show enhanced ulcerogenicity with NSAIDs), that ZMG exhibited a dose-response reduction in gastric ulcerogenicity from NSAIDs which was about comparable with that of the histamine H_2 antagonist, cimetidine [56]. Data on the protective effects of ZMG in cold-stressed arthritic rats given aspirin are shown in Figure 10 from which it can be seen that the effects of this complex were comparable to zinc sulphate and superior to zinc oxide. Our studies also showed that the protective effects of ZMG were time-related, i.e. the timing of the dose of ZMG was defined to be within a narrow time period with respect to the dose of the NSAID and to be protective both the ZMG and NSAID have to be given orally [55,56], thus showing the specificity of protection. There was no reduction in the anti-inflammatory activity of the NSAIDs when

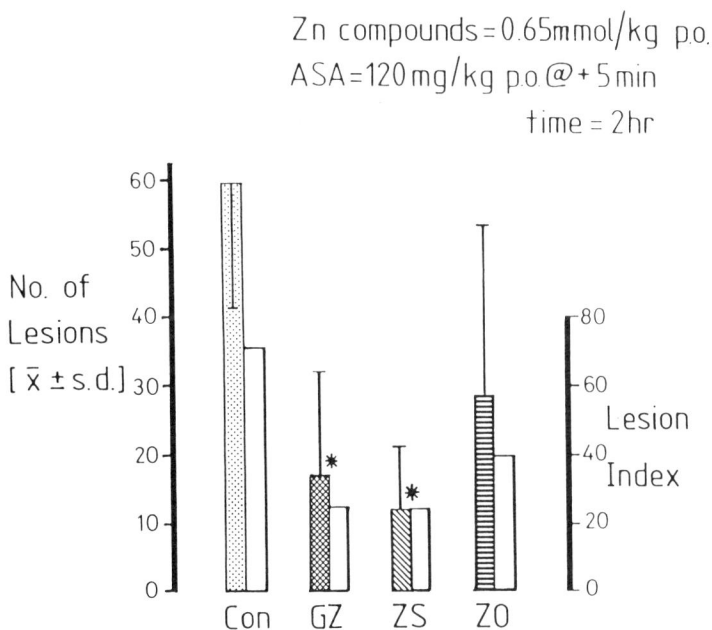

Figure 10: Effects of zinc monoglycerolate (GZ) compared with zinc sulphate (ZS) and zinc oxide (ZO) given concurrently with aspirin on the gastro-ulcerogenic effects of the latter 2 h after oral administration of these compounds to arthritic rats exposed to −18°C for 35 min. The number of lesions and their area were measured by visual image analysis [31].

given in combination with ZMG [56], and no demonstrable toxicity has been observed even with large oral doses of ZMG in laboratory animals (unpublished observations, K.D. Rainsford and M.W. Whitehouse).

CONCLUSIONS

In this review a number of different strategies have been explored for reducing the ulcerogenicity of NSAIDs in the GI tract. Some have already shown promise while others still require further exploration and persistent investigation to determine their suitability for clinical use. In the meantime we are beginning to understand further the role of NSAID effects on specific mucosal defence prcesses in the genesis of GI injury by these drugs.

REFERENCES

1. Doherty C. Non-steroidal anti-inflammatory drugs in patients with peptic ulcer diseases: to be considered in certain circumstances. Br Med J. 1989;298:176-9.
2. Hawkey C. Non-steroidal anti-inflammatory drugs in patients with peptic ulcer diseases: rarely justified in terms of cost or benefit. Br Med J 1989; 298:177-8.
3. Roth SH. NSAID gastropathy - the central issue. Drugs 1990;40:25-28.
4. Fries JF. NSAID gastropathy; the second most deadly rheumatic disease? Epidemiology and risk appraisal. J Rheumatol. 1991;18 (suppl. 28): 6-10.
5. Griffin MR, Piper JM, Daugherty JR, Snowden M, Ray, WA. Nonsteroidal anti-inflammatory drug use and increased risk for peptic ulcer disease in elderly persons. Ann Intern Med. 1991; 114:257-63.
6. Soll AH, Weinstein WM, Kurata J, McCarthy D. Nonsteroidal anti-inflammatory drugs and peptic ulcer disease. Ann Intern Med, 1991; 114:307-19.
7. Bjarnason I, Fehilly B, Smethurst P, Menzies IS, Levi AJ. Importance of local versus systemic effects of non-steroidal anti-inflammatory drugs in increasing intestinal permeability in man. Gut 1991; 32: 275-7.
8. Jenkins AP, Trew DR, Crump BJ, Nukajam WS, Foley JA, Menzies IS, Creamer B. Do non-steroidal anti-inflammatory drugs increase colonic permeability. Gut 1991; 32:66-9.
9. Rainsford KD. Mechanisms of gastric contrasted with intestinal damage by non-steroidal anti-inflammatory drugs. In: Rainsford KD, Velo GP. (eds.) Side Effects of Anti-inflammatory Drugs. Part 2. Studies in Major Organ Systems. Lancaster, MTP Press,1987:3-26.
10. Whittle BJR, Vane JR. A biochemical basis for the gastrointestinal toxicity of non-steroidal antirheumatoid drugs. Arch Toxicol 1984; 7 (Suppl.): 315-22.
11. Rainsford KD. Toxicity of currently used anti-inflammatory and anti-rheumatic drugs. In: Lewis AJ, Furst DE (eds.) Newer Anti- Inflammatory Drugs. New York, Marcel Dekker, 1987: 215-44.
12. Rainsford KD. Side-effects of anti-inflammatory/analgesic and anti-rheumatic drugs. In: Williamson WRN (ed). Anti-Inflammatory Drugs. New York, Marcel Dekker, New York, 1978: 359-406.
13. Rainsford KD Current concepts of the mechanisms of side effects of non-steroidal anti-inflammatory drugs as a basis for establishing research priorities: an experimentalists view. J Rheumatol 1988; 15 (Suppl. 17): 63-70.
14. Rainsford KD. Mechanisms of NSAID-induced gastrointestinal mucosal injury: a basis for preventing ulceration and symptoms from these agents. Aliment Pharmacol Therap 1988; 2S: 43-55.

15. Rainsford KD. Interplay between anti-inflammatory drugs and eicosanoids in gastro-intestinal damage. In: Hillier K (ed.) Eicosanoids and the Gastrointestinal Tract. Lancaster, MTP Press, 1988: 111-128.
16. Szabo S, Spill WF, Rainsford KD. Nonsteroidal anti-inflammatory drug-induced gastropathy: mechanisms and management. Medical Toxicol 1989; 4: 77-94.
17. Rainsford KD. Mechanisms of gastrointestinal damage by non- steroidal anti-inflammatory drugs. In: Szabo S, Pfeiffer CJ (eds).Ulcer Disease: New Aspects of Pathogenesis and Pharmacology. Boca Raton (FL), CRC Press, 1989: 3-13.
18. Price AH, Fletcher M. Mechanisms of NSAID-induced gastroenteropathy. Drugs 1990; 40: 25-8.
19. Rainsford KD. Microvascular injury during gastric mucosal damage by anti-inflammatory drugs in pigs and rats. Agents Actions. 1983;13:457–460.
20. Rainsford KD, Willis CM, Walker SA, Robins PG. Electron microscopic observations comparing the gastric mucosal damage induced in rats and pigs by benoxaprofen with aspirin, reflecting their differing actions as prostaglandin synthesis inhibitors. Br J Exp Pathol. 1982;63:25–34.
21. Rainsford KD, Willis C. Relationship of gastric mucosal damage induced in pigs by anti-inflammatory drugs to their effects on prostaglandin production. Dig Dis Sci. 1982;27:624–635.
22. Rainsford KD. Effects of 5-lipoxygenase inhibitors and leukotriene antagonists on the development of gastric mucosal lesions induced by nonsteroidal anti-inflammatory drugs in cholinomimetic treated mice. Agents Actions. 1987;21:316-319.
23. Whitehouse MW, Rainsford, KD. Esterification of acidic anti-inflammatory drugs suppresses their gastro-toxicity without adversely affecting their anti-inflammatory activity in rats. J Pharm Pharmacol. 1980;32:795–796.
24. Whitehouse MW, Rainsford, KD. Comparison of the ulcerogenic actions of different salicylates. In: Pfeiffer, CJ (ed.), Boca Raton (Florida), CRC Press, 1982; 127-141.
25. Rainsford, K.D. Novel non-steroidal anti-inflammatory drugs. In: Brooks, P.M. (ed) Bailliere's Clinical Rheumatology, vol.2. London, Bailliere-Tindall 1988; 485-511.
26. Jeremy JY, Williams JD. Drug development report (5): Prodrugs: the answer to NSAID-induced gastropathy? J Drug Dev 1990; 3:93–107.
27. Rainsford KD, Fox SA, Osborne DJ. Comparative effects of some non-steroidal anti-inflammatory drugs on the ultrastructural integrity and prostaglandin levels in the rat gastric mucosa: relationship to drug uptake. Scand J Gastroenterol 1984: 19 (Suppl. 101): 55-68.
28. Rainsford KD, Fox SA, Osborne DJ. Relationship between drug absorption, inhibition of cyclooxygenase and lipoxygenase pathways and the development of gastric mucosal damage by non-steroidal anti-inflammatory drugs in rats and pigs. In: Bailey, MJ (ed). New York, Plenum Press, 1985; 639-653.
29. Rainsford KD. Comparison of the gastric ulcerogenic activity of new non-steroidal anti-inflammatory drugs in stressed rats. Br J Pharmacol. 1981;73:79c–80c.
30. Rainsford KD. An analysis of the gastrointestinal side-effects of non-steroidal anti-inflammatory drugs, with particular reference to comparative studies in man and laboratory species. Rheumatol Int. 1982;2:1–10.
31. Rainsford KD. Gastric ulcerogenicity of non-steroidal anti-inflammatory drugs in mice with mucosa sensitized by cholinomimetic treatment. J Pharm Pharmacol. 1987;39:669–672.
32. McCormack K, Brune K. The amphiprotic character of azapropazone and its relevance to the gastric mucosa. Arch Toxicol. 1991;64:1–6.
33. McCormack, K. Mathematical model for assessing risk of gastrointestinal reactions to NSAIDs. In: Rainsford KD (ed). Azapropazone. 20 years of clinical use. Lancaster, Kluwer, 1989; 81-93.
34. Rainsford KD. Structure-activity relationships of non-steroidal anti-inflammatory drugs. I. Gastric ulcerogenic activity. Agents Actions 1978; 8:587-605.
35. Whittle BJR. Protection of the gastric mucosa by prostaglandins and their analogs. ISI Atlas of Science: Pharmacology 1987; 1: 168-172.
36. Agrawal NM, Dajani EZ. Options in the treatment and prevention of NSAID-induced gastroduodenal mucosal damage. J Rheumatol 1990; (suppl. 20) 17:7-11.

37. Ligumsky M, Golanska EM, Hansen DG, Kauffman GL. Aspirin can inhibit gastric mucosal cyclo-oxygenase without causing lesions in rat. Gastroenterology 1983; 84:756-761.

38. Goldin E, Stalnikowicz R, Wengrower D, Eliakim R, Fich A, Ligumsky M, Karmeli F, Rachmilewitz D. No correlation between indomethacin-indiced gastrodudenal damage and inhibition of gastric prostanoid synthesis. Aliment Pharmacol Therap 1988; 2:369-375.

39. Rainsford KD. Comparative effects of oxaprozin on the gastrointestinal tract of rats and mice: relationship to drug uptake and effects in vivo on eicosanoid metabolism. Aliment Pharmacol Therap 1988; 2:439-450.

40. Tavares IA, Collins PO, Bennett A. Inhibition of prostanoid synthesis by human gastric mucosa. Aliment Pharmacol Therap 1987; 1:617-625.

41. Carty TJ, Stevens JS, Lombardino JG, Parry MJ, Randall MJ. Piroxicam, a structurally novel anti-inflammatory compound. Mode of prostaglandin synthesis inhibition. Prostaglandins 1980; 19:671-682.

42. Dahlen S-E, Bjrk J, Hedqvist P, Arfors K-E, Hammerstrm S, Lindgren J-A, Samuelson B. Leukotrienes promote plasma leakage and leukocyte adhesion in postcapillary venules:In vivo effects with relevance to the acute inflammatory response. Proc Natl Acad Sci USA 1981; 78:3887-3891.

43. Peskar BM, Hoppe U, Lange K, Peskar BA. Effects of non-steroidal anti-inflammatory drugs on rat gastric mucosal leukotriene C_4 and prostanoid release – relation to ethanol injury. Br J Pharmacol 1988; 93:937-943.

44. Pendleton RG, Stavorski JR. Evidence for differing leukotriene receptors in gastric mucosa. Europ J Pharmcol 1986; 125:297-299.

45. Salvati P, Whittle BJR. Investigation of the vascular actions of arachidonate lipoxygenase and cyclooxygenase products. Prostaglandins 1981; 22:141-156.

46. Wallace JL, Keenan CM, Granger DN. Gastric ulceration induced by non-steroidal anti-inflammatory drugs is a neutrophil dependent process. Am J Physiol 1990; 259:G462-G467.

47. Wallace JL, Arfors KE, Webb-McKnight G. A monoclonal antibody against the CD18 leukocyte adhesion molecule prevents indomethacin-induced gastric damage in the rabbit. Gastroenterology 1991; 100:878-883.

48. Kuehl FA Jr, Dougherty HW, Ham EA. Interactions between prostaglandins and leukotrienes. Biochem Pharmacol 1984; 33:1-5.

49. Waisman Y, Marcus H, Ligumski M, Dinari G. Modulation by opiates of small intestinal prostaglandin E_2 and $3',5'$-cyclic adenosine monophosphate levels and of indomethacin-induced ulceration in the rat. Life Sci 1991; 48:2035-2042.

50. Rainsford KD, Whitehouse MW. Biochemical gastro-protection from acute ulceration induced by aspirin and related drugs. Biochem Pharmacol 1980; 29:1281-1289.

51. Rainsford KD. Prevention of indomethacin induced gastro-intestinal ulceration in rats by glucose-citrate formulations: role of ATP in mucosal defences. Br J Rheumatol 1987; 26:(Abstr Suppl. 2) 81.

52. Walker FS, Pritchard MH, Jones JM, Owen GM, Rainsford KD. Inhibition of indomethacin-induced gastrointestinal bleeding, both immediate and persistent, in man by citrate-glucose formulations. Br J Rheumatol 1987; 26:(Abstr Suppl. 2) 12.

53. Whitehouse MW, Rainsford-Koechli V, Rainsford KD. Aspirin gastrotoxicity: protection by various strategems. In: Rainsford KD, Velo GP (eds.). Side Effects of Anti-inflammatory/ Analgesic Drugs. New York, Raven Press,1984; 77-87.

54. Rainsford KD, Dieppe PA, Pritchard MH, Rhodes J, Leach H, Russell RI, Walker FS, Hort JF. Protection from gastrointestinal side-effects by azapropazone by its incorporation into a glucose-sodium citrate formulation. Aliment Pharmacol Ther. 1991;5:.

55. Rainsford KD, Whitehouse MW. Anti-ulcer activity of zinc monoglycerolate (Glyzinc (R)): a slow-release zinc formuulation. Clin Expt Physiol Pharmacol. 1987.

56. Rainsford KD, Whitehouse MW. Anti-ulcer activity of a slow-release zinc complex, zinc monoglycerolate [Glyzinc(R)]. J. Pharm. Pharmacol. 1991; accepted.

57. Rainsford KD. Mechanisms of gastrointestinal toxicity of non-steroidal anti-inflammatory drugs. Scand J Gastroenterol 1989; 24:(Suppl 163) 9-16.

15

Novel strategies of gastric and duodenal mucosal protection against NSAID injury: role of protease inhibitors, muscle relaxants and growth factors

S. Szabo, E. Gyomber, R.E. Morales, L. Nagy and P. Vattay

Chemical Pathology Research Division, Department of Pathology, Brigham and Women's Hospital, Harvard Medical School, Boston, MA 02115, USA

The pathogenesis of gastroduodenal mucosal lesions induced by non-steroidal anti-inflammatory drugs (NSAIDs) is a complex and multi-factorial process [1–3]. Since these lesions involve a spectrum of alterations including single ulcers, multiple localized haemorrhagic erosions and diffuse mucosal changes whose pathogenesis is poorly understood, the term NSAID gastropathy is often used as a group designation [3]. The NSAID gastropathy has certain similarities and differences with non-specific 'peptic' ulcers, e.g. the natural history of both lesions is incompletely understood and while NSAID gastropathy is more frequent in females and localized mostly in the stomach, 'peptic' ulcers are more prevalent in males and in the duodenum [2].

The standard treatment for both groups of disorders has been acid-oriented, i.e. use of antacids and antisecretory agents, although as a recent review of the literature points out [3], the response of NSAID gastropathy to acid-suppressing agents has been at best equivocal.

A second generation of preventive agents became available with the introduction of the concept of gastric cytoprotection [4–6] and with new biochemically based pharmacological approaches for the prevention and treatment of NSAID-induced gastroduodenal mucosal lesions [7,8]. Although this approach produced some clinically tested and promising compounds such as misoprostol [5], most of the compounds, e.g. prostaglandins (PG), sulphydryls (SH) and non-SH anti-oxidants [9,10] need further work at basic research and clinical level.

Side-effects of Anti-inflammatory Drugs 3. Rainsford KD, Velo GP (eds), Inflammation and Drug Therapy Series, Volume V.

In the meantime, a third generation of compounds became available for the prevention and treatment of chemically induced gastroduodenal ulcers. These agents do not suppress gastric acid secretion, hence, they act more physiologically; in agreement with the multifactorial pathogenesis of NSAID-induced gastroduodenal lesions, they affect several pharmacological parameters. Furthermore, in addition to prophylaxis, some of the compounds also accelerate the healing of chronic ulcers. Since some of these results originate from our recent investigations, we thus briefly review our recent findings on the role of enzyme inhibitors, smooth muscle relaxants and growth factors in NSAID-induced gastric and duodenal acute and chronic ulcers. These novel strategies are summarized in Table 1.

Table 1. Novel strategies for the prevention and treatment of NSAID-induced gastric and duodenal mucosal injury

Acute erosions and ulcers
        – cysteine (thiol) protease inhibitors
        – angiotensin converting enzyme (ACE) inhibitors
        – smooth muscle relaxants (pinaverium)
Chronic ulcer healing
        – growth factors (bFGF, PDGF)

PROTEASE INHIBITORS

These enzyme inhibitors were implicated in the pathogenesis and pharmacology of chemically induced acute gastric mucosal lesions based on our previous work on the prevention of ethanol- or aspirin-induced haemorrhagic gastric erosions by SH compounds [3,9–12]. Subsequently, we found that pretreatment of rats with low doses of SH alkylators such as N-ethylmaleimide (NEM) or iodoacetate administered intragastrically (i.g.) also offered dose- and time-dependent gastroprotection [13–16]. The following experiments were performed as follow-up to these preliminary studies.

Cysteine protease inhibitors

Cysteine or thiol proteases are one of the four major classes of proteinases which possess SH group(s) at the catalytic site or SH groups are crucial for their enzymatic activity [17]. These proteases are localized in the cytoplasm, plasma membrane and lysosomes in high concentrations especially in the kidney, gastric mucosa and spleen [13,17].

We proposed that one of the main mechanisms of mucosal protection by NEM and iodoacetate is the inhibition of gastric cysteine (thiol) proteases which contribute to the development of chemically induced tissue damage [13–16]. These enzymes, especially cathepsin B, exhibit prominent tissue destructive properties and are important in the metastatic invasion of malignant tumours [18], activation of pro-collagenase and in the degradation of membrane glycoproteins in adult organs and during embryogenesis [19].

The hypothesis about cysteine proteases was a follow-up to our previous demonstration that the common biochemical element in the mechanism of action of diverse gastroprotective agents such as metals, SH-containing compounds, diethyl maleate (DEM) which depletes glutathione, and PG is not glutathione but rather a decrease in the concentration of gastric mucosal protein SH [9,20]. This decrease in total protein cysteine SH concentration might be beneficial in the gastric mucosa for at least two reasons: (a) a decrease in protein cysteine and increase in cysteine disulphides enhance the stability of proteins [6] and presumably make the membrane proteins more resistant to damage; (b) the diminished protein SH levels may be associated with reduced release and activity of cysteine proteases such as cathepsin B [11,13].

The last possibility has been tested in our and other laboratories. We demonstrated histochemically and biochemically that cysteine proteases such as cathepsin B are localized in large concentrations in the top third of the gastric mucosa and these cells released large amounts of cathepsin B after intragastric infusion of 50% ethanol [13,16]. A single small i.g. dose of iodoacetate or NEM completely prevented the release of thiol proteases and abolished the alcohol-induced haemorrhagic gastric mucosal lesions [13,16]. Pretreatment of rats with NEM or chloroacetate also decreased the area and extent of acute haemorrhagic gastric erosions caused by acidified aspirin (Table 2) or HCl. These results suggest that protease inhibitors exert gastroprotection of wide spectrum which includes, besides NSAIDs, ethanol and HCl.

Subsequent pharmacological and structure-activity studies revealed that new derivatives of NEM and iodoacetate represent a novel group of very potent gastroprotective agents with long duration of action and low

Table 2. Effect of iodoacetate and chloroacetate on aspirin-induced gastric erosions in the rat

Group	Treatment	Area of mucosal lesions (% of glandular stomach)
1	Aspirin	0.7 ± 0.4
2	Iodoacetate + aspirin	$0.3 \pm 0.1*$
3	Chloroacetate + aspirin	$0.06 \pm 0.03*$

* $= p < 0.05$
Iodoacetate (1 mg/100 g) or chloroacetate (5 mg/100 g, i.g.) was administered 30 min before acidified aspirin (10 mg/100 g in 1% methylcellulose prepared with 0.2 N HCl), and the animals were killed 1 h after aspirin

Table 3. Time-dependent effect of the cysteine protease inhibitor N-ethylmaleimide (NEM) on ethanol-induced gastric erosions in the rat

Group	Treatment[+] Name	Time between NEM and ethanol	Area of mucosal lesions (% of glandular stomach)
1	Vehicle	–	22.6±4.8
2	NEM	1 min	0.0±0 ***
3	NEM	5 min	0.8±0.4 ***
4	NEM	15 min	0.7±0.6 ***
5	NEM	30 min	0.9±0.7 ***
6	NEM	1 h	3.3±1.4 **
7	NEM	2 h	2.1±0.6 **
8	NEM	4 h	8.2±3.7 *
9	NEM	8 h	4.9±0.9 **
10	NEM	12 h	7.7±3.0 *
11	NEM	24 h	7.6±1.9
12	NEM	48 h	20.1±4.6

* = $p < 0.05$; ** = $p < 0.01$; *** = $p < 0.005$

[+] In addition, rats of all groups were given 1 ml of 100% ethanol by gavage, and the animals were killed 1 h later. Vehicle solvent or NEM (0.1 mg/100 g) were adminstered i.g. at times indicated

toxicity. Namely, the mucosal protective effects of a single dose of NEM was lost only after 48 h (Table 3). In comparison, adaptive cytoprotection exerted by low concentration of damaging agents last only for 30–60 min, while gastroprotection by PG and SH derivatives is usually demonstrable for 4–6 h [4,6,11]. Thus, these studies indicate that cysteine protease inhibitors are novel agents for the prevention of NSAID-induced acute gastric mucosal lesions, but further investigations are needed to define their mode of action and identify new derivatives with high therapeutic index.

Angiotensin converting enzyme inhibitors

Since SH compounds offering gastroprotection and vascular factors (e.g. prevention of vascular injury and maintenance of blood flow) play a role in gastric mucosal injury and protection, we recently tested the hypothesis that SH and non-SH containing inhibitors of angiotensin converting enzyme (ACE) might also exert gastroprotection because of their SH content and/or effect on microvasculature. These studies were published recently [21] and are briefly summarized here.

The results obtained in fasted Sprague–Dawley female rats revealed that the acute gastric erosions induced by 1 ml of 100% ethanol were completely prevented by 30 min pretreatment of SH-containing captopril in the dose of 50 mg/100 g and were reduced dose-dependently from 16.7±2.2% in controls to 11.4±0.6 and 0.5±0.2% of the glandular stomach by 10 and 30 mg/100 g, respectively.

Zofenoprilat, which is also an SH-containing compound, proved to be the next effective in reducing gastric mucosal lesions at 50 mg/100 g. Among the non-SH ACE inhibitors significant but less gastroprotection was exerted by fosenopril, while lisinopril and enalapril were inactive.

The haemorrhagic mucosal lesions caused by HCl were decreased significantly from 7.4±3.4 to 0.6±0.1 and 1.6±1.2% by 50 mg/100 g of lisinopril and enalapril pretreatment, respectively (Figure 1). We tested the effects of the same two drugs on the aspirin-induced gastric mucosal damage. Administered at the same dose, lisinopril and enalapril also reduced significantly the mucosal erosions from 1.2±0.1 to 0.3±0.2 and 0.1±0.1% of the glandular stomach, respectively (Figure 1).

In addition to the treatment of hypertension, ACE inhibitors may have a role in the prophylaxis and treatment of NSAID gastropathy. Local tissue concentration of ACE inhibitors may act as antioxidants and more importantly as regulators of mucosal vascular endothelia and blood flow. This is strongly supported by the recent finding that endothelin, a potent vasoconstrictor released from vascular endothelium, stimulates angiotensin I conversion to angiotensin II *in vitro* [22] and activates the renin–angiotensin system *in vivo* [23]. Our laboratory showed that endothelin induced gastric vascular and mucosal lesions, enhanced the damaging effect of aspirin, HCl and ethanol and that the antibody exerts gastroprotection [24]. These results, and many new studies demonstrate that development and prevention of vascular injury in the stomach play a role in the mucosal damage and protection.

These results indicate that the SH-containing ACE inhibitors captopril and zofenoprilat exerted more gastroprotection against ethanol than non-SH inhibitors. However, the non-SH containing lisinopril and enalapril

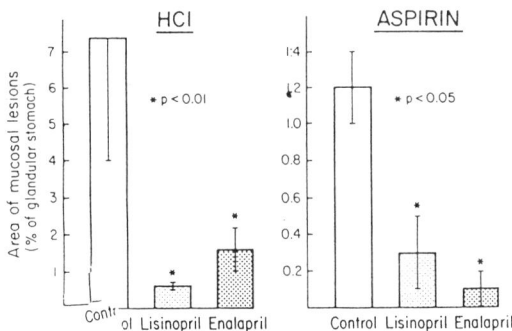

Figure 1. Effect of lisinopril and enalapril pretreatment on HCl and aspirin-induced gastric haemorrhagic mucosal lesions (reprinted with permission from Acta Biomed Hung Am. 1990;2:4–6)

diminished gastric erosions induced by aspirin or HCl. We conclude that ACE inhibitors could serve as new pharmacological agents in the protection of gastric mucosa against NSAID injury.

SMOOTH MUSCLE RELAXANTS

It is now well documented that early endothelial injury, increased vascular permeability and congestion in the gastric mucosa are key elements in the pathogenesis of acute mucosal lesions induced by ethanol, aspirin or indomethacin [6,25–29]. The new recognition is that in addition to direct or indirect (e.g. via release of endogenous mediators such as endothelin and leukotrienes) endothelial injury, vascular compression by constricting smooth muscles of the glandular stomach may also contribute to early congestion in the gastric mucosa [30–32]. Okabe and Takeuchi have actually proposed that one of the main mechanisms of gastroprotection by PG, SH and their derivatives is the gastric relaxation induced by the protective agents [31]. Indeed, Ruppin and Domschke demonstrated that papaverine prevented the chemically induced acute gastric erosions, and the protection in part was mediated by endogenous PG [33]. Although these authors did not implicate smooth muscle relaxation, we hypothesized that direct or indirect smooth muscle relaxation might be one of the pathways of gastroprotection. This, in part, may be due to the easy compressibility of thin-walled venules and veins which often run obliquely through muscularis mucosae and muscularis propria of the glandular stomach [34].

Based on these findings and on our preliminary results concerning muscle contraction, elevation of intravenous pressure and localization of chemically induced mucosal lesions [32], we tested the hypothesis that a calcium antagonist selective for the gastrointestinal tract pinaverium [35] might exert gastroprotection. Pinaverium bromide (Dicetel), unlike verapamil, nifedipine and diltiazem which block L-type voltage-gated Ca^{++} channels in cardiovascular systems [36], acts as a specific antagonist of influx of Ca^{++} through voltage-dependent channels on the surface of smooth muscle cells [35]. It is poorly absorbed and essentially selective for the gastrointestinal tract, causing relaxation in the oesophagus and stomach, with a slight increase in gastric emptying [37].

Our dose–response studies performed in fasted rats demonstrate that pinaverium administered i.g. by gavage at 1 but not at 0.2 mg/100 g 30 min before 1 ml of 100% ethanol offered more than 50% reduction in haemorrhagic mucosal lesions. Doses 5 mg/100 g or higher virtually abolished the development of haemorrhagic erosions caused by ethanol. To characterize the duration of gastroprotection by pinaverium, we performed extensive time-course studies. Surprisingly, pinaverium was very effective in decreasing the ethanol-induced gastric erosions if administered

5 or 15 min before alcohol. This effect was demonstrable for 6 h, and was hardly detectable with the 8 or 12 h pretreatment. Thus, judged by the duration of gastroprotection, pinaverium is equal or superior to most of the PG or SH derivatives.

To demonstrate that the protective effect of pinaverium is not specific against ethanol, we also used other damaging agents such as aspirin, indomethacin, HCl and NaOH. These results demonstrate that pinaverium exerted a dose-dependent protection against the haemorrhagic mucosal lesions caused by the i.g. administration of acidified aspirin (Table 4), indomethacin, or 1 ml of 0.6 N HCl or 0.2 N NaOH. It is thus apparent that pinaverium is a potent gastroprotective agent with long duration of action and wide substrate specificity.

Table 4. Dose-dependent effect of pinaverium on aspirin-induced haemorrhagic gastric mucosal injury in the rat

Group	Treatment[1]		Area of mucosal lesions (% of glandular stomach)
	Compound	Dose (mg/100 g)	
1.	Saline	–	1.1 ± 0.4
2.	Pinaverium	2	0.4 ± 0.1
3.	Pinaverium	10	0.1 ± 0.1 *
4.	Pinaverium	50	0.02 ± 0.01 *

* = $p < 0.05$
[1] In addition, rats of all groups were given 10 mg/100 g of aspirin in 0.2 N HCl i.g. for 30 min after pretreatment with saline or pinaverium. The animals were killed 1 h after aspirin

Histological examination of gastric sections from rats treated with pinaverium revealed that the grossly and stereomicroscopically evident gastroprotection was associated with reduction or absence of haemorrhagic or anaemic necrosis in the gastric mucosa. The superficial epithelial injury was still apparent in the presence or absence of protective agents, although the rapid epithelial restitution seems to repair faster the NSAID- or ethanol-induced superficial injury in rats given pinaverium or its active derivative. By the degree of correlation between macroscopic and microscopic gastroprotection, Dicetel is similar to the quality and quantity of protection by PG, SH and protease inhibitors.

GROWTH FACTORS

Growth factors are candidates for the treatment of chronic gastric and duodenal ulcers caused by NSAIDs. Epidermal growth factor (EGF) administration reduced the chemically induced acute gastric erosions as well [38], but its main effect might have been due, in part, to a decrease in

121

gastric acid secretion. Instead of the acid-oriented approach to treat chronic ulcers, we selected growth factors which directly stimulate the proliferation of several cell types and, especially, induce angiogenesis without reducing gastric secretion. We then used basic fibroblast growth factor (bFGF) which is the most potent endothelial mitogen which also stimulates the proliferation of fibroblasts, epithelial and smooth muscle cells [39] and platelet-derived growth factor (PDGF) which affects several mesenchymal cells and granulation tissue production. Since NSAIDs cause only gastric and not duodenal ulcers in rodents, we used the cysteamine-induced chronic duodenal ulcer model to test the hypothesis that stimulation of angiogenesis and granulation tissue might accelerate ulcer healing.

Normally fed female rats received three doses of cysteamine-HCl, 25 mg/100 g i.g. at about 4 h intervals. Three days later, rats with penetrating duodenal ulcers (as determined by laparotomy under ether anaesthesia) were randomized into vehicle control and treatment groups. Rats received: (a) vehicle alone; (b) wild type recombinant human bFGF; (c) acid-resistant mutein CS23 (Takeda Chemical Industries, Ltd) at 100 ng/100 g, PDGF (Creative BioMolecules) at 100 or 500 ng/100 g or, for comparison, (d) the histamine H_2 receptor antagonist cimetidine (Smith Kline & Beecham), 10 mg/100 g by gavage twice daily until autopsy on day 21, when ulcers were measured and histological sections taken [40,41].

The results indicate that the incidence, i.e. rats with ulcers, was decreased only by bFGF-CS23 and PDGF during the 3-week treatment (Table 5). The ulcer crater was reduced at marginal significance by cimetidine, and markedly by bFGF-w, the acid resistant bFGF-CS23 and dose-dependently by PDGF. Histology of bFGF-treated rats revealed: prominent angiogenesis, mild mononuclear cell infiltration, dense granulation tissue in the ulcer bed and healed ulcer which were completely epithelized. Morphometric analysis of angiogenesis in histological sections after immunohistochemical staining for endothelial cell-specific factor VIII revealed hypovascular ulcer craters in comparison with adjacent normal mucosa, and about a 10-fold increase in angiogenesis in ulcer craters of rats treated with CS23. PDGF increased granulation tissue production with a slight influence on angiogenesis.

In fasted rats with 1 h pyloric ligature neither bFGF nor PDGF decreased gastric acid and pepsin secretion. We concluded that oral administration of an angiogenic polypeptide made acid-stable by recombinant site-specific mutagenesis significantly accelerated the healing of chronic duodenal ulcers produced by cysteamine. Treatment with bFGF-CS23 caused a 10-fold increase in angiogenesis in the ulcer bed. These findings demonstrate the important role of angiogenesis in ulcer healing and that in addition to the acid-oriented approach, direct cellular pharmacological treatment of ulcer itself is now also possible.

Table 5. Influence of bFGF, PDGF or cimetidine on the healing of cysteamine-induced chronic duodenal ulcers in rats

Therapy	Dose	Size of ulcer crater	Rats with ulcers
Vehicle	–	100%	93%
bFGF-wild	100 ng/100 g	22.8% ($p < 0.05$)	80%
bFGF-CS23	100 ng/100 g	17.4% ($p < 0.01$)	40%
PDGF	100 ng/100 g	14.8% ($p = 0.051$)	50%
PDGF	500 ng/100 g	11.8% ($p = 0.048$)	29%
Cimetidine	10 mg/100 g	39.0% ($p = 0.072$)	86%

Rats were given cysteamine on the first day to induce duodenal ulcer as described in the text. Animals with severe, penetrating or perforating duodenal ulcer (verified by laparotomy) were randomized into vehicle or treatment groups and treated orally twice daily with doses listed until day 21 when autopsy was performed, ulcer crater measured and histological sections taken

ACKNOWLEDGEMENTS

These studies were supported in part by grants from Kali-Chemie Pharma and Takeda Chemical Industries, Ltd. The contributions of Drs N. Ramos and W. Spill and Ms Susan DiPietro are greatly appreciated.

We also thank companies which provided free drug samples for these studies: Bristol-Myers-Squibb (captopril), Ciba, Creative BioMolecules, Inc. (PDGF), Kali-Chemie Pharma (pinaverium), Merck Sharp & Dohme (lisinopril), Smith Kline & Beecham (cimetidine) and Takeda Chemical Industries Ltd (bFGF and bFGF-CS23).

REFERENCES

1. Rainsford KD. Uncoupling the toxicological morass in the development of new antirheumatic drugs – is there any hope? Br J Rheumatol. 1991;30:161–166.
2. Roth SH. Nonsteroidal anti-inflammatory drug gastropathy. Arch Intern Med. 1986;146:1075–1076.
3. Szabo S, Spill WF, Rainsford KD. Non-steroidal anti-inflammatory drug-induced gastropathy. Mechanisms and management. Med Tox Adv Drug Exp. 1989;4:77–94.
4. Robert A. Cytoprotection by prostaglandins. Gastroenterology. 1979;77:761–767.
5. Graham DY, Agrawal N, Roth SH. Prevention of NSAID-induced gastric ulcer with the synthetic prostaglandin misoprostol – a multicenter, double-blind, placebo-controlled trial. Lancet. 1988;2:1277–1280.
6. Szabo S. Critical and timely review of the concept of gastric cytoprotection. Acta Physiol Hung. 1989;73:115-127.
7. Rainsford KD, Whitehouse MW. Biochemical gastro-protection from acute ulceration induced by aspirin and related drugs. Biochem Pharmacol. 1980;29:1281.
8. Mozsik Gy, Javor I. A biochemical and pharmacological approach to the genesis of ulcer disease. A model study of ethanol-induced injury to gastric mucosa in rats. Dig Dis Sci. 1988;33:92–105.
9. Dupuy D, Raza A, Szabo S. The role of endogenous nonprotein and protein sulfhydryls in gastric mucosal injury and protection. In: Szabo S, Pfeiffer CG, eds. Ulcer disease: new aspects of pathogenesis and pharmacology. Boca Raton, FL: CRC Press; 1989.

10. Mozsik Gy, Pihan G, Szabo S et al. Free radicals, nonsulfhydryl antioxidants, drugs and vitamins in acute gastric mucosal injury and protection. In: Szabo S, Mozsik Gy, eds. New pharmacology of ulcer disease. New York: Elsevier; 1987.

11. Szabo S, Trier JS, Frankel PW. Sulfhydryl compounds may mediate gastric cytoprotection. Science. 1981;214:200–202.

12. Strubelt O. The role of sulfhydryls in the ulcerogenic action of non-steroidal antirheumatics. In: Szabo S, Mozsik Gy, eds. New pharmacology of ulcer disease. New York: Elsevier; 1987.

13 Szabo S, Pihan G, Raza A, Muller EA, Hauschka PV. Multiple mechanisms of cell injury in the gastric mucosa. Fed Proc. 1987;46:1152.

14. Robert A, Lancaster C, Olfsson AS, Gilbertson DK. N-Ethylmaleimide (NEM) either protects or damages the gastric mucosa depending on route and duration of administration. Gastroenterology. 1988;94:A377.

15. Szabo S. Proteinase inhibitors for treatment of gastrointestinal ulcer disease. US Patent No. 4,891,356; 1990.

16. Nagy L, Johnson BR, Saha B, LeQuesne P, Neumeyer JL, Plebani M, Szabo S. Correlation between gastroprotection and inhibition of cysteine proteases by new maleimide derivatives. Dig Dis Sci. 1990;35:1037.

17. Polgar L. The different mechanisms of protease action have a basic feature in common: proton transfer from the attacking nucleophil to the substrate leaving group. Acta Biochim Biophys Hung. 1988;23:207–213.

18. Chung S, Kawai K. Protease activities in gastric cancer tissues. Clin Chem Acta 1990;189:205–210.

19. Okada Y, Yokota Y. Purification and properties of cathepsin B from sea urchin eggs. Comp Biochem Physiol. 1990;96B:381–386.

20. Dupuy D, Szabo S. Protection by metals against ethanol-induced gastric injury in the rat: comparative biochemical and pharmacological studies implicate protein sulfhydryls. Gastroenterology. 1986;91:966–974.

21. Gyomber E, Vattay P, Johnson BR, Szabo S. Effect of sulfhydryl and non-sulfhydryl containing angiotensin converting enzyme inhibitors on chemically induced gastric mucosal lesions. Acta Biomed Hung Am. 1990;2:4–6.

22. Kawaguchi H, Sawa H, Yasuda H. Endothelin stimulates angiotensin I to angiotensin II conversion in cultured pulmonary artery endothelial cells. J Mol Cell Cardiol. 1990;22:839–842.

23. Rakug H, Tauchi Y, Nakamura M, Nagano M, Higashimori K, Mikami H, Ogihara T. Endothelin activates the vascular renin angiotensin system in rat mesenteric arteries. Biochem Int. 1990;21:867–872.

24. Morales RE, Johnson BR, Szabo S. Endothelin-induced vascular and mucosal lesions are enhanced by ethanol and HCl, not reduced by nitrendipine or indomethacin but the antibody exerts gastroprotection. Gastroenterology. 1990;98:A663.

25. Szabo S, Trier JS, Brown A et al. Early vascular injury and increased permeability in gastric mucosal injury caused by ethanol in rat. Gastroenterology. 1985;88:228–236.

26. Guth PH. Vascular factors in gastric mucosal injury. In: Szabo S, Pfeiffer CJ, eds. Ulcer disease: new aspects of pathogenesis and pharmacology. Boca Raton, FL: CRC Press; 1989.

27. Robins PG. Ultrastructural observations of the pathogenesis of aspirin-induced gastric erosions. Br J Exp Pathol. 1980;61:497.

28. Woods KL, Smith JL, Graham DY. Intragastric accumulation of Evan's blue as a method for assessing aspirin-induced acute gastric mucosal injury in humans. Dig Dis Sci. 1988;33:769–773.

29. Gyomber E, Vattay P, Szabo S. Role of early vascular lesions in the pathogenesis of gastric hemorrhagic mucosal lesions caused by indomethacin in rats. Gastroenterology. 1991;100:A826.

30. Szabo S, Folkman J, Morales RE, Vattay P, Pinkus G, Kato K. Vascular factors in mucosal injury, protection and ulcer healing. In: Garner A, O'Brien PE, eds. Mechanisms of injury, protection and repair of the upper gastrointestinal tract. West Sussex: Wiley; 1991.

31. Takeuchi J, Furukawa O, Nishiwaki H, Okabe S. 16,16-Dimethyl prostaglandin E2 aggravates gastric mucosal injury induced by histamine in rats. Gastroenterology. 1987;93:1276–1286.
32. Janicek M, Hollenberg NK, Lin YS, Szabo S. Area of congestion in angiography and rise of intravenous pressure determine the localization and extent of chemically-induced gastric mucosal injury. Gastroenterology. 1988;94:A206.
33. Ruppin H, Hagel J, Kachel G, Domschke S, Domschke W. Gastric cytoprotection in rat and man by various drugs: contrasting and competitive results. In: Szabo S, Mozsik Gy, eds. New pharmacology of ulcer disease. New York: Elsevier; 1987.
34. Piasecki C, Wyatt C. Patterns of blood supply to the gastric mucosa. A comparative study revealing an end-artery model. J Anat. 1986;149:21–39.
35. Christen MO, Tassignon JP. Dicetel (pinaverium bromide): a calcium antagonist selective for the gastrointestinal tract. In: Christen MO, Godfraind T, McCallum RW, eds. Calcium antagonism in gastrointestinal motility. Paris: Elsevier; 1989.
36. Godfraind R, Morel N, Salomone S, Wibo M. Tissue selectivity of calcium antagonists: pharmacological aspects. In: Christen MO, Godfraind T, McCallum RW, eds. Calcium antagonism in gastrointestinal motility. Paris: Elsevier; 1989.
37. McCallum RW. Role of calcium antagonists in digestive disorders. In: Christen MO, Godfraind T, McCallum RW, eds. Calcium antagonism in gastrointestinal motility. Paris: Elsevier; 1989.
38. Konturek SJ, Grzozowski T, Dembinski A, Warzecha Z, Yamazaki J. Gastric protective and ulcer-healing action of epidermal growth factor. In: Garner A, Whittle BJR, eds. Advances in drug therapy of gastrointestinal ulceration. Chichester: Wiley; 1989.
39. Folkman J, Klagsburn M. Angiogenic factors. Science. 1987;235:442–447.
40. Folkman J, Szabo S, Vattay P, Morales RE, Pinkus G, Kato K. Effect of orally administered bFGF on healing of chronic duodenal ulcers, gastric secretion and acute mucosal lesions in rat. Gastroenterology. 1990;98:A44.
41. Vattay P, Gyomber E, Morales RE, Szabo S. Effect of orally administered platelet-derived growth factor (PDGF) on healing of chronic duodenal ulcers and gastric secretion in rats. Gastroenterology. 1991;100:A180.

16

The role of misoprostol in preventing NSAID-induced damage to the gastrointestinal tract

Paul A. Nicholson

G.D. Searle, 4901 Searle Parkway, Skokie, IL 60077, USA
Now at: SmithKline Beecham Pharmaceuticals, PO Box 1510,
King of Prussia, PA 19406, USA

INTRODUCTION

Soll [1] has recently reviewed the pathogenesis of gastric and duodenal ulcers caused by NSAIDs. These drugs, their prodrugs or enteric coated formulations damage the stomach and duodenum directly or indirectly (systemically). They share at least one common pharmacological property, namely, inhibition of cyclo-oxygenase, and it is by this mechanism that they reduce the ability of the mucosa to produce those prostaglandins which play a pivotal role in mucosal defence. The specific pathological pathways by which damage is induced remain speculative.

However, a direct correlation between NSAID-induced acute mucosal damage and inhibition of mucosal prostaglandin content or production has not been shown, possibly because of methodological difficulties. Nevertheless, the administration of antibodies to prostaglandins to rabbits has been shown to produce marked ulceration of the whole gastrointestinal tract, and the administration of synthetic prostaglandins to man prevents NSAID-induced damage of the stomach and duodenum in excess of that produced by acid inhibition alone.

The effects of NSAIDs on the lower gastrointestinal tract are less well defined. However, the majority of patients who receive NSAIDs over long periods develop asymptomatic inflammation of the small intestine often associated with the loss of blood and protein and measurable ileal dysfunction [2].

Less common is the development of diaphragm-like strictures which have been observed in association with NSAID use. More recently use of a Sonde enteroscope has revealed erosions or ulcers of the jejunum or ileum as possible sources of bleeding in patients with anaemia associated with NSAID use [3].

Side-effects of Anti-inflammatory Drugs 3. Rainsford KD, Velo GP (eds),
Inflammation and Drug Therapy Series, Volume V.

PHARMACOLOGICAL EFFECTS OF MISOPROSTOL

Mucus secretion

Misoprostol has been shown to produce increases in soluble and adherent mucus in Wistar rats [4]. Consistent with this result Wilson et al. [5] have shown in man that soluble mucus, determined by measurement of N-acetylneuraminic acid in gastric aspirate, is increased in a dose-dependent way by misoprostol in doses of 200, 400, and 800 µg, in the basal and pentagastrin-stimulated state.

Bicarbonate secretion

Smedfors and Johanssen [6] compared the effects of misoprostol and cimetidine on bicarbonate secretion in rats in isolated duodenal loops. Basal bicarbonate secretion was significantly increased when misoprostol 10^{-10} mol/L was added to the perfusate, an effect which was subsequently shown to be dose-dependent between concentrations 1×10^{-12} to 1×10^{-4} mol/L. The addition of cimetidine to the perfusate was without effect at doses 1×10^{-7} to 1×10^{-4} mol/L. In man, Selling et al. [7] showed that doses of misoprostol up to 400 µg administered by perfusion significantly increased mean basal bicarbonate secretion in isolated proximal and distal duodenal segments, a result confirmed in a second study in patients with duodenal ulcer.

Blood flow

Blood flow was measured in dogs in a canine fundic chambered preparation. Misoprostol increased blood flow almost 4 times above baseline measurements [8]. In a Heidenhain pouch preparation in dog, misoprostol increased the clearance ratio of ^{14}C-aminopyrine while significantly inhibiting acid secretion indicating that its effect upon acid secretion is not secondary to diminished blood flow [9]. Leung et al. [10] have also shown that misoprostol reduced acid output, but maintained mucosal blood flow in pentagastrin-stimulated rats.

In man and in rat Sato and others [11] have shown that misoprostol produces a modest increase in mucosal blood volume throughout the stomach without change in mucosal blood haemoglobin oxygen saturation. Their technique (reflectance spectrophotometry) has been shown to correlate with the several measurements of gastric blood flow (hydrogen gas clearance, aminopyrine clearance, flow meter studies).

EFFECTS OF MISOPROSTOL IN MODELS OF NSAID DAMAGE

Animal studies

Misoprostol has been shown to protect the rat gastrointestinal mucosa challenged with aspirin and other NSAIDs, and in a study reported by Bauer et al. [12] was compared with cimetidine and sucralfate.

Misoprostol protected against the damaging effects of indomethacin, ibuprofen, piroxicam, and naproxen. Cimetidine protected against only indomethacin, and sucralfate was not active against indomethacin and not tested against the other three NSAIDs.

Studies in man

The protective effect of misoprostol has been tested against a diverse range of NSAIDs in healthy volunteers and in patients (Table 1). The methods of assessment have included measuring blood loss in gastric aspirate, measuring blood loss in faeces, and assessing endoscopic findings in the stomach and duodenum. To ensure that results were not due to pharmacokinetic interactions, formal pharmacokinetic studies have also been conducted with a number of representative NSAIDs (Table 1). The effects of misoprostol have also been studied in patients with rheumatoid arthritis or osteoarthritis.

Table 1. The kinetic and protective studies performed with misoprostol and six NSAIDs

Class	Agent	Pharmaco-kinetics	Volunteers	Patients
Indole	Indomethacin	+	+	−
Proprionic acid derivative	a) Ibuprofen	+	+	+
	b) Naproxen	−	+	+
Oxicam	Piroxicam	−	−	+
Phenylacetic acid derivative	Diclofenac	+	+	+
Salicylate	Aspirin	+	+	+

Studies in healthy subjects

Low doses of misoprostol (25 μg or 50 μg qid) given 30 minutes before aspirin (975 mg qid) reduced blood loss in the stomach as measured in gastric aspirates [13], but only the larger doses of misoprostol reduced bleeding significantly in comparison to placebo.

128

Also in comparison to placebo, misoprostol 25 µg qid significantly reduced faecal blood caused by aspirin 650 mg qid assessed by measurement of ^{51}Cr-labelled red cells in the stools [14]. In both of these studies protection occurred at doses with minimal effect upon acid secretion.

Using a single 1300 mg dose of aspirin as a mucosal challenge and assessing effects by endoscopy Silverstein et al. [15] were able to show that the protective effect of misoprostol was dose-related (Figure 1). In studies of one week's duration and also using endoscopic assessment Silverstein (Figure 2) was able to show that protection against aspirin 975 mg given qid was dose-related although the differences between the two highest doses of misoprostol (100 µg qid, 200 µg qid) did not achieve statistical significance.

In similar endoscopic studies Lanza et al. showed that misoprostol protected against ibuprofen better than placebo [16], against aspirin better than sucralfate or placebo [17], and against tolmetin better than cimetidine or placebo [18,19]. Aadlund et al. showed that misoprostol 200 µg given twice daily protected against damage due to naproxen better than placebo [20].

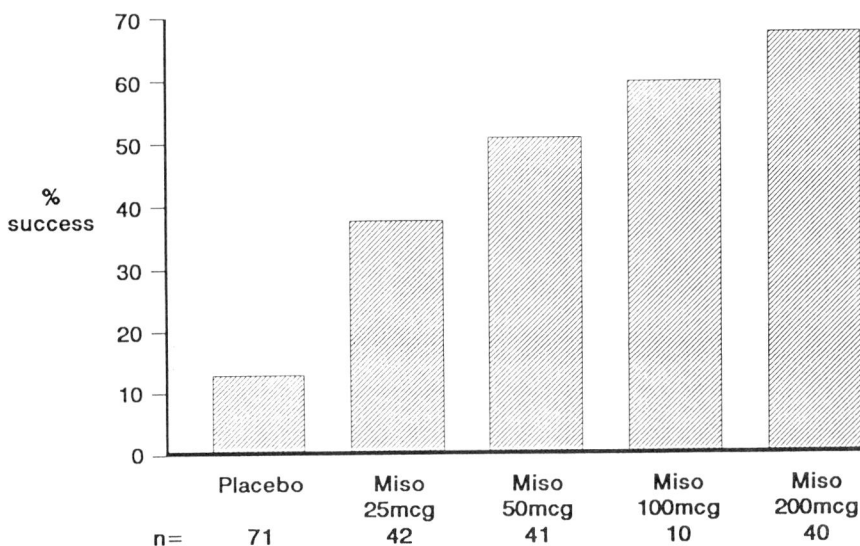

Figure 1. Composite results from three separate studies assessing efficacy of misoprostol versus a single challenge with aspirin 1300 mg [15]

Studies in patients

Two hundred and forty-one patients with rheumatoid arthritis who had developed gastroduodenal lesions while taking aspirin in doses of 2.6 g to 5.2 g per day for one month, were randomly allocated to receive misoprostol 200 µg qid or placebo concomitantly. In the following eight weeks, in spite of continuing with aspirin at the same constant dose, significantly more gastric lesions (70% versus 25%) and duodenal lesions (86% versus 53%) healed in patients receiving misoprostol. Although the study was not designed for the purpose, it showed that significantly fewer new ulcers developed in the misoprostol group than in the placebo group [21], a finding which stimulated further study.

Graham et al. [22] showed that misoprostol prevented the development of gastric ulcers in a study of 420 patients with osteoarthritis who were being treated with naproxen, piroxicam or ibuprofen. This randomized double-blind study compared the effect of misoprostol 200 µg qid or 100 µg qid with placebo. Misoprostol reduced the incidence of ulcers significantly, but the difference between the incidence in the misoprostol groups (which favoured the higher dose) did not achieve statistical significance (Figure 3). In a similar, but single-blind randomized study Agrawal and Saggioro compared the protective effect of misoprostol 200 µg qid with sucralfate

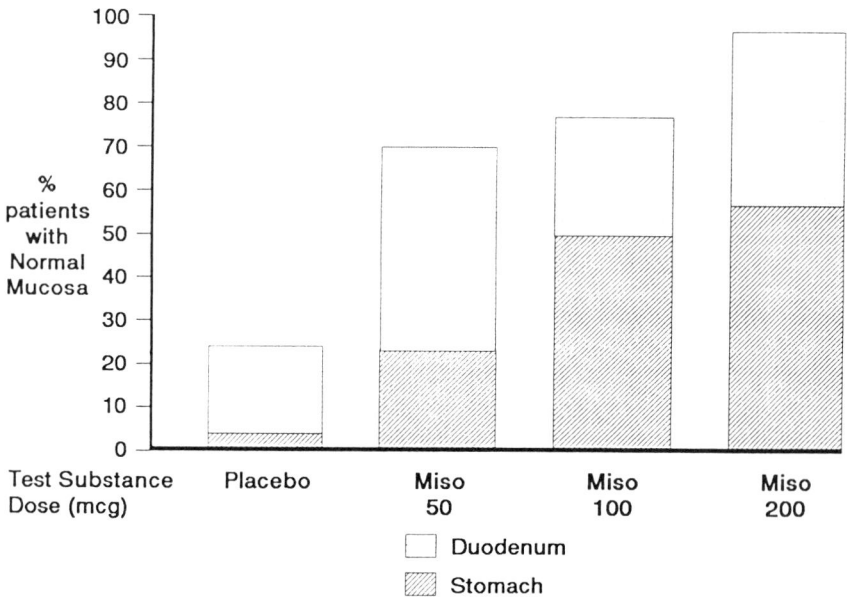

Figure 2. Percent of patients with normal mucosa analysed by dose and by anatomical site [15]

1.0 g qid [23]. Over the three month period of the study 21 of 131 patients (16%) who received sucralfate developed ulcers, compared with 2 of 122 patients (1.6%) who received misoprostol.

Three double-blind randomized studies have been conducted to show that misoprostol prevents the emergence of clinically significant mucosal lesions caused by diclofenac [24–26]. Geis et al. [24] reported on 382 patients with either rheumatoid or osteoarthritis who received misoprostol (200 µg bid or tid) or placebo in addition to diclofenac 50 mg bid or tid over a period of 6 months, and showed that misoprostol produced a significant and sustained reduction in upper gastrointestinal lesions (Figure 4).

Melo Gomes et al. [25] studied 361 patients with osteoarthritis treated with diclofenac 50 mg bid or tid, and misoprostol 200 µg bid or tid or placebo for 1 month. Those receiving misoprostol developed significantly fewer lesions or ulcers. Stead and Geis [26] reported similar results in 339 patients with rheumatoid arthritis treated with diclofenac and misoprostol or placebo.

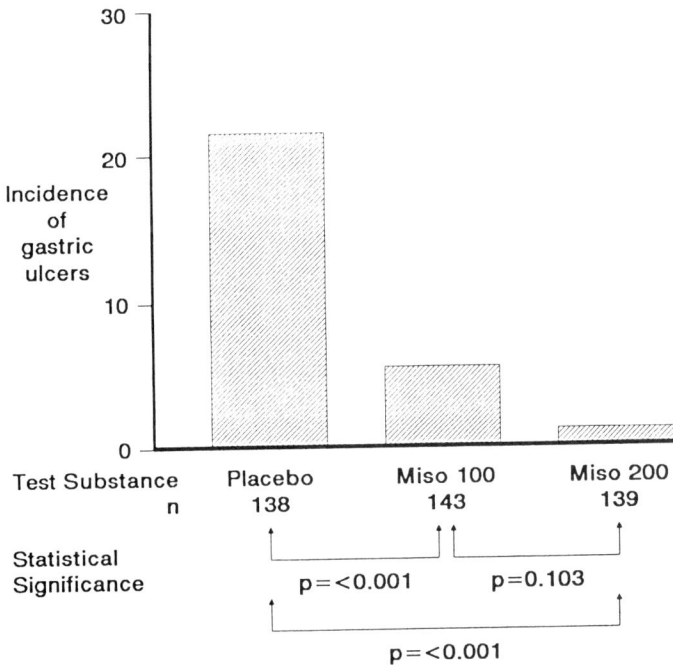

Figure 3. Incidence of gastric ulcers by treatment group [22]

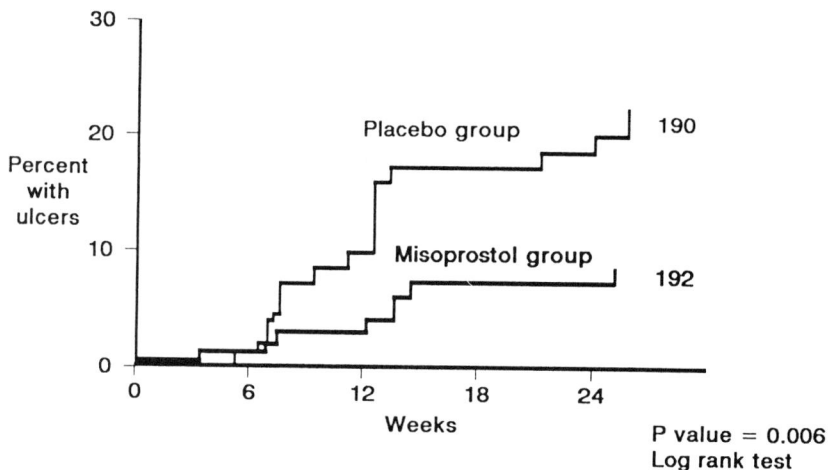

Figure 4. Cumulative incidence of ulcers over 6 months by treatment group [24]

The efficacy of misoprostol has therefore been shown in patients treated in the short term (one month), in the intermediate term (three months), or the long term (six months). It has been shown to prevent damage due to a range of chemically diverse NSAIDs, and to be equally effective in patients with rheumatoid arthritis or osteoarthritis.

DISCUSSION

NSAIDs reduce mucosal blood flow in areas that eventually ulcerate. Kitahora and Guth [27] reported the development of white thrombi on the walls of the mucosal vasculature prior to ulceration, suggesting a role for circulating leucocytes. In rats, previous depletion of neutrophils has been shown to reduce gastric damage due to NSAIDs [28].

The adherence of leucocytes to the vascular endothelium is often critical in models of gastrointestinal ulceration, and depends upon the interaction of adhesion molecules on both the leucocyte and the endothelium. The monoclonal antibody IB-4 is directed against the common beta submit (CD 18) of adhesion molecules on the leucocyte. Wallace et al. [29] have shown that pretreatment of rabbits with this antibody reduces vasocongestion, leucocyte margination and subsequent haemorrhagic damage caused by indomethacin.

Levi and colleagues [30] have shown in man that NSAIDs inhibit the regeneration of epithelial cells adjacent to gastric ulcers. They have shown in rats that indomethacin not only increases the size of cryoprobe-induced ulcers, but also delays healing and reduces mitotic activity in glands adjacent to the ulcers. Furthermore, they have shown that misoprostol reverses the inhibition of healing and also restores the proliferative rate. The effects of indomethacin therefore appear to be prostaglandin-related. Local effects of prostaglandin on mucosal blood flow could explain the phenomena and the effects of misoprostol on the microcirculation may therefore be of paramount importance in its efficacy in preventing NSAID-induced ulcers.

The evidence that misoprostol does prevent NSAID-induced lesions including ulcers in the stomach and duodenum accrues from animal studies, studies in healthy subjects and studies in patients. The results of these are broadly consistent and explicable in pharmacological terms.

Dose–response studies in human models [15] have shown that maximal efficacy is achieved between doses of 100 μg qid and 200 μg qid. In patients Graham et al.[22] showed that doses of 100 μg qid and 200 μg qid prevented ulcers due to naproxen, ibuprofen and piroxicam significantly better than placebo, but not significantly different from each other. In three separate controlled studies where misoprostol has been compared with placebo in patients treated with diclofenac, total daily doses of 400 to 600 μg have significantly reduced the frequency of lesions including ulcers of the stomach and duodenum.

With the majority, but not all NSAIDs, the freedom to titrate the dosage of misoprostol while on the dose response plateau and within the recommended dose range simplifies its administration, allowing one 200 μg dose of misoprostol to be taken with each dose of NSAID.

REFERENCES

1. Soll AH. The pathogenesis of ulcers caused by non-steroidal anti-inflammatory drugs, pp. 307–309. In: Soll AH, moderator. Nonsteroidal anti-inflammatory drugs and peptic ulcer disease. Ann Intern Med. 1991;114:307–319.

2. Bjarnason I, Smethurst P, Fenn CG, Lee CE, Menzies IS, Levi AJ. Misoprostol reduces indomethacin-induced changes in human small intestinal permeability. Dig Dis Sci. 1989;34:407–411.

3. Morris AJ, Madhok R, Sturrock RD, Capell HA, MacKenzie JF. Enteroscopic diagnosis of small bowel ulceration in patients receiving non-steroidal anti-inflammatory drugs. Lancet. 1991;337:520.

4. Sellars LA, Carroll NJ, Allen A. Misoprostol-induced increases in adherent gastric mucus thickness and luminal mucus output. Dig Dis Sci. 1986;31:91S–95S.

5. Wilson DE, Quadros E, Rajapaksa T et al. Effects of misoprostol on gastric acid and mucus secretion in man. Dig Dis Sci. 1986;31:126S–129S.

6. Smedfors B, Johansson C. Stimulation of duodenal bicarbonate secretion by misoprostol. Dig Dis Sci. 1986;2:96S–100S.

7. Selling JA, Hogan DL, Koss MA et al. Prostaglandin E₁ misoprostol stimulates human duodenal mucosal bicarbonate secretion (abstract). Gastroenterology. 1985;88(5 pt 2):1580.

8. Larsen KR, Jensen NF, Davis EK et al. The cytoprotective effects of (±) 15-deoxy-16-α,β-hydroxy-16-methyl PGE₁, methyl ester (SC-29333) versus aspirin-shock gastric ulcerogenesis in the dog. Prostaglandins. 1981;21(Suppl):119–124.

9. Colton DG, Driskill DR, Phillips EL et al. Effect of SC-29333 an inhibitor of gastric secretion on canine gastric mucosal blood flow and serum gastrin levels. Arch Int Pharmacodyn Ther. 1978;236:86–95.

10. Leung FW, Miller JC, Guth PH. Dissociated effects of misoprostol on gastric acid secretion and mucosal blood flow. Dig Dis Sci. 1986;31:86A–90S.

11. Sato N, Kawano S, Kamada T et al. Hemodynamics of gastric mucosa and gastric ulceration in rats and in patients with gastric ulcer. Dig Dis Sci. 1986;31:35S–41S.

12. Bauer RF, Bianchi RG, Casler J et al. Comparative mucosal protective properties of misoprostol, cimetidine and sucralfate. Dig Dis Sci. 1986;31:81S–85S.

13. Hunt JN, Smith JL, Jiang CL, Kessler L. Effect of synthetic prostaglandin E_1 analog on aspirin-induced gastric bleeding and secretion. Dig Dis Sci. 1983;28:897–902.

14. Cohen MM, Clark L, Armstrong L, D'Souza A, D'Souza J. Reduction of aspirin-induced fecal blood loss with low-dose misoprostol tablets in man. Dig Dis Sci. 1985;30:605–611.

15. Silverstein FE, Kimmey MB, Saunders DR, Levine DS. Gastric protection by misoprostol against 1300 mg of aspirin, an endoscopic study. Dig Dis Sci. 1986;31:137S–141S.

16. Lanza FL, Fakouhi D, Rubin A et al. A double-blind placebo controlled comparison of the efficacy and safety of 50, 100 and 200 µg of misoprostol qid in the prevention of ibuprofen induced gastric and duodenal mucosal lesions and symptoms. Am J Gastroenterol. 1989;84:633–636.

17. Lanza FL, Peace KE, Gustitis L et al. A blinded endoscopic comparative study of misoprostol versus sucralfate and placebo in the prevention of aspirin induced gastric and duodenal ulceration. Am J Med. 1987;83(1A):37–40.

18. Lanza FL. Prophylactic effect of misoprostol on lesions of the gastric mucosa induced by oral administration of tolmetin in healthy subjects. Dig Dis Sci. 1986;31:131S–136S.

19. Lanza FL, Aspinall R, Swabb E et al. Double-blind placebo controlled endoscopic comparison of the mucosal protective effects of misoprostol versus cimetidine on tolmetin-induced mucosal injury in the stomach and duodenum. Gastroenterology. 1988;95:289–294.

20. Aadlund E, Fausa O, Vatn M et al. Protection by misoprostol against naproxen induced gastric mucosal damage. Am J Med. 1987;83(1A):37–40.

21. Roth S, Agrawal N, Mahouald M et al. Misoprostol heals gastroduodenal injury in patients with rheumatoid arthritis receiving aspirin. Arch Intern Med. 1989;149:775–779.

22. Graham DY, Agrawal NM, Roth SH. Prevention of NSAID-induced gastric ulcer with misoprostol: multicentre double-blind placebo-controlled trial. Lancet. 1988;1:1277–1286.

23. Agrawal NM, Saggioro A. Treatment and prevention of NSAID-induced gastroduodenal mucosal damage. J Rheumatol. 1991;(in press).

24. Geis GS, Erhardt LJ, Stead H. Prevention of diclofenac induced gastroduodenal mucosal lesions by misoprostol: a multinational placebo controlled parallel group study. Proceedings of the XII European Congress of Rheumatology; 1991 June 30–July 6; Budapest, Hungary.

25. Melo Gomes JA, Bolton W, Stead H, Geis S. The gastroduodenal safety and efficacy of the fixed combination of diclofenac, an NSAID, and misoprostol, a mucosal protective agent, in the treatment of osteoarthritis. Br J Rheumatol. 1991;(in press)

26. Stead H, Geis GS. Diclofenac/misoprostol fixed combination in patients with osteoarthritis. Proceedings of the XII European Congress of Rheumatology; 1991 June 30–July 6; Budapest, Hungary.

27. Kitahora T, Guth PH. Effect of aspirin plus hydrochloric acid on the gastric mucosal microcirculation. Gastroenterology. 1987;93:810–817.

28. Wallace JL, Keenan CM, Granger DN. Gastric ulceration induced by nonsteroidal anti-inflammatory drugs is a neutrophil dependent process. Am J Physiol. 1990;259:G462–G467.

29. Wallace JL, Arfors KE, Webb-McKnight G. A monoclonal antibody against the CD18 leucocyte adhesion molecule prevents indomethacin-induced gastric damage in the rabbit. Gastroenterology. 1991;100:878–883.

30. Levi S, Goodlad RA, Lee CY et al. Inhibitory effect of non-steroidal anti-inflammatory drugs on mucosal cell proliferation associated with gastric ulcer healing. Lancet. 1990;336:840–843.

17

Possible factors involved in the protective effects of interleukin-1 in aspirin- and indomethacin-induced gastric damage

Kenneth G. Mugridge, Mauro Perretti, John L. Wallace*
and Luca Parente

Sclavo Research Centre, via Fiorentina 1, 53100 Siena, Italy and
*Gastrointestinal Research Group, University of Calgary, Alberta,
TN2 4NI, Canada

INTRODUCTION

Interleukin-1 (IL-1) is a polypeptide cytokine that has been described as possessing a wide variety of immunogenic and non-immunogenic activities [1]. Recently another important facet of this cytokine's biological activity has emerged concerning its protective effects against gastroduodenal damage in several animal models. This was first shown in the studies of Wallace et al. [2] which demonstrated IL-1 to potently reduce the gastric damage caused in rats by indomethacin and ethanol as well as the duodenal damage caused by the noxic agent cysteamine. Subsequent studies by Robert et al. [3] confirmed the cytokine's protective effects in the ethanol model and also showed IL-1 to reduce the gastric damage caused by another non-steroidal anti-inflammatory drug (NSAID), aspirin. However, the mechanisms underlying the protective actions of IL-1 are not entirely clear. The cytokine is a potent stimulator of prostaglandin (PG) synthesis in many cell types [4–6] including rat forestomach [7] and rabbit colon [8]. The later study by Robert et al. [3] also indicated that administration of IL-1 to rats could increase the capacity of the gastric mucosa to synthesize PGE_2. Since a number of PGs have the ability to protect the upper gastrointestinal tract [9] it is feasible that their increased synthesis caused by IL-1 may contribute to the reduced mucosal injury. Another factor which may contribute towards the gastroprotective actions of IL-1 is its ability to potently inhibit gastric acid secretion [2,3,10–15]. In this review, we consider the relative importance and contribution of prostaglandin synthesis and inhibition of gastric acid secretion towards the

Side-effects of Anti-inflammatory Drugs 3. Rainsford KD, Velo GP (eds),
Inflammation and Drug Therapy Series, Volume V.

gastroprotective actions of IL-1 in experimental NSAID-gastropathy. Subsequent attention will be turned to other possible factors involved in IL-1 protection of the gastric mucosa.

PROSTAGLANDINS: DO THEY CONTRIBUTE TOWARDS THE GASTROPROTECTIVE ACTIONS OF IL-1 IN NSAID-GASTROPATHY?

The studies of Wallace et al. [2] observed that IL-1 protected the gastric mucosa from the damage caused by the oral instillation of 100% ethanol to rats. This action of IL-1 is dose-dependent and is completely abrogated by indomethacin pretreatment of animals. This later observation, confirmed by a subsequent study [3], suggested a mediatory role for endogenous PGs in the IL-1 protective actions. IL-1 is able to rapidly increase, within 20 minutes, PGE_2 synthesis from rat forestomach *in vitro* possibly through stimulation of phospholipase A_2 activity [7]. This factor may account for the rapid onset of action, within 15 minutes, observed for IL-1 in the ethanol model. Although the ethanol studies suggest that endogenous PGs have an important role in the protective effects of IL-1, it remained unclear whether this factor could also be of importance in the NSAID models. To understand further this question, studies using both aspirin- and indomethacin-induced gastric damage models were conducted.

Human recombinant IL-1β (0.1 and 3 μg/kg) was administered intraperitoneally (i.p.) or intragastrically (i.g.) to 24 h fasted Wistar rats immediately after their treatment with aspirin (200 mg/kg i.g.) or indomethacin (5 mg/kg i.p.). Assessment of gastric damage was carried out after 2 h and 3 h respectively. Additionally, segments of the muscular forestomach and corpus mucosa were dissected out and processed for their ability to synthesize 6-oxo $PGF_{1\alpha}$, used as an index of cyclo-oxygenase activity, using a 'chop and vortex' procedure similar to that described originally [16]. As shown in Figures 1 and 2, treatment of rats with the lower dose of IL-1 by either route of administration reduces the extent of gastric damage caused by indomethacin or aspirin (37–66%) without any modification of 6-oxo $PGF_{1\alpha}$ synthesis. Using the higher dose of IL-1, a better degree of protection (73–96%) is observed against both NSAIDs which is accompanied by a significant increase in the ability of the forestomach to synthesize 6-oxo $PGF_{1\alpha}$. The major observation from these studies is that IL-1 can exert a substantial part of its gastroprotective actions through PG-independent mechanisms. However, whether or not the increased protection obtained with the higher dose of IL-1 is actually dependent on the elevated capability for PG formation is unclear. A number of indications point against the likelihood of this involvement. Firstly, it has to be stressed that in both models the restoration of 6-oxo $PGF_{1\alpha}$ synthesis in the forestomach following IL-1 treatment is small

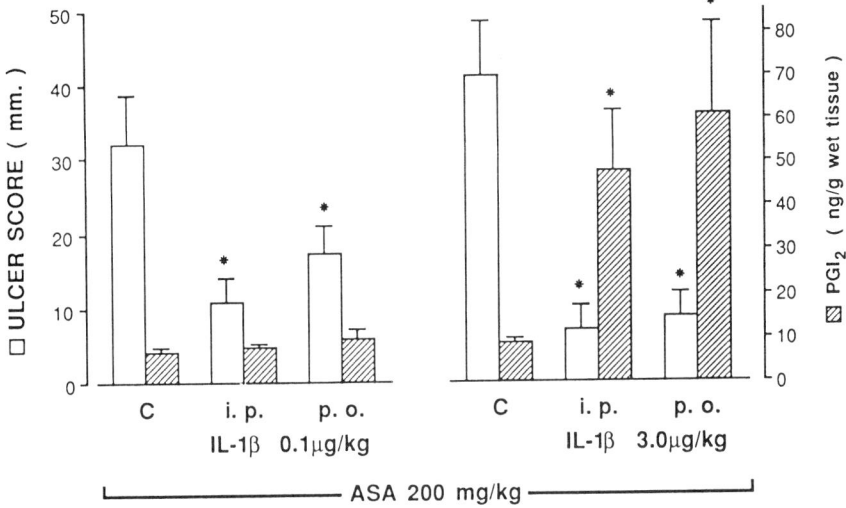

Figure 1. Effects of Il-1 on the formation of gastric damage in rats caused by i.g. administration of aspirin (ASA) and the *ex vivo* synthesis of PGI_2 from the forestomach. IL-1 was administered immediately after aspirin treatment. The extent of macroscopically visible damage was measured 2 h later and expressed as the sum length (mm) of each individual lesion. PGI_2 synthesis was measured by specific radioimmunoassay of the stable metabolite 6-oxo $PGF_{1\alpha}$. Results are expressed as mean $\pm$ SEM ($n = 10$–15) where * denotes a significant ($p < 0.05$) difference from the aspirin treated group. Synthesis of PGI_2 in tissues from animals not receiving aspirin or IL-1 was 529.2 ± 65.6 ng/g wet tissue ($n = 11$).

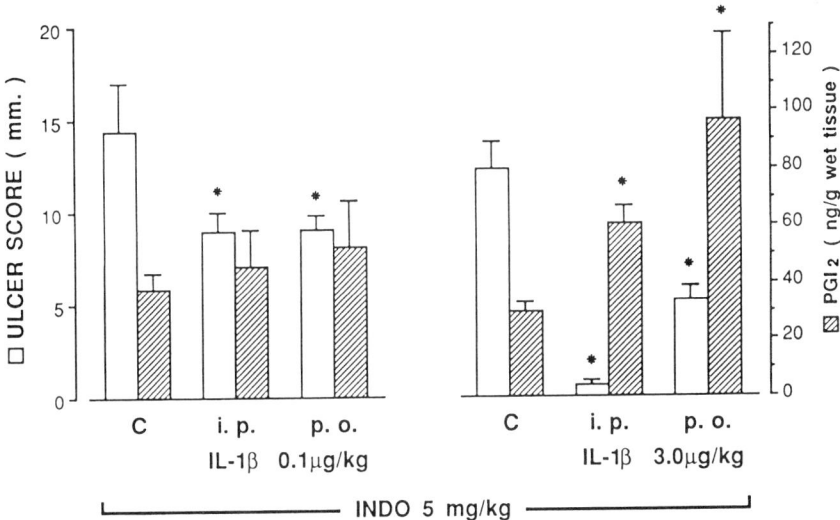

Figure 2. Effects of Il-1 on the formation of gastric damage in rats caused by the i.p. administration of indomethacin (INDO) and the *ex vivo* synthesis of PGI_2 from the forestomach. Experimental procedure is described previously in figure 1 excepting that analysis of gastric damage and PGI_2 synthesis was carried out 3 h after indomethacin treatment. Results are shown as mean $\pm$ SEM ($n = 5$–15) where * denotes a significant ($p < 0.05$) difference from the aspirin treated group. Synthesis of PGI_2 in tissues from animals not receiving aspirin or IL-1 was 453.0 ± 37.0 ng/g wet tissue ($n = 30$)

137

($\sim 10\%$). Secondly, no significant increases in this prostanoid's synthesis can be observed from segments of the corpus mucosa (data not shown), the region of the stomach where the formation of haemorrhagic lesions is most prominent. This has also been confirmed in other studies which have shown IL-1, at a dose which gives almost complete protection against the gastric damage induced by a much higher dose of indomethacin (20 mg/kg i.g.), fail to increase 6-oxo $PGF_{1\alpha}$ synthesis from the gastric corpus (Wallace JL, Keenan CM, Cucala M, Mugridge KG, Parente L, manuscript submitted). It is also speculative as to whether the small increase in the capacity of the forestomach to synthesize PGs can influence events occuring in the corpus mucosa.

It is noteworthy from these studies to observe the oral efficacy of IL-1 in these models. This is at variance with the results obtained by Robert et al. [3] which demonstrate that orally administered IL-1 did not protect against the gastric damage caused by ethanol. The reasons for this differential activity are not very clear although such are the plethora of biological actions exhibited by IL-1, it is likely that the mechanisms underlying its gastroprotective actions in the various experimental models will be diverse rather than common. This is exemplified by the fact that the protective effects of IL-1 in the ethanol model appear to be modulated by PG-dependent mechanisms whereas in the NSAID models this dependence is unlikely. The question therefore remains as to how IL-1 protects the gastric mucosa from NSAID-induced injury. An obvious line of approach was to examine the relevance of the potent antisecretory activity of the cytokine in these models.

IS THE ANTISECRETORY ACTIVITY OF IL-1 IMPORTANT FOR ITS GASTROPROTECTIVE ACTIONS?

It is now well established that IL-1 is a potent inhibitor of gastric acid secretion [2,3,10–15]. The study by Uehara et al. [10] was the first to observe that the antisecretory activity of IL-1 could be reversed by the pretreatment of rats with indomethacin suggestive of a mediatory role for PGs although later studies observed that the cytokine could reduce acid production caused by pentagastrin independent of PG involvement [14,15]. In the light of all these various reports, the question of whether this potent antisecretory activity could be responsible for the gastroprotective effects of IL-1 was of paramount importance. The first negative indication was provided by Wallace et al. [2] who proposed that since ethanol produces damage independent of the presence of luminal acid it is unlikely that IL-1 could exert its protective effects through its effects on gastric acid secretion. In the later study by Robert et al. [3] it was proposed that the protective effects of IL-1 in the ethanol model were probably not related to its antisecretory actions in view of the fact that other antisecretory drugs such as H_2-receptor antagonists or acetylcholine-receptor antagonists do not offer enhanced protection. In contrast the gastric damage produced by both aspirin and indomethacin is dependent upon the presence of luminal acid [17,18] and feasibly the antisecretory actions of IL-1 could be of more relevance in these models.

To investigate the possible inter-relationship between the gastro-protective effects of IL-1 in NSAID-induced gastropathy and its ability to inhibit gastric acid secretion, a study was carried out specifically using the aspirin model. It was a consistent observation in the previous studies investigating the putative relationship between IL-1 and gastric PG formation, that the administration of aspirin (200 mg/kg i.g.) to rats caused not only the formation of haemorrhagic lesions but also the accumulation of luminal fluid within the stomach. This fluid is not found in vehicle treated animals and although too viscous to titrate it is acidic (pH 3.4 ± 0.1; $n = 3$). This model therefore provides an ideal situation to investigate the putative relationship between the two elements of IL-1 action, viz inhibition of gastric damage and acid secretion. The results from this study, shown in Table 1, demonstrate both i.p. and i.g. administration of IL-1 to reduce the formation of gastric erosions caused by aspirin. In the case of its i.p. administration, significant reduction of damage (66%) is observed with the lower dose of IL-1 (0.1 µg/kg) which is accompanied by inhibition of luminal fluid accumulation (70%). Treatment of rats with the higher dose of IL-1 (3 µg/kg i.p.) causes a further decrease in lesion formation (85%) without any further modification of fluid accumulation. In contrast, oral treatment with the 0.1 µg/kg dose of the cytokine reduces the incidence of gastric erosions (62%) similar to that obtained by its corresponding i.p. administration, without any effect on luminal fluid volume. At the higher concentration (3 µg/kg) given by the i.g. route, significant decreases (66%) of luminal fluid accumulation are obtained although the protective effects of this dose increased only marginally (72%). The indication from these studies is that IL-1 can offer the major part of its gastroprotective effect without affecting gastric secretion. It is also of interest that the antisecretory actions of IL-1 in this model can be effected even though gastric cyclooxygenase activity is substantially ($\sim 90\%$) inhibited. Coupled with the pentagastrin studies mentioned previously [14,15], it is evident that IL-1 can exert antisecretory activity through PG-dependent and PG-independent mechanisms. Other evidence also points against the antisecretory activity of IL-1 being instrumental in its gastroprotective actions. Table 2 demonstrates that using adrenalecto-mized rats, the gastric damage caused by i.p. administration of aspirin (200 mg/kg) is not inhibited to any extent by a dose of IL-1 (3 µg/kg i.p.) which in normal animals is seen to exert substantial protection. However, IL-1 was still able to retain a very high inhibition (86%) of luminal fluid accumulation in these animals confirming the previous observation by

Table 1. Effect of IL-1 on gastric lesion formation and accumulation of luminal fluid caused by the administration of aspirin to rats

Treatment	Gastric damage score (mm)	Gastric fluid volume (ml)
Aspirin	33.1 ± 2.9	2.30 ± 0.15
Aspirin + IL-1 (0.1 µg/kg i.p.)	11.0 ± 2.2*	0.67 ± 0.15*
Aspirin + IL-1 (3.0 µg/kg i.p.)	5.1 ± 1.1*	0.73 ± 0.16*
Aspirin + IL-1 (0.1 µg/kg i.g.)	12.5 ± 4.9*	2.00 ± 0.29
Aspirin + IL-1 (3.0 µg/kg i.g.)	9.3 ± 2.5*	0.80 ± 0.34*

IL-1 was given to rats immediately after the i.g. administration of aspirin (200 mg/kg). Measurement of gastric damage and luminal fluid volume was assessed 2 h later. Results are expressed as mean ± SEM where * denotes a significant ($p < 0.05$) difference from aspirin-treated animals. Sample size for Il-1 treated rats was 18 and that for aspirin was 58

Table 2. Influence of adrenalectomy on IL-1 induced inhibition of gastric lesion formation and luminal fluid accumulation caused by administration of aspirin to rats

Treatment	Gastric damage score (mm)	Gastric fluid volume (ml)
Aspirin	131.6 ± 10.4	0.65 ± 0.21
Aspirin + IL-1	115.7 ± 10.6	0.09 ± 0.08*

IL-1 (3 µg/kg i.p.) was given to rats immediately after the administration of aspirin (200 mg/kg i.g.). Analysis of gastric damage, measured as described in figure 1, and luminal fluid accumulation was assessed 2 h later. Results are expressed as mean ± SEM ($n = 8$) where * denotes a significant ($p < 0.05$) difference from the aspirin-treated group

Saperas et al. [11]. Taken together it appears that the retention of its antisecretory activity in adrenalectomized animals is not sufficient for IL-1 to reduce gastric damage. More recent studies have shown doses of IL-1 to produce ~50% reduction of indomethacin-induced damage in rats without any significant effect on the volume or acid content of gastric juice [Wallace JL, Keenan CM, Cucala M, Mugridge KG, Parente L, manuscript submitted].

The indications from the studies described above, suggest that the involvement of PGs or the inhibition of gastric acid secretion is likely to account for only a minor part, if any, of IL-1 protective actions against NSAID-induced damage. In view of the wide number of biological effects that are attributable to IL-1 [1], much speculation concerning the mechanisms by which it exerts its protective actions, at least in the NSAID models, could be made. In this light, a number of recent findings may limit this speculation and these are discussed in the following section.

WHAT OTHER FACTORS COULD BE INVOLVED IN IL-1 PROTECTIVE ACTIONS AGAINST NSAID-INDUCED GASTRIC DAMAGE?

Recent studies suggest that NSAID-gastropathy may be a neutrophil-dependent process. Rats rendered neutropenic by pre-treatment with anti-neutrophil serum or methotrexate [19] or rabbits treated with a monoclonal antibody which prevents neutrophil adherence to the vascular endothelium [20], are more resistant to the damaging effects of indomethacin on the gastric mucosa. The question of whether the beneficial effects of IL-1 in the indomethacin model could be related to effects on neutrophil function is therefore of importance. Positive evidence now supports this concept. IL-1 has been shown to reduce the magnitude of LTB_4-induced neutropenia in rats and also to inhibit the migration of neutrophils in response to LTB_4 as well as FMLP (Wallace JL, Keenan CM, Cucula M, Mugridge KG, Parente L, manuscript submitted). It is of relevance that this same study by Wallace et al. demonstrates dexamethasone, another agent which can interfere with neutrophil adherence to the vascular endothelium [21,22], to also inhibit both LTB_4-induced neutropenia and the extent of indomethacin-induced gastric damage. In fact previous studies have also observed glucocorticoids to reduce indomethacin-induced intestinal damage in rats [23]. The question that now arises from the studies described above is whether IL-1 exerts its protective effects in the NSAID models through some interaction with or release of endogenous corticosteroids. In this context, IL-1 is known to activate the hypothalamic-pituitary-adrenal axis by stimulating the secretion of hypothalamic corticotropin-releasing factor [24,25]. The release of adrenocorticotropin itself by IL-1 has been recently demonstrated [26] whereas another study has also shown the cytokine to cause the release of corticosteroids by direct stimulation of the adrenal cortex [27]. If the release of corticosteroids by IL-1 is important in its reduction of NSAID-induced gastropathy, the inability of the cytokine to stimulate the release of these hormones in adrenalectomized rats may explain the disappearance of its protective effects. It is also of possible importance to note that in adrenalectomized rats the extent of damage caused by aspirin is much greater, approximately 4-fold, than in normal animals. It is speculative to suggest that in these animals, without the controlling influence of corticosteroids, the adherence of neutrophils to the vascular endothelium and their migration into damaged tissue may be higher. Since it appears that NSAID-gastropathy is dependent upon the presence of neutrophils [19,20], it is feasible that the presence of elevated numbers of these cells could evoke greater damage.

Another possibility which may account for IL-1 actions could arise from its ability to directly alter neutrophil functions such as the secretion of mediators [28,29] or phagocytosis [30]. Direct effects on the vascular

141

endothelium to release substances which interfere with neutrophil migration or function may also represent a means for IL-1 to exert its effects. The cytokine is well known to release prostacyclin from endothelial cells [31] although the indications from the various studies discussed previously suggest that the release of PGs is not totally involved in the protective effects of IL-1 in the NSAID models. Other endothelium-derived substances include nitric oxide. The endogenous production of this labile vasodilator has been proposed to be an important factor modulating the regulation of gastric mucosal integrity [32]. In this light, it has been shown to significantly inhibit ethanol-induced damage [33] and has been suggested to reduce HCl-induced gastric damage in rats [34]. Nitric oxide also inhibits FMLP-induced stimulation of neutrophils *in vitro* [35] and inhibitors of its formation increase leucocyte adherence [36]. IL-1 also causes the release of nitric oxide from vascular smooth muscle cells [37]. However, it has to be stressed that in this latter study, the induction of nitric oxide synthase by IL-1 requires a period of time, at least 6 hours, before any significant increases in nitric oxide can be detected. Relevant to this point is the fact that endotoxin, a potent stimulator of IL-1 production [38], does not increase the constitutive nitric oxide synthase found in endothelial cells but, like IL-1, induces this enzyme in the smooth muscle cells of the vascular wall [39]. Since the protective effects of IL-1 are clearly evident within 2 or 3 hours of aspirin or indomethacin administration respectively, it is doubtful whether the cytokine could induce sufficient levels of nitric oxide synthase in this period. Inasmuch that the protective effects of IL-1 against indomethacin-induced gastric damage are demonstrable even after 12 hours (Wallace JL, Keenan CM, Cucula M, Mugridge KG, Parente L, manuscript submitted), it is feasible that increased nitric oxide synthesis caused by the cytokine may be more important in maintaining the protective effect rather than initiating it. This interesting possibility warrants further investigation.

REFERENCES

1. Dinarello CA. Interleukin-1 and its biologically related cytokines. Adv Immunol. 1989;44:153–205.
2. Wallace JL, Keenan CM, Mugridge KG, Parente L. Reduction of the severity of experimental gastric and duodenal ulceration by interleukin-1β. Eur J Pharmacol. 1990;186:279–284.
3. Robert A, Olafsson AS, Lancaster C, Zhang W-R. Interleukin-1 is cytoprotective, stimulates PGE_2 synthesis by the stomach, and retards gastric emptying. Life Sci. 1991;48:123–134.
4. Dayer JM, Stephens MI, Schmidt E, Karge W, Krane SM. Purification of a factor from human blood monocyte-macrophages which stimulates the production of collagenase and prostaglandin E_2 by cells cultured from rheumatoid synovial tissues. FEBS Lett. 1981;12:253–256.
5. Whiteley PJ, Needleman P. Mechanism of enhanced fibroblast arachidonic acid metabolism by mononuclear cell factor. J Clin Invest. 1984;74:2249–2253.

6. Chang J, Gilman SC, Lewis AJ. Interleukin-1 activates phospholipase A_2 in rabbit chondrocytes: a possible signal for IL-1 action. J Immunol. 1986;136:1283–1287.

7. Mugridge KG, Donati D, Silvestri S, Parente L. Arachidonic acid lipoxygenation may be involved in interleukin-1 induction of prostaglandin biosynthesis. J Pharmacol Exp Ther. 1989;250:714–720.

8. Cominelli F, Nast CC, Dinarello CA, Gentilini P, Zipser RD. Regulation of eicosanoid production in rabbit colon by interleukin-1. Gastroenterology. 1989;97:1400–1405.

9. Hawkey CJ, Rampton DS. Prostaglandins and the gastrointestinal mucosa: are they important in its function, disease or treatment? Gastroenterology. 1985;89:1162–1188.

10. Uehara A, Okumura T, Sekiya C, Okumura K, Takasugi Y, Namika M. Interleukin-1 inhibits the secretion of gastric acid in rats: possible involvement of prostaglandin. Biochem Biophys Res Commun. 1989;162:1578–1584.

11. Saperas ES, Yang H, Rivier C, Tache Y. Central action of recombinant interleukin-1 to inhibit acid secretion in rats. Gastroenterology. 1990;99:1599–1606.

12. Ishikawa T, Nagata S, Ago Y, Takahashi K, Karibe M. The central inhibitory effect of interleukin-1 on gastric acid secretion. Neurosci Lett. 1990;119:114-117.

13. Uehara A, Okumura T, Kitamori S, Takasugi Y, Namika M. Interleukin-1: a cytokine that has potent antisecretory and anti-ulcer actions via the central nervous system. Biochem Biophys Res Commun. 1990;173:585–590.

14. Cucala M, Mugridge K, Parente L, Wallace JL. Interleukin-1 is a potent inhibitor of gastric acid secretion. Gut. 1990;31:A1184–A1185.

15. Wallace JL, Cucala M, Mugridge KG, Parente L. Secretagogue-specific effects of interleukin-1 on gastric acid secretion. Am J Physiol. 1991;261: (in press)

16. Whittle BJR, Higgs GA, Eakins KE, Moncada S, Vane JR. Selective inhibition of prostaglandin production in inflammatory exudates and gastric mucosa. Nature. 1980;284:271–273.

17. Gerkins JF, Shand DG, Flexner C, Nies AS, Oates JA, Data JL. Effect of indomethacin and aspirin on gastric blood flow and acid secretion. J Pharmacol Exp Ther. 1977;203:646–652.

18. Levine RA, Schwartzel EH Jr. Effect of indomethacin on basal and histamine-stimulated human gastric acid secretion. Gut. 1984;25:718–722.

19. Wallace JL, Keenan CM, Granger DN. Gastric ulceration induced by non-steroidal anti-inflammatory drugs is a neutrophil dependent process. Am J Physiol. 1990;259:G462–G467.

20. Wallace JL, McKnight GW, Arfors KE. A monoclonal antibody against the CD18 leukocyte adhesion molecule prevents indomethacin-induced gastric damage in the rabbit. Gastroenterology. 1991;100:878–883.

21. Scheimer RP. The mechanisms of antiinflammatory steroid action in allergic diseases. Annu Rev Pharmacol Toxicol. 1985;25:381–412.

22. Bowen DL, Fauci AS. Adrenal corticosteroids. In: Gallin JI, Goldstein IM, Snyderman R, eds. Inflammation: basic principles and clinical correlates. New York: Raven Press; 1988:877–895.

23. Derelanko MJ, Long JF. Effect of corticosteroids on indomethacin-induced intestinal ulceration in the rat. Dig Dis Sci. 1980;25:823–829.

24. Sapolsky R, Rivier C, Yamamoto G, Plotsky P, Vale W. Interleukin-1 stimulates the secretion of hypothalamic corticotropin-releasing factor. Science. 1987;238:522–524.

25. Berkenbosch F, Van Oers J, Del Rey A, Tilders F, Besodovsky H. Corticotropin-releasing factor-producing neurons in the rat activated by interleukin-1. Science. 1987;238:524–526.

26. Rivier C, Vale W, Brown M. In the rat, interleukin-1α and -β stimulates adrenocorticotropin and catecholamine release. Endocrinology. 1989;125:3096–3102.

27. Roh MS, Drazenovich KA, Barbose JJ, Dinarello CA, Cobb CF. Direct stimulation of the adrenal cortex by interleukin-1. Surgery. 1987;102:140–146.

28. Borish L, Rosenbaum R, McDonald B, Rosenwasser LJ. Recombinant interleukin-1β interacts with high-affinity receptors to activate neutrophil leukotriene B_4 synthesis. Inflammation. 1990;14:151–162.

29. Smith RJ, Speziale SC, Bowman BJ. Properties of interleukin-1 as a complete secretagogue for human neutrophils. Biochem Biophys Res Commun. 1985;130:1233–1240.

30. Ogle JD, Noel JG, Balasurbramaniam A, Sramkoski RM, Ogle CK, Alexander JW. Comparison of abilities of recombinant interleukin-1α and -β and non-inflammatory IL-1β fragment 163–171 to upregulate C3b receptors (CR1) on human neutrophils and to enhance their phagocytic capacity. Inflammation. 1990;14:185–194.
31. Rossi V, Breviario F, Ghezzi P, Dejana E, Mantovani A. Prostacyclin synthesis induced by vascular cells by interleukin-1. Science. 1985;229:174–176.
32. Whittle BJR, Lopez-Belmonte J, Moncada S. Regulation of gastric mucosal integrity by endogenous nitric oxide: interactions with prostanoids and sensory neuropeptides in the rat. Br J Pharmacol. 1990;99:607–611.
33. MacNaughton WK, Wallace JL. Endothelium-derived relaxing factor (nitric oxide) has protective actions in the stomach. Life Sci. 1989;45:1869–1876.
34. Kitagawa H, Takeda F, Kohei H. Effect of endothelium-derived relaxing factor on the gastric lesion induced by HCl in rats. J Pharmacol Exp Ther. 1990;253:1133–1137.
35. McCall T, Whittle BJR, Boughton-Smith NK, Moncada S. Inhibition of FMLP-induced aggregation of rabbit neutrophils by nitric oxide. Br J Pharmacol. 1988;95:517P.
36. Kubes P, Suzuki M, Granger DN. Nitric oxide: an endogenous mediator of leukocyte adhesion. Proc Natl Acad Sci USA. 1991;88:4651–4655
37. Beasley D, Schwartz JH, Brenner BM. Interleukin-1 induces prolonged L-arginine-dependent cyclic guanosine monophosphate and nitrate production in rat vascular smooth muscle cells. J Clin Invest. 1991;87:602–608.
38. Dinarello CA. Interleukin-1. Rev Infect Dis. 1984;6:51–95.
39. Knowles RG, Salter M, Brooks SL, Moncada S. Anti-inflammatory glucocorticoids inhibit the induction by endotoxin of nitric oxide synthase in the lung, liver and aorta of the rat. Biochem Biophys Res Commun. 1990;172:1042–1048.

18

Prevention and treatment of NSAID-gastroduodenal damage: the role of H₂-receptor antagonists

G. Bianchi Porro and S. Ardizzone

Gastroenterology Unit, L. Sacco Hospital, Milan, Italy

INTRODUCTION

Non-steroidal anti-inflammatory drugs (NSAIDs) are the most common and universally prescribed group of drugs, and remain the standard treatment for pain and inflammation associated with various forms of arthritis and other musculoskeletal discomforts. While NSAIDs can relieve pain and inflammation they can also cause gastrointestinal symptoms, ulceration, perforation, gastrointestinal bleeding and in rare cases, death [1].

Generally, NSAID-therapy is discontinued when lesions are diagnosed endoscopically or when gastrointestinal symptoms become manifest. These measures, however, especially in patients with rheumatoid arthritis, can lead to the return of articular pain and significant functional limitation. In these cases, it may be prudent not to interrupt NSAID-therapy but to add an anti-ulcer drug to prevent the development of the gastroduodenal damage or to treat the established NSAID-induced gastroduodenal lesion.

This paper reviews the role of H₂-receptor antagonists in the prevention and treatment of gastric and duodenal mucosal lesions, and asks if these drugs are effective in reducing the chance of perforation or haemorrhage in patients at risk of NSAID-induced ulcer.

THE PREVENTION OF NSAID INJURY

Before reviewing the studies on the prevention of NSAID-induced gastroduodenal damage, it is appropriate to consider the problems emerging from available trials.

Side-effects of Anti-inflammatory Drugs 3. Rainsford KD, Velo GP (eds), Inflammation and Drug Therapy Series, Volume V.

Definition of mucosal protection

There appears to be a wide choice of 'effective drugs' available to provide 'protection' against the damaging effects of NSAIDs. However, the protection afforded by the drug may be of little – if any – clinical significance. The majority of studies have used elaborate scoring systems to describe grades of injury (erythema, haemorrhage, erosion and acute ulcer). A reported improvement, using cytoprotective and antisecretory drugs and based on the reduction of the degree of erythema or the number of haemorrhages is of questionable significance as these injuries are thought to be quickly reversible and not necessarily associated with clinical manifestations.

Lack of correlation between acute injury and chronic complications

As Figure 1 illustrates, most patients who ingest NSAIDs develop acute mucosal injury. Many patients also experience gastrointestinal intolerance (some with acute injury, either with or without symptoms). A very small number of these ulcer patients develop complications again with and without gastrointestinal symptoms. Therefore, symptoms and the presence of acute mucosal injury are not predictive of the presence of a chronic ulcer and its complications. Most trials have studied ways in which to prevent acute gastric or duodenal injury following single or short-term doses of NSAIDs. These studies assume that acute gastric injury is the precursor of chronic ulceration. This assumption may well be false. Prevention of acute damage due to NSAIDs does not necessarily predict the prevention of chronic ulceration and the risks of bleeding or perforation.

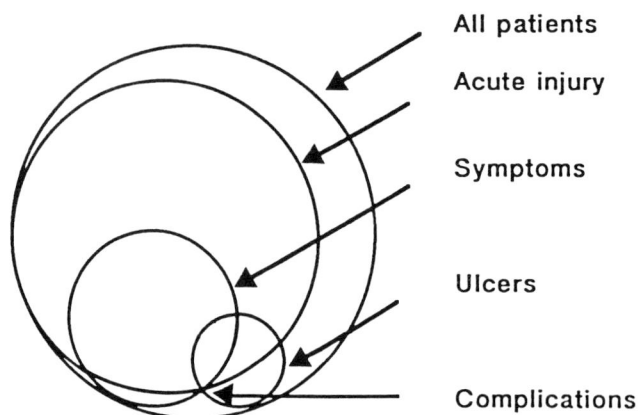

Figure 1. Venn diagram of side-effects in patients taking NSAIDs. This illustrates the lack of predictive value of acute mucosal NSAID-induced injury and gastrointestinal symptoms for the development of chronic ulcer and its complications (2)

Risk of ulcer perforation or haemorrhage

The use of NSAIDs is associated with a risk of developing a life-threatening gastrointestinal complication.

In case-controlled studies of patients presenting with perforated ulcers or admitted for bleeding duodenal or gastric ulcers, there is a highly significant association between perforation and the use of NSAIDs in comparison with a hospital-control population [3–5].

Low incidence of significant ulcer complications

The incidence of severe complications due to NSAID use is low, approximately one case per 10,000 patient-months of NSAID use [6]. Therefore a trial designed to study the prevention of the NSAID complications, would require an enormous number of subjects to provide any meaningful data. The presence of an ulcer could be a logical alternative conclusion as ulcers occur more frequently than their complications.

Unfortunately, no study has looked at the prevention of ulcerative complications. Bearing in mind that NSAIDs do carry a significant risk of ulceration and its complications, the physician must use this scant information to make decisions concerning patients on NSAIDs.

Identification of patients at risk of NSAID-induced ulceration

Several studies have shown that elderly people are at particular risk of developing gastrointestinal ulceration on NSAID treatment [3–5,7]. In the study of Jick et al. [8], the adjusted rate ratio of risk for a patient 60–79 years old taking NSAIDs was 20 times greater than for a similar patient 10–39 years old. The risk for a patient over 80 years was more than twice that of a 60–79 years old patient. This increased risk is of particular importance given the more frequent occurrence of certain kinds of arthritis and resultant NSAID use with increasing age. No other risk factors for the development of NSAID-induced gastrointestinal damage have been clearly established.

Randomized, double-blind, placebo-controlled studies with H₂-receptor antagonists in the prevention of NSAID-induced gastroduodenal damage

There is little doubt that the H_2-receptor antagonists reduce the NSAID-induced gastrointestinal mucosal lesions by acute administration of aspirin and other NSAIDs [9,10]. The effects of H_2-receptor antagonists on the prevention of gastroduodenal mucosal lesions after prolonged use of

NSAIDs are less evident. In studies dealing with this topic, the gastric and duodenal mucosal damage was assessed according to a numerical rating scale (Table 1).

Berkowitz et al. [12] examined whether concomitant administration of ranitidine could protect against the gastroduodenal mucosal damage associated with aspirin therapy in healthy men. Twenty-four subjects received ranitidine (150 mg b.i.d.), and 19 received placebo b.i.d. plus aspirin (650 mg b.i.d.) for four weeks. Gastric and duodenal injury were assessed separately at baseline and after four weeks of treatment. The ranitidine/aspirin group had significantly less mucosal damage in the stomach and duodenum than the placebo/aspirin group. The maximum mucosal damage scores after treatment were significantly lower in subjects receiving ranitidine for both gastric and duodenal mucosa (Table 2).

We conducted a prophylactic study [13] with the co-administration of ranitidine on 332 patients with rheumatic disease treated with one or more NSAIDs. After submitting the patients to an upper gastrointestinal endoscopy, 246 (75%) were found to have a normal gastric mucosa and

Table 1. Table of scores for mucosal lesions at endoscopic examinations (adapted from Lanza et al. [12])

Lesion	Score
None	0
Erythema	1
1–4 punctate haemorrhages	1
5–10 punctate haemorrhages	2
11–20 punctate haemorrhages	3
1–4 erosions	2
5–9 erosions	3
10–20 erosions	4
Ulcer	4
Confluent haemorrhages	4

Table 2. Maximum mucosal damage after treatment

	Stomach No. (%) of patients*		Duodenum No. (%) of patients**	
Grade	Ranitidine (n=24)	Placebo (n=19)	Ranitidine (n=24)	Placebo (n=19)
0	4 (17)	0	14 (58)	6 (32)
1	1 (4)	1 (5)	0	1 (5)
2	10 (42)	4 (21)	8 (33)	5 (26)
3	7 (29)	4 (21)	2 (8)	5 (26)
4	2 (8)	10 (53)	0	2 (11)

*$p < 0.01$ for comparison of the distribution of maximum grades between groups for stomach
**$p = 0.02$ for comparison of distribution of maximum grades between groups for duodenum

were therefore randomized to receive, in a double-blind fashion, either ranitidine 150 mg b.i.d. or placebo, in association with their prescribed NSAID for four weeks. Results are shown in Table 3. No difference between ranitidine and placebo was observed in relation to the incidence of gastric lesions.

Table 3. Endoscopic results after 4 weeks of co-administration of ranitidine 300 mg per day or placebo in 246 rheumatic patients on NSAID-therapy

	Ranitidine	Placebo	p value
Normal	64 (53.8%)	70 (55.11%)	> 0.05
Gastric erosions	46 (38.7%)	46 (36.2%)	> 0.05
Drop-outs	9 (7.6%)	11 (8.7%)	> 0.05
Total	119 (100%)	127 (100%)	

Roth et al. [14] evaluated the use of cimetidine 300 mg q.i.d. in 94 patients with endoscopically proven NSAID gastropathy. No reduction in the percentage of patients with gastric mucosal damage was seen with cimetidine after eight weeks of treatment.

In a trial by Ehsanullah et al. [15] in 263 patients receiving NSAIDs and with a normal pre-treatment endoscopy, there was a reduction in the number of duodenal ulcers but not gastric ulcers occurring during the eight weeks when ranitidine 150 mg b.i.d. daily was given, compared with placebo-treated patients.

Robinson et al. [16] evaluated the effect of ranitidine in preventing mucosal damage caused by various NSAIDs in 144 patients with normal endoscopic findings at baseline. Patients were randomly assigned to receive either ranitidine 150 mg b.i.d. or placebo for eight weeks, in association with their prescribed NSAID. Duodenal damage was significantly less in the ranitidine group compared with the placebo group by weeks 4 and 8 ($p < 0.01$). Duodenal ulcers did not develop in any patient on ranitidine (0/57) compared to 4/49 (8%) patients on placebo ($p = 0.02$). No significant difference was found in gastric damage between treatment groups: 6/60 (10%) in the ranitidine group and 6/50 (12%) in the placebo group developed gastric ulcers.

Comment

These trials suggest that co-administration of full-dose H_2-receptor antagonists with NSAIDs protect against chronic duodenal ulcer but is not of significant benefit in the prophylaxis of NSAID-induced gastric ulceration. These studies were looking at relatively short-term and

149

probably innocuous ulcers. Whether histamine H_2-receptor antagonists prevent the development of life-threatening haemorrhage or perforation remains to be determined.

THE TREATMENT OF ESTABLISHED NSAID-INDUCED ULCERATION

In this section we review those studies wherein the efficacy of H_2-receptor antagonists, in the treatment of established NSAID-induced ulceration, was evaluated.

In a sophisticated trial, Manniche et al. [17] evaluated 67 patients with rheumatic disease being treated with NSAIDs, who entered a controlled trial with an ulcer diagnosis of duodenal ($n = 51$), gastric ($n = 14$), or gastric and duodenal ($n = 2$). The main study objectives were to compare ranitidine to sucralfate in ulcer treatment and to observe the influence of continued NSAID administration during peptic ulcer therapy. Ulcers healed within 9 weeks in 52 patients. The mean healing time was similar in 27 patients given ranitidine 150 mg b.i.d. (4.9 weeks) and 25 patients given sucralfate 1 g q.i.d. (4.6 weeks). Of the 30 patients who continued taking NSAIDs during the treatment with either ranitidine or sucralfate, 23 ulcers healed (mean healing time = 5.0 weeks). Of the 32 patients who stopped NSAIDs intake, ulcer healing was documented in 29 (mean healing time = 4.6 weeks). The difference in healing rates was not statistically significant ($p > 0.10$).

An international multi-centre trial [18] was recently conducted comparing the therapeutic efficacy of two different dosages of omeprazole (40 mg/day and 20 mg/day) with ranitidine 150 mg b.i.d. in patients with benign gastric ulcer. With almost 200 patients on each drug, a minority continued to take NSAIDs during treatment. Although the difference failed to reach significance, omeprazole 40 mg/day was superior to omeprazole 20 mg/day at 4 and 8 weeks and achieved over twice the healing rate of ranitidine during the same 4 and 8 week periods ($p = 0.02$).

We conducted a trial [19] to evaluate the therapeutic efficacy of cimetidine in comparison to colloidal bismuth subcitrate (CBS) for their respective effects in promoting healing of gastric and duodenal ulcers in rheumatoid arthritic patients undergoing chronic antirheumatic treatment with NSAIDs that could not be discontinued. Forty-seven patients with duodenal ulcer and 44 with gastric ulcer were admitted to the study and randomly allocated to receive either cimetidine 400 mg t.i.d. or colloidal bismuth subcitrate 120 mg q.i.d. without discontinuing the NSAID treatment being taken at the initial endoscopic examination. An endoscopic control was planned at weeks 4 and 8 of therapy. Without interrupting their anti-rheumatic drug therapy, patients with unhealed ulcers at 8 weeks of therapy were treated for a further 4–8 weeks with the alternative anti-ulcer study drug. Endoscopic controls were scheduled at weeks 12 and 16 of therapy. Tables 4 and 5 illustrate the respective ulcer healing rates. No statistical difference was found between the healing activities of cimetidine and colloidal bismuth subcitrate in rheumatoid arthritis.

Table 4. Healing rates after 4 and 8 weeks of therapy*

	Cimetidine		CBS	
	4	8	4	8
DU	4/24 (58%)	15/24 (62.5%)	12/20 (60%)	14/20 (70%)
GU	9/20 (45%)	12/20 (60%)	10/20 (45%)	13/22 (60%)

$+p > 0.05$

Table 5. Healing rates in the sub-group of patients with unhealed ulcers after 8 weeks of therapy and assigned to the alternative anti-ulcer drug for a further 4–8 week period*

	Cimetidine		CBS	
	12	16	12	16
DU	3/6 (50%)	5/6 (83.3%)	4/8 (50%)	6/8 (75%)
GU	3/7 (42.8%)	4/7 (57.1%)	4/8 (50%)	5/8 (62%)

In a multi-centre study [20], the effect of ranitidine on healing NSAID-associated peptic ulcers was compared in a group of patients who had stopped NSAID treatment with another group who had continued their NSAID therapy. A total of 190 patients with confirmed ulcers were randomized to continue or stop NSAID administration. All patients in addition received ranitidine 150 mg b.i.d. Patients were endoscopically controlled at 4, 8 and 12 weeks. Gastric ulcers at 8 weeks had healed in 63% of those patients taking NSAIDs compared to 95% of those who had stopped NSAID treatment. For duodenal ulcer patients, the healing rates at week 8 were 84% in the group continuing with NSAIDs compared to 100% in those who had discontinued NSAIDs. The differences in healing rates were statistically significant for both gastric ulcer ($p = 0.001$) and for duodenal ulcer ($p = 0.006$). At 12 weeks, 79% of gastric ulcers and 92% of duodenal were healed in the group continuing with NSAIDs. All patients with gastric and duodenal ulcers who stopped taking NSAIDs were healed at 12 weeks.

Comment

These studies indicate that no statistical difference was found between the healing activities of H_2-receptor antagonists and GI protective drugs. Even if NSAID treatment is continued, substantial healing rates are achieved albeit at a slower pace, particularly in the case of gastric ulcers.

CONCLUSIONS

Histamine H_2-receptor antagonists, effective in reducing acute injury when taken before or with non-steroidal anti-inflammatory drugs, are inexplicably ineffective in chronic prophylaxis for 4 weeks or more in preventing gastric ulcers, although the number of duodenal ulcers is reduced. No study has looked at the prevention of complications of ulceration and there is therefore no data as to whether or not continued NSAID administration leads to an increase in complications.

Given the rarity of complication and the incompleteness of our knowledge with regard to the prevention of ulcer complications, there is little indication for widespread use of any of the available drugs for prophylaxis against NSAID injury.

REFERENCES

1. Holvoet J, Terriere L, Van Hee W, Verbist L, Fierens E, Hautekeete ML. Relation of upper gastrointestinal bleeding to non-steroidal anti-inflammatory drugs and aspirin: a case–control study. Gut. 1991;32:730–734.
2. Howard JM, Le Riche NGH. The management of NSAID gastropathy. Bailliere's Clinical Rheumatology. 1990;4:269–291.
3. Somerville K, Faulkner G, Langman M. Non-steroidal anti-inflammatory drugs and bleeding peptic ulcer. Lancet. 1986;1:462–464.
4. Walt R, Katschinski B, Logan R, Ashley J, Langman M. Rising frequency of ulcer perforation in elderly people in the United Kingdom. Lancet. 1986;1:489–492.
5. Armstrong CP, Blower AL. Non-steroidal anti-inflammatory drugs and life threatening complications of peptic ulceration. Gut. 1987;28:527–532.
6. Langman MJS. Epidemiological evidence on the association between peptic ulceration and anti-inflammatory drug use. Gastroenterology. 1989;96:640–644.
7. Collier DJ, Pain JA. Non-steroidal anti-inflammatory drugs and peptic ulcer perforation. Gut. 1985;26:359–363.
8. Jick SS, Perera DR, Walker AM, Jick H. Non-steroidal anti-inflammatory drugs and hospital admission for perforated peptic ulcer. Lancet.1987;2:380–382.
9. Berkowitz JM, Adler SN, Sharp JT, Warner CW. Reduction of aspirin-induced gastroduodenal mucosal damage with ranitidine. J Clin Gastroenterol. 1986;8:377–380.
10. Kimmey MB, Silverstein FE. Role of H2-receptor blockers in the prevention of gastric injury resulting from nonsteroidal anti-inflammatory agents. Am J Med. 1988;84(Suppl.2A):49–52.
11. Lanza FL, Royer GL, Nelson RS. Endoscopic evaluation of the effects of aspirin, buffered aspirin, and enteric-coated aspirin on gastric and duodenal mucosa. N Engl J Med. 1980;303:136–138.

12. Berkowitz JM, Rogenes PR, Sharp J, Warner CW. Ranitidine protects against gastroduodenal mucosal damage associated with chronic aspirin therapy. Arch Intern Med. 1987;147:2137–2139.

13. Bianchi Porro G, Pace F, Caruso I. Why are non-steroidal anti-inflammatory drugs important in peptic ulceration? Aliment Pharmacol Ther. 1987;1:540S–547S.

14. Roth SH, Bennet RE, Mitchell CS, Hartman RJ. Cimetidine therapy in non-steroidal anti-inflammatory drug gastropathy. Double-blind long-term evaluation. Arch Intern Med. 1987;147:1798–1801.

15. Ehsanullah RSB, Page MC, Tildesley G, Wood JR. Prevention of gastroduodenal damage induced by non-steroidal anti-inflammatory drugs: controlled trial of ranitidine. Br Med J. 1988;297:1017–1021.

16. Robinson MG, Griffin JW, Bowers J, Kogan FJ, Kogut DG, Lanza F, Warner CW. Effect of ranitidine gastroduodenal mucosal damage induced by non-steroidal anti-inflammatory drugs. Dig Dis Sci. 1989;34:424–428.

17. Manniche C, Malchow-Moller A, Andersen JR, Pedersen C, Hansen TM, Jess P, Helleberg L, Rasmussen SN, Tage-Jensen U, Nielsen SE. Randomised study of the influence of non-steroidal anti-inflammatory drugs in the treatment of peptic ulcer in patients with rheumatic disease. Gut. 1987;28:226–229.

18. Walan A, Bader JP, Classen M, Lamers CBHW, Piper DW, Rutgersson K, Eriksson S. Effect of omeprazole and ranitidine on ulcer healing and relapse rates in patients with benign gastric ulcer. N Engl J Med. 1989;320:69–75.

19. Petrillo M, Ardizzone S, Bianchi Porro G. Cimetidine versus colloidal bismuth subcitrate (De-Nol) in peptic ulcer therapy of patients with rheumatoid arthritis undergoing chronic non-steroidal anti-inflammatory drug treatment. Eur J Gastroenterol Hepatol. 1990;2(Suppl.1):S82–S83.

20. Lancaster-Smith MJ, Jaderberg ME, Jackson DA. Ranitidine in the treatment of non-steroidal anti-inflammatory drug-associated gastric and duodenal ulcers. Gut. 1991;32:252–255.

19

Omeprazole in the prevention and therapy of gastroduodenal lesions on NSAID therapy

C.B.H.W. Lamers

Department of Gastroenterology–Hepatology,
University Hospital Leiden, Leiden, The Netherlands

INTRODUCTION

Omeprazole inhibits the final step in the formation of hydrochloric acid by blocking the enzyme H^+–K^+-ATPase on the secretory membrane of the parietal cell [1]. It is a highly effective inhibitor of acid secretion and has been shown to promote the healing of duodenal ulcer, gastric ulcer and reflux oesophagitis [1–3]. The compound is also effective in healing peptic ulcer resistant to high doses of H_2-receptor antagonists, in healing ulcers and alleviating symptoms of diarrhoea and malabsorption in patients with Zollinger–Ellison syndrome and enhancing the efficacy of pancreatic enzyme replacement therapy in patients with cystic fibrosis [1–4]. However, little is known of the effect of H^+–K^+-ATPase inhibitors in the prevention of NSAIDs-induced acute gastric lesions and in the healing of peptic ulcer in patients on continuous NSAID therapy.

PREVENTION OF ACUTE NSAID-INDUCED GASTRIC LESIONS BY OMEPRAZOLE

Animal studies

Konturek et al. studied the effect of various doses of omeprazole on acute gastric lesions induced by intragastric instillation of acidified aspirin in rats [5]. The authors showed that omeprazole dose-dependently inhibited the mean ulcer area induced by aspirin. There was no difference when the drug was administered intragastrically or subcutaneously. This finding is in contrast with gastric lesions induced by absolute alcohol, where the intragastric application of omeprazole induced markedly better protection than the subcutaneous administration of the drug [5]. The finding that both intragastric and subcutaneous administration of omeprazole prevents

Side-effects of Anti-inflammatory Drugs 3. Rainsford KD, Velo GP (eds),
Inflammation and Drug Therapy Series, Volume V.

aspirin-induced gastric lesions suggests that the protection of such lesions by omeprazole is mediated by acid inhibition and not by a topical mucosal protective action. The observation that the inhibition of gastric PGI_2 production by acidified aspirin was not prevented by omeprazole further supports the importance of acid inhibition in the prevention of acute aspirin-induced gastric mucosal lesions. It was further shown that only antisecretory doses of 2 to 200 µmol/kg omeprazole were protective, whereas the 0.2 µmol/kg dose of omeprazole did neither significantly inhibit gastric acid secretion nor the acute lesions of the gastric mucosa induced by acidified aspirin. Similar prevention of acidified aspirin induced gastric lesions was found by Mattsson et al. applying doses between 10 and 80 µmol/kg of omeprazole orally to rats [6].

Human studies

In human studies NSAID-induced acute gastric lesions are assessed by either an endoscopic score or quantification of gastric blood loss. Daneshmend et al. showed in a randomized, double blind, placebo-controlled cross-over study in healthy subjects that antisecretory doses of omeprazole significantly inhibited gastic mucosal blood loss induced by aspirin [7]. Omeprazole (20 mg o.d. or 40 mg b.i.d.) or placebo were given for 7 days while aspirin (900 mg b.i.d.) was given for the last 2 days. Gastric blood loss was measured in gastric aspirates by the ortho-tolidine reaction. Gastric mucosal blood loss was 3.4 µmol/10 min on aspirin and omeprazole 20 mg o.d., 2.4 µmol/10 min on aspirin and omeprazole 40 mg b.i.d. compared to 16.1 µmol/10 min on aspirin alone and 1.4 µmol/10 min on placebo. Bigard and Isal studied the effect of 4 days treatment with omeprazole or placebo on acute gastric lesions induced by 1000 mg aspirin by endoscopy in healthy subjects [8]. Gastric lesions were scored according to the method of Lanza. An endoscopy score of 3 or 4 was considered clinically significant. In the first part of the study 60 mg omeprazole o.d. decreased the incidence of significant gastric lesions from 93% on placebo to 0% [8]. In the second part of the study the investigators showed that the incidence of clinically significant endoscopic lesions was inhibited from 83% on placebo to 8% by 40 mg o.d. omeprazole and to 33% by 20 mg o.d. omeprazole [8]. Interestingly, Muller et al. found that lower doses of 5 and 10 mg o.d. omeprazole for 5 days orally induced only a modest non-significant decrease of acute gastric mucosal lesions induced by a solution of 1500 mg aspirin as assessed by endoscopy [9]. Taking the studies of Bigard et al. and Muller et al. it can be concluded that antisecretory doses of omeprazole are needed to significantly prevent aspirin-induced gastric mucosal lesions.

155

Oddsson et al. investigated in a randomized double-blind study the effect of omeprazole 40 mg o.d. or placebo for 7 days on naproxen 500 mg b.i.d. induced gastropathy administered orally on days 3 through 7 by endoscopy in 5 healthy volunteers [10]. Omeprazole significantly decreased the endoscopy score for duodenal mucosal lesions from 1.93 to 0.27, whereas the improvement of the naproxen-induced gastropathy, from 1.53 to 0.93, failed to reach statistical significance. Dorta et al. investigated by endoscopy in a double-blind, placebo-controlled study the effect of omeprazole 40 mg o.d. for 2 weeks on gastroduodenal mucosal lesions, on endoscopic biopsy site healing, and on histology of gastroduodenal mucosal biopsies after oral treatment with diclofenac 50 mg b.i.d. during the second week of the study in 12 healthy volunteers [11]. Omeprazole did not prevent the development of endoscopical and histological mucosal lesions in the stomach and duodenum and did not improve healing rates of mucosal biopsy sites in the stomach and duodenum.

When summarizing the various studies in healthy humans, it can be concluded that omeprazole in antisecretory doses diminishes aspirin-induced gastric mucosal lesions, but does not unequivocally decrease gastroduodenal mucosal lesions induced by the NSAIDs naproxen and diclofenac.

HEALING OF ULCERS DURING CONTINUOUS NSAID THERAPY

Animal studies

Wang et al. studied the effect of omeprazole on the delay by indomethacin of the healing of gastric ulcers induced by submucosal gastric injection of 0.03 ml 20% acetic acid in rats [12]. Indomethacin in a daily dose of 1 mg/ kg s.c. during the whole study period increased the mean ulcerated area from 6.6 to 16.0 mm^2 in a 2-week study and from 3.8 to 11.2 mm^2 in a 4-week experiment. In both studies omeprazole in doses ranging from 10 to 100 mg/kg daily per os dose-dependently reduced the mean ulcerated area. In the 2-week experiments the prevention amounted to 28, 60 and 76% for the 10, 30 and 100 mg/kg/day doses of omeprazole, respectively. The prevention in the 4-week study was 34 and 55% for the two higher doses of omeprazole. The latter doses of omeprazole abolished basal and histamine-stimulated gastric acid secretion when measured 0.5 hour after administration of the drug and significantly inhibited basal and stimulated acid secretion 20 hours after the final administration of omeprazole. Thus, antisecretory doses of omeprazole significantly and dose-dependently prevent the delayed healing of acetic acid-induced gastric ulcers in response to repeatedly administered indomethacin in rats.

Human studies

In a study comparing the endoscopically observed healing of benign gastric ulcer by omeprazole 20 mg o.d., omeprazole 40 mg o.d. and ranitidine 150 mg b.i.d. in 602 patients, 69 patients received this therapy during continuous treatment with NSAIDs [13]. At 4 weeks 61%, 81% and 32% of patients had healed ulcers with omeprazole 20 mg o.d., omeprazole 40 mg o.d. and ranitidine 150 mg b.i.d., respectively. The healing rates at 8 weeks were 82% and 95% after treatment with 20 mg and 40 mg omeprazole daily compared to 53% with ranitidine. When the healing rates of the patients on NSAIDs were compared to those of all gastric ulcer patients in the study it turned out that NSAID therapy significantly reduced the healing rates by ranitidine, but not by the two doses of omeprazole (Table 1).

Table 1. Effect of omeprazole and ranitidine on endoscopical ulcer healing in patients with gastric ulcer (entire group) and in a subgroup with gastric ulcer on continuing NSAID therapy (NSAID group)

	Omeprazole		Ranitidine 150 mg b.i.d.
	20 mg o.d.	40 mg o.d.	
4 weeks			
entire group	117/170 (69%)	131/164 (80%)	103/175 (59%)
NSAID group	11/18 (61%)	17/21 (81%)	6/19 (32%)
8 weeks			
entire group	153/172 (89%)	164/171 (96%)	144/169 (85%)
NSAID group	14/17 (82%)	21/22 (95%)	9/17 (53%)

Bianchi Porro et al. compared the efficacy of omeprazole 20 mg o.d. with the mucosa protective drug sucralfate 1 g q.i.d. in 30 rheumatic patients with either gastric, duodenal or combined gastric and duodenal ulcers [14]. At 4 weeks 100% of patients had healed ulcer on omeprazole compared to 64% on sucralfate.

It is concluded that omeprazole therapy is superior to both ranitidine and sucralfate treatment of patients with peptic ulcer during continuous NSAID therapy. Thus, powerful acid inhibition is of great value in the therapy of ulcers in patients on NSAIDs.

REFERENCES

1. Clissold SP, Campoli-Richards DM. Omeprazole. Drugs. 1986;32:15–47.
2. Lamers CB. Clinical impact of H^+, K^+-ATP-ase inhibitors. Digestion. 1989;S1:1–95.
3. Maton PN. Omeprazole. N Engl J Med. 1991;324:965–975.
4. Heyerman HG, Lamers CB, Bakker W. Omeprazole enhances the efficacy of pancreatin (pancrease) in cystic fibrosis. Ann Intern Med. 1991;114:200–201.

5. Konturek SJ, Brzozowski T, Radecki T. Protective action of omeprazole, a benzimidazole derivative, on gastric mucosal damage by aspirin and ethanol in rats. Digestion. 1983;27:159–164.
6. Mattsson H, Andersson K, Larsson H. Omeprazole provides protection against experimentally induced gastric mucosal lesions. Eur J Pharmacol. 1983;91:111–114.
7. Daneshmend TK, Stein AG, Bhaskar NK, Hawkey CJ. Abolition by omeprazole of aspirin induced gastric mucosal injury in man. Gut. 1990;31:514–517.
8. Bigard MA, Isal JP. Prevention of aspirin-induced gastric lesions by omeprazole in healthy subjects. Gastroenterology. 1989;96:A44.
9. Muller P, Dammann HG, Simon B. Akute Schädigung der Magenschleimhaut durch Acetylsalicylsäure. Arzneim Forsch. 1986;36:265–268.
10. Oddsson E, Gudjonsson H, Thjodleifsson B. Protective effect of omeprazole or ranitidine against naproxen induced damage to the human gastroduodenal mucosa. Proceedings of the World Congress of Gastroenterology, Sydney, 1990, August 26–31; FP22.
11. Dorta G, Sarga E, Nicolet M, Schnegg JF, Vouillamoz D, Amstrong D, Blum AL. Influence of omeprazole on healing and prevention of gastroduodenal mucosal lesions during administration of NSAIDs. Gastroenterology. 1991;100:A55.
12. Wang JY, Nagai H, Okabe S. Effect of omeprazole on delayed healing of acetic acid-induced gastric ulcers in rats. Jpn J Pharmacol. 1990;54:82–85.
13. Walan A, Bader JP, Classen M, Lamers CBHW, Piper DW, Rutgersson K, Eriksson S. Effect of omeprazole and ranitidine on ulcer healing and relapse rates in patients with benign gastric ulcer. N Engl J Med. 1989;320:69–75.
14. Bianchi Porro G, Santalucia F, Petrillo M. Omeprazole versus sucralfate in the treatment of NSAID-induced gastric and duodenal ulcer. Gut. 1990;31:A1175.

20

Sucralfate in the prevention of NSAID-induced gastric ulceration

Poul J. Ranløv and Axel Malchow-Møller

The Division of Medical Gastroenterology, Department of Internal Medicine B, Central Hospital, DK-3400 Hillerød and The Department of Internal Medicine, Svendborg Hospital, DK-5700 Svendborg, Denmark

SUCRALFATE

Sucralfate is an aluminium salt of sulphated sucrose. The sucrose backbone carries a varying number of sulphated aluminium salts which, in an acid environment, releases free $Al_2(OH)_5^+$ which by polymerization leads to the formation of a gel with an affinity for mucous surfaces, especially with damaged epithelium (Figure 1). Sucralfate competes with and deactivates pepsin by preventing the binding of the pepsin molecule to the mucous surface. The aluminium salt is weakly alkaline and adsorbs willingly bile acids and trypsin. Sucralfate stimulates the normal gastric mucosa to the secretion of prostaglandin E_2, an effect which is blocked by indomethacin

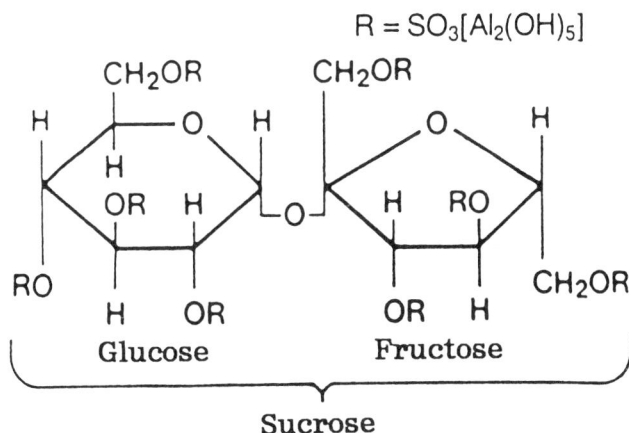

Figure 1. The chemical structure of sucralfate. In an acidic environment dissociation of $Al_2(OH)_5^+$ occurs, leading to polymerization of the substance and formation of a gel binding to the gastric mucosal surface

Side-effects of Anti-inflammatory Drugs 3. Rainsford KD, Velo GP (eds), Inflammation and Drug Therapy Series, Volume V.

[1]. Sucralfate binds the highly GI protective epidermal growth factor (EGF) and concentrates EGF in ulcerated areas [2]. Sucralfate increases mucosal blood flow [3]. It also stimulates bicarbonate secretion and epithelial restitution. All these virtues may be summarized: sucralfate is a largely acid-independent cytoprotective drug.

About 0.5–2% of ingested sucralfate is absorbed systemically. Toxic accumulation of aluminium in the body has not been reported but remains a possibility in patients with renal insufficiency. Sucralfate reduces bioavailability of warfarin and phenytoin by impaired absorption. Side-effects are few and inconspicuous: slight constipation, borborrhygmia, and dry mouth. It is a relatively inexpensive drug.

Sucralfate is definitely superior to placebo in ulcer healing: 80% of duodenal ulcers will heal within 4 weeks; 75% of gastric ulcers within 8 weeks. These figures are comparable to those of H_2-antagonists. Ulcer relapse after sucralfate healing comes later than after cimetidine. Sucralfate has obtained a certain merit in the maintenance treatment of reflux oesophagitis [4].

SUCRALFATE AND NSAID-INDUCED GASTROPATHY

Clinical experience and available data from the literature all point towards a characteristic clinical entity related to NSAID-intake: The Non-Steroidal Anti-Inflammatory Drug Gastropathy, a term originally coined by Roth [5]. This syndrome of NSAID-induced gastropathy (Table 1) differs in several respects from the traditional concept of Peptic Ulcer Disease: the latter is acid-mediated, mainly duodenal with a predominant occurrence in younger male persons; NSAID-induced gastropathy locates mainly in the antral-prepyloric region as small, shallow, and silent ulcers, preferentially in elderly females. In peptic ulcer disease the presenting symptom may be bleeding or perforation.

Table 1. Definition of NSAID-induced gastropathy versus classical peptic ulcer disease. (After Roth [5])

NSAID-induced gastropathy	Peptic ulcer disease
Restricted to the antral or pre-pyloric region	Over 90% localized to the duodenal bulb
Related to NSAID intake	Unknown aetiology
Acid-related	H^+-reducing therapy effective
Prostaglandin synthesis low Elderly females	Prostaglandins unaffected Younger males

That blocking by NSAIDs of the cyclo-oxygenases leads to reduction of the cytoprotective prostaglandins makes the cytoprotective drug sucralfate seem a rational choice for treatment or prevention of NSAID-induced gastric (and intestinal) damage. Roth and Bennett [6] lament that 'the previous literature has been confounded with short-term studies on healthy volunteers and animals that emphasize the resiliency of normal gastric adaptation to heal such gastropathy'. Likewise, endoscopic studies comparing the effect of acute administration of NSAIDs on the gastroduodenal mucosa in normal volunteers failed to predict which NSAIDs would be safest when administered chronically.

SUCRALFATE WITH NSAIDS: ACUTE STUDIES

There are several reports on short-term gastric expositions to chemical and toxic agents in man and experimental animals in which the modifying potential of sucralfate has been explored. Stapleton et al. [7] employed the bile duct-ligated pig to test the cytoprotective activity of sucralfate and found – with sucralfate – only minimal gastric lesions in two out of seven operated pigs while seven out of seven pigs of the control groups (pretreated with saline, famotidine or misoprostol) within 48 hours developed severe macroscopic ulceration. The results were regarded as evidence that acid inhibition is not the only important factor in ulcer healing.

Stern et al. [8] found, in healthy human subjects, that aspirin produced endoscopic changes that were significantly inhibited by sucralfate given 30 minutes before the ASA (Table 2). They also found that pretreatment with indomethacin abolished this sucralfate protection. Their findings seem to corroborate the notion that sucralfate stimulates endogenous prostaglandin formation. Their sole investigative parameter was mean endoscopic lesion score.

Konturek et al. [9] found sucralfate treatment in a dose of 1 g four times daily for 4 days significantly reduced spontaneous gastric microbleeding in untreated volunteers and, later, significantly prevented blood loss from the stomach in those same volunteers when given aspirin

Table 2. Mean endoscopic lesion scores in normal persons treated with aspirin with and without simultaneous sucralfate (After Stern et al. [8])

Study I	
Aspirin + placebo	2.75 ± 0.49
Aspirin + sucralfate	1.13 ± 0.44
Study II	
Aspirin + placebo + indomethacin	2.88 ± 0.55
Aspirin + sucralfate + indomethacin	1.88 ± 0.40

2.5 g for 2 days. Konturek measured gastric bleeding by a gastric lavage technique and his findings were probably in accordance with the lowered mean endoscopic lesion score reported by Stern et al. [8], estimated through a gastroscope. That is: fewer visible gastric lesions, lesser gastric bleeding.

An apparent discrepancy is presented by a somewhat similar acute study published by us [10]: 16 healthy male volunteers took part in a double blind, double-dummy cross-over study with one week of ASA + sucralfate and one week of ASA + placebo with a two weeks wash-out period in between. Daily total faecal blood loss was measured by the ^{51}Cr erythrocyte labelling technique (Figure 2). The study failed to demonstrate any obvious effect of sucralfate in preventing or reducing aspirin-induced gastrointestinal bleeding. The test persons were not subjected to endoscopic examination, while their mean endoscopic lesion scores were not known. In retrospect, it could be speculated that the gastric mucosa of our test persons was protected and the gastric bleeding as such reduced; however, sucralfate might not have protected the distal intestine, which is why the total faecal blood loss monitored might represent intestinal rather than gastric bleeding.

This explanation finds some support in the observations of Aabakken et al. [11] who studied the protective effects of sucralfate on naproxen-induced mucosal lesions both in the proximal and in the distal

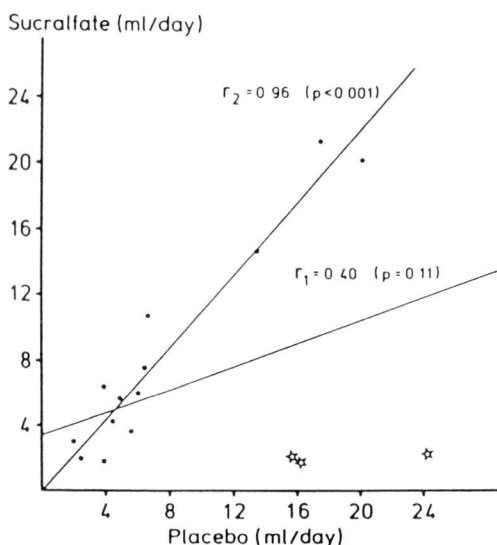

Figure 2. Correlation of acetylsalicylic-acid-induced faecal blood loss in 16 male volunteers receiving 1 g sucralfate four times daily or placebo. r_1 is the overall correlation coefficient; r_2 is calculated after exclusion of three persons with minimal bleeding after sucralfate but pronounced bleeding after placebo (indicated with stars). (Malchow-Møller and Ranlov (10))

162

gastrointestinal tract. Their design was comparable to ours in that their drug periods were one week and wash-out 3 weeks. They estimated gastric lesions by endoscopy and distal gut lesions by ^{51}Cr-EDTA absorption and found sucralfate offering protection against NSAID-induced damage in the stomach and proximal duodenum, but not in the distal gut where sucralfate failed to alleviate the NSAID-induced pathologic increase in ^{51}Cr-EDTA absorption signifying distal gut mucosal damage.

Which goes to show that acute studies on NSAID-protective measures, if such studies should be done at all, must take the whole gastrointestinal tract into account.

SUCRALFATE WITH NSAIDS: LONG-TERM STUDIES

Stern and co-workers, in a later publication [12] examined the effects of two weeks of aspirin ingestion in humans using a common clinical dosage. Using an endoscopic grading score of mucosal damage they found that sucralfate failed to ameliorate aspirin-induced damage to the gastric mucosa compared with placebo. These results were in contrast to their earlier findings in a similar, but acute study. However, others [13] in previous studies employing similar protocols have reached different conclusions: that sucralfate provided complete or partial gastric mucosal protection from the gastrotoxic effects of aspirin, compared with placebo. The discrepancies cannot be explained from the available data. Again, others [14,15] reached totally different conclusions on identical protocols. Attempts to explain the varying results include: the timing of sucralfate administration (prior to or concurrent with the NSAID?); formulation of sucralfate (tablets or granulate, or suspension?); dosage of sucralfate; should 'predosing' over several days be employed?; the role of a possible adaptive mucosal response; etc.

SUCRALFATE WITH NSAIDS: TREATMENT AND PREVENTION STUDIES

Side-effects related to the stomach and the intestines have limited and compromised the usefulness of ASA and NSAIDs for many rheumatic patients and led to discontinuing of an otherwise beneficial therapy. As a result, an effective method of controlling NSAID-induced gastric complaints while maintaining the therapeutic benefits of these drugs has been much in demand. As NSAID-induced gastropathy is acid-independent a rational pharmacological approach to the problem suggests the exclusion of antacids and H$_2$-receptor antagonists. Thus, cytoprotection seems a natural answer, limiting the prospective drugs to be investigated to sucralfate and misoprostol.

One such study was designed by Caldwell et al. [16] who, in a randomized, double-blind trial compared sucralfate with placebo in 143 symptomatic patients to assess their relative efficacy in the treatment of gastric mucosal damage associated with NSAIDs. The follow-up covered six months, on a fixed regimen of NSAIDs, half the patients receiving additional sucralfate, the other half placebo. The results indicate that sucralfate used in conjunction with NSAIDs may allow patients to continue therapy by relieving gastrointestinal symptoms and mucosal damage associated with NSAIDs. Improvement in the gastric mucosa was maintained in the long-term follow-up. Thus, according to the authors, patients may be allowed to continue receiving NSAIDs when a cytoprotective agent such as sucralfate is used as an adjunct.

The investigation by Shepherd and collaborators [17] substantiates the findings of Caldwell's group: in their (pilot) study 26 patients with rheumatoid arthritis and a stable NSAID treatment regimen were identified as having 'fully developed gastric and duodenal mucosal lesions' (not ulcers). Consequently, they were put on a single-blind regimen with sucralfate or cimetidine for 6 weeks. 11/14 taking sucralfate and 8/12 taking cimetidine improved their endoscopic lesions scores significantly (Figure 3). All had been established in a treatment regimen of NSAIDs for at least three months and had developed dyspepsia, iron-deficiency anaemia, or both (but no ulcers). Shepherd and co-workers further demonstrated enhanced prostaglandin synthesis in the antrum and body of the stomach in spite of continued NSAID consumption. Before that, Roth and co-workers [18] had treated a total of 104 patients with NSAID-induced gastropathy (without ulcers) for 8 weeks in a controlled trial of cimetidine against placebo. They concluded, that their patients fared no better with cimetidine than with placebo; a strong suggestion that NSAID-induced gastropathy bears no or little relation to gastric acidity.

In a prospective study involving the greater Copenhagen area [19] we consecutively included 67 patients with rheumatic disease necessitating continued and regular daily medication with NSAIDs. At the time of entry into the controlled trial all patients had endoscopy-verified gastric ($n = 14$), duodenal ($n = 51$), or both gastric and duodenal ulcer ($n = 2$). Sixty-two patients completed the study which involved control endoscopy every three weeks. The main objective was to observe the influence of continued NSAID administration during anti-ulcer therapy while 30 patients were randomized to continued NSAID treatment (Table 3). Of these 23 ulcers healed (77%, mean: 5 weeks), half of them after sucralfate treatment. Virtually, the same healing rate and mean healing time were found for ranitidine and sucralfate. The main conclusion drawn from the study was that the outcome of treatment of a rheumatic patient for a peptic ulcer is not affected by concurrent treatment with NSAIDs. Between those who stopped NSAID intake and those who continued we were unable to detect

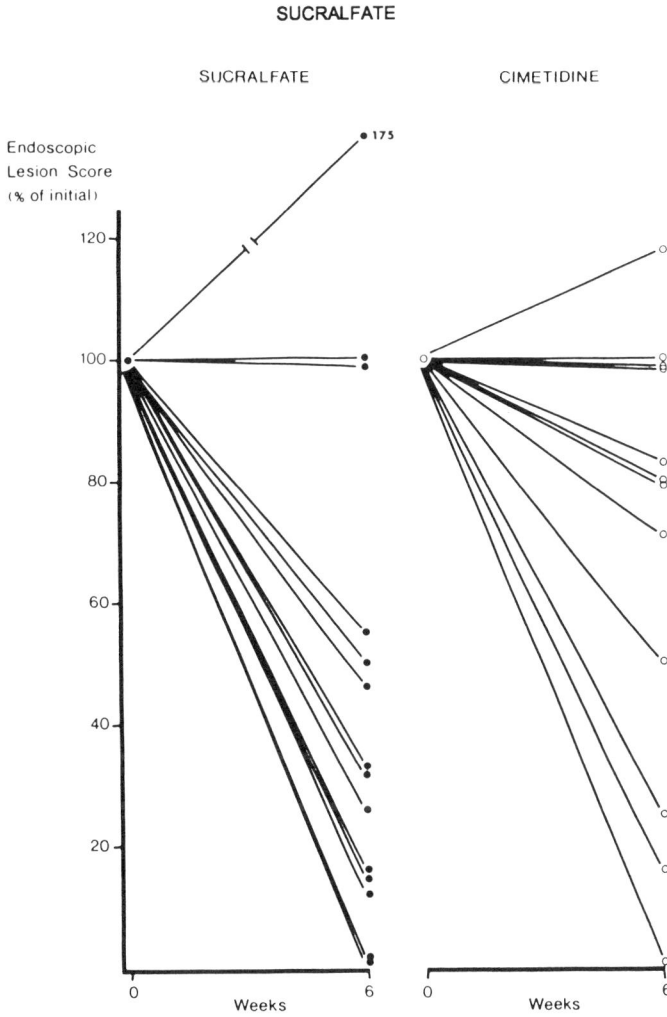

Figure 3. Results of a comparative study of sucralfate and cimetidine in 26 patients with NSAID-induced gastropathy followed for 6 months in a single-blind design. (Shepherd et al. (17))

any significant differences, either in percent ulcers healed or in time necessary to achieve complete endoscopic ulcer healing. Thus, sucralfate appeared effective in healing NSAID-related stomach ulcers.

However, other studies suggest that in those starting NSAID therapy, prophylactic cotreatment with H_2-receptor antagonists or sucralfate has minimal or no effect in preventing the development of NSAID-induced gastric ulcers, although the incidence of duodenal ulcers may be reduced

Table 3. NSAID and peptic ulcer treatment. Influence of NSAID on peptic ulcer treatment in 62 patients with rheumatic disease. No statistically significant differences between maingroups or subgroups (after Manniche et al. [19])

	Continued NSAID				Withdrawal of NSAID			
	Ratio of healed ulcers		Mean time to healing (weeks)		Ratio of healed ulcers		Mean time to healing (weeks)	
	GU	DU	GU	DU	GU	DU	GU	DU
Small ulcers (diam < 1.0 cm)	1/2 (50%)	14/15 (93%)	9.0	4.0	3/3 (100%)	12/12 (100%)	3.0	3.0
Large ulcers (diam ≥ 1.0 cm)	2/4 (50%)	6/9 (67%)	7.5	6.0	3/4 (75%)	11/13 (85%)	8.0	5.7
Subtotal	3/6 (50%)	20/24 (83%)			6/7 (86%)	23/25 (92%)		
Total: GU + DU	23/30 (77%)		5.0		29/32 (91%)		4.6	

GU = gastric ulcer; DU = duodenal ulcer

[20]. It seems difficult to visualize a rational explanation to the phenomenon that a drug may show efficiency in healing a specific lesion and at the same time demonstrate impotence in preventing it.

CONCLUSIONS AND SUGGESTIONS

In spite of contradicting reports and confusing evidence regarding the efficacy of sucralfate and its role in managing gastrointestinal complications to NSAID therapy, we believe – based on sound judgement and our clinical experience – with Tytgat [21] that the above-mentioned studies warrant an embarkation on a large-scale program evaluating the usefulness of long-term sucralfate therapy in the prevention and healing of NSAID-induced gastrointestinal mucosal damage. In particular whether such combined treatment may be instrumental in decreasing the incidence of gastric bleeding and perforation which – rather than the more innocent NSAID-induced gastropathy – are the major threats to this population of elderly rheumatic patients.

However, as it seems that much of the available literature is loaded with selection bias and retrospective data collection, the risks are too often presented exaggerated. Therefore

we suggest

a redefinition of terms: assume that **two** distinct gastrointestinal disease entities may complicate chronic rheumatic disease:

1. *NSAID-induced gastropathy* (5) characterized by signs and symptoms from the antrum: mucosal hyperaemia with petecchial lesions and erosions. If ulcers do occur, they are prepyloric and shallow, often silent, with subclinical bleeding and iron-deficiency anaemia. All in all, a benign condition mainly responsible for the upper abdominal dyspepsia complicating NSAID administration and clearly brought about by it. This syndrome is acid-unrelated. Treatment: sucralfate or misoprostol. Prevention: sucralfate.

2. *Peptic ulcer disease* linked to a preexisting disposition; in ways not fully understood its course is modified by NSAID-treatment without being caused by it. One such modifying mechanism is the muffling of ulcer pains due to the analgesic effects of the NSAIDS, explaining the common occurrence of 'silent ulcers'. It is likely to be responsible for the serious or fatal cases of gastric bleeding and perforation. It is acid-related. Treatment: H_2-receptor antagonists or omeprazole. Prevention: H_2-receptor antagonists or sucralfate.

167

To bring us any further in the management of gastrointestinal disease in chronic rheumatic patients

we need

1. Cohort studies on well-defined groups of rheumatic patients.
2. Prospectively planned data collections.
3. Identification of risk groups.
4. Clinical studies aiming towards involuntary end-points such as major bleeding; perforation; or death.
5. Proper epidemiological methods employed in assessing the occurrence and distribution of gastrointestinal signs and symptoms in groups of rheumatic patients.
6. Pharmacological studies on the side-effects of NSAIDs involving the whole gastrointestinal tract, not only the stomach.

We don't need

1. More acute studies
2. More studies on healthy persons
3. More retrospective pill-counting in surgical departments

We recommend

careful questioning of patients about to embark on a long-term NSAID treatment with a particular view to identification of the risk group with pre-existing peptic ulcer disease. Whenever possible to perform an endoscopy in an elderly rheumatic patient before starting long-term treatment with NSAIDs. To investigate GI-symptoms occurring during a (necessary) NSAID treatment with an endoscopy, before deciding to stop it. Do not start NSAID in a patient with a pre-existing ulcer; heal it first and then consider NSAID with an adjunct and planned regular endoscopic controls. When an ulcer develops during an otherwise beneficial NSAID treatment consider continuing NSAID concurrent with sucralfate if prepyloric or gastric, H_2-receptor antagonists or omeprazole if duodenal. Continue with long-term prevention with either, under endoscopic control for silent ulcers.

We conclude

'. . . the problem with non-steroidal anti-inflammatory drugs is not that they are particularly dangerous but that they are so widely used' [22].

REFERENCES

1. Hollander D, Tarnawski A, Gergely H, Zipser RD. Sucralfate protection of the gastric mucosa against ethanol-induced injury: a prostaglandin-mediated process? Scand J Gastroenterol. 1984;19(Suppl. 101):97–102.

2. Nexø E, Poulsen SS. Does epidermal growth factor play a role in the action of sucralfate. Scand J Gastroenterol. 1987;22(Suppl. 127):45–49.

3. Tarnawski A, Hollander D, Stachura J, Mach T, Bogdal J. Effect of sucralfate on the normal human gastric mucosa. Endoscopic, histological and ultrastructural assessment. Scand J Gastroenterol. 1987;22:111–123.

4. Elsborg L. Sucralfate in the treatment of reflux-esophagitis. Scand J Gastroenterol. 1987;22(Suppl. 127):101–110.

5. Roth SH. Nonsteroidal anti-inflammatory drug gastropathy. Arch Intern Med. 1986;146:1075–1076.

6. Roth SH, Bennett RE. Nonsteroidal anti-inflammatory drug gastropathy. Recognition and response. Arch Intern Med. 1987;147:2093–2099.

7. Stapleton GN, Marks IN, Fourie AJ, McLeod H, Hickman R, Mall A, Terblanche J. Sucralfate in the prevention of porcine experimental peptic ulceration. Am J Med. 1989;86(Suppl. 6A):21–22.

8. Stern AI, Ward F, Hartley G. Protective effect of sucralfate against aspirin-induced damage to the human gastric mucosa. Am J Med. 1987;83(Suppl. 3B):83–85.

9. Konturek SJ, Kwiecien N, Obtulowicz W, Oleksy J. Gastroprotection by sucralfate against acetylsalicylic acid in humans. Role of endogenous prostaglandins. Scand J Gastroenterol. 1987;22(Suppl. 140):19–22.

10. Malchow-Møller A, Ranløv PJ. Does sucralfate reduce acetylsalicylic-acid-induced gastric mucosal bleeding? Scand J Gastroenterol. 1987;22:550–552.

11. Aabakken L, Larsen S, Osnes M. Sucralfate for prevention of naproxen-induced mucosal lesions in the proximal and distal gastrointestinal tract. Scand J Rheumatol. 1989;18:361–368.

12. Stern AI, Ward F, Sievert W. Lack of gastric mucosal protection by sucralfate during long-term aspirin ingestion in humans. Am J Med. 1989;86(Suppl. 6A):66–69.

13. Tesler MA, Lim ES. Protection of gastric mucosa by sucralfate from aspirin-induced erosions. J Clin Gastroenterol. 1981;3(Suppl. 2):175–179.

14. Wu WC, Castell DO. Does sucralfate protect against aspirin induced mucosal lesions? Yes and no! (abstract). Gastroenterology. 1984;86:1303.

15. Lanza FL, Pearce K, Gustitus L, Rack MF, Dickson B. A blinded endoscopic comparative study of misoprostol versus sucralfate and placebo in the prevention of aspirin-induced gastric and duodenal ulceration. Am J Gastroenterol. 1988;83:143–146.

16. Caldwell JR, Roth SH, Wu WC, Semble EL, Castell DO, Heller MD, Marsh WH. Sucralfate treatment of nonsteroidal anti-inflammatory drug-induced gastrointestinal symptoms and mucosal damage. Am J Med. 1987;83(Suppl. 3B):74–82.

17. Shepherd HA, Fine D, Hillier K, Jewell R, Cox N. Effect of sucralfate and cimetidine on rheumatoid patients with active gastroduodenal lesions who are taking nonsteroidal anti-inflammatory drugs: a pilot study. Am J Med. 1989;86(Suppl. 6A):49–54.

18. Roth SH, Bennett RE, Mitchell CS, Hartmann RJ. Cimetidine therapy in nonsteroidal anti-inflammatory drug gastropathy. Arch Intern Med. 1987;147:1798–1801.

19. Manniche C, Malchow-Møller A, Anderson JR, Pedersen C, Hansen TM, Jess P, Helleberg L, Rasmussen SN, Tage-Jensen U, Nielsen SE. Randomised study of the influence of non-steroidal anti-inflammatory drugs on the treatment of peptic ulcer in patients with rheumatic disease. Gut. 1987;28:226–229.

20. Graham DY. Prevention of gastroduodenal injury induced by chronic nonsteroidal antiinflammatory drug therapy. Gastroenterology. 1989;96(2 Pt Suppl. 2):675–681.

21. Tytgat GNJ. Future potential applicability of sucralfate in gastroenterology. Scand J Gastroenterol. 1990;25(Suppl. 173):34–38.

22. Hawkey CJ. Non-steroidal anti-inflammatory drugs and peptic ulcers. Facts and figures multiply, but do they add up? Br Med J. 1990;300:278–284.

21

Ketotifen – a novel approach to the prevention of damage in the gastrointestinal tract

Rami Eliakim, Fanny Karmeli and Daniel Rachmilewitz
Department of Medicine, Hadassah University Hospital, Mount Scopus, Jerusalem, Israel

INTRODUCTION

Ketotifen is a benzocycloheptathrophene derivative effective in the long term management of asthma, allergic and anaphylactic reactions [1]. Ketotifen interferes with several components of the inflammatory process, including recruitment and activation of effector cells and release of mediators. Its main action in asthma is to block the production and prevent the release and/or action of inflammatory mediators, e.g. histamine, platelet activating factor (PAF), leukotrienes B4, C4 (LTB$_4$, LTC$_4$) and prostaglandin E2 (PGE$_2$) in mast cells and eosinophils [1]. Other important effects of ketotifen include inhibition of calcium influx and stabilization of the cell membrane in mast cells, increase of β_2 adrenoreceptor density, as well as cAMP levels [1].

In diseases of the gastrointestinal tract, the use of ketotifen has so far been limited and confined mainly to prevention of food allergies. Mast cells are a major source of histamine, eicosanoids and PAF in the gastrointestinal tract. Mucosal mast cells of the human stomach contain chondroitin sulphate E and, therefore, differ from connective tissue – heparin containing mast cells [2]. The two types of mast cells also differ in content as well as in response to mast cell stabilizers, e.g. disodium cromoglycate, to which mucosal mast cells are not responsive [3]. Mast cells are involved in the pathogenesis of ethanol-induced gastric mucosal injury [4]. The extent of ethanol induced gastric injury correlates with the number of activated mast cells [4]. Taking all these factors into account, it seemed logical to evaluate whether ketotifen is effective in the prevention and/or modulation of gastric mucosal damage induced by irritants such as indomethacin, 25% NaCl and 0.6 N HCl.

Side-effects of Anti-inflammatory Drugs 3. Rainsford KD, Velo GP (eds), Inflammation and Drug Therapy Series, Volume V.

Mast cells and eosinophils are also involved in induction and amplification of inflammatory processes in the intestine [5] and are found in increased numbers in the active site in inflammatory bowel disease [6–8]. On the other hand, the effects of a mast cell stabilizer, disodium cromoglycate, on patients with ulcerative colitis is controversial [9]. We tested the protective effects of ketotifen, a drug which we found to be one hundred times more effective than cromoglycate in protecting the gastric mucosa, in the modulation of two experimental models of inflammatory bowel disease – the acetic acid and the trinitrobenzene sulphonic acid (TNB) models in the rat.

METHODS

Upper gastrointestinal experiments

Methods are given in detail above [10,11]. Briefly, male rats (Hebrew University strain), 150–200 g were fasted overnight and allowed free access to water. One ml 96% ethanol was administered intragastrically (i.g.), control rats receiving 0.5% NaCl. In some experiments, either substance P $(1 \, \mu mol \, L^{-1} \, (100 \, g)^{-1})$ intraperitoneally (i.p.) or vasoactive intestinal peptide (VIP) $(10^{-7} \, mol \, L^{-1} \, (100 \, g)^{-1})$ intravenously (i.v.) were given immediately prior to or simultaneously with the 1 ml of ethanol. Rats were killed 10 minutes after ethanol administration. Other irritants used were 1 ml 0.6 N HCl or 25% NaCl, which were given i.g. or indomethacin (30 mg/kg) subcutaneously (s.c.). In the first two experiments rats were killed 60 minutes after irritant administration while in the latter, rats were killed 3 hours after administration of indomethacin. Rats were killed by cervical dislocation, the stomach washed with ice cold 0.15 mol/L NaCl and the extent of haemorrhagic erosions assessed (sq mm area involved). To evaluate the effect of irritants on inflammatory mediators, the mucosa was washed and extracted for determination of PAF, LTC_4 and LTB_4, as previously described. To evaluate the protective effects of ketotifen, it was administered i.g. (100 μg/100 g) 30 minutes prior to damage induction by the various irritants.

Experimental colitis

TNB model

Non-fasted male rats were used. Inflammation was induced by a single intracolonic administration of 0.25 ml of 50% ethanol containing 30 mg TNB, as previously described [12]. Rats were killed 24 hours and 21 days after damage induction, colons isolated and a 10 cm segment of distal colon resected, washed and weighed. Mucosal damage was assessed by the scoring system described by Wallace et al. [12] or expressed as sq mm of area involved. The mucosa was scraped and processed for determination of PGE_2, TXB_2, LTB_4, LTC_4 and myeloperoxidase (MPO) activity, as previously described [10,11].

Acetic acid model

Under light ether anaesthesia a midline incision was made, the colon isolated and the junction of the caecum-ascending colon ligated. Two ml of 5% acetic acid were injected into the lumen of the colon at its proximal part, followed by 3 ml of air, after which the midline incision was closed. Control rats were injected with 0.9% NaCl. Twenty-four hours later rats were killed, their colons removed and processed, as in the TNB model above.

In both experimental models treated rats were given ketotifen (100 µg/ 100 g) twice daily 48 hours prior to induction of damage and throughout the experiment. Data are expressed as mean $\pm$ SE. Statistical analysis for significance was performed according to the Student t test for unpaired data.

RESULTS

All the irritants tested induced significant injury to the gastric mucosa. Ketotifen almost totally prevented the mucosal damage induced by ethanol alone or in combination with substance P or VIP, as well as that induced by 0.6 N HCl, 25% NaCl or indomethacin (Table 1). In almost all instances tested, the protection provided by a single dose of ketotifen was accompanied by decreased mucosal levels of PAF, LTB_4 and LTC_4 (Table 1).

Pretreatment with ketotifen (100 µg/100 g rat) significantly decreased mucosal lesion score and lesion area both 1 and 21 days after damage induction with TNB and 24 hours after damage induction in the acetic acid model. The protective effect of ketotifen was accompanied by a significant decrease in mucosal TXB_2, LTC_4 and PGE_2 levels in the TNB model, and in MPO activity, PGE_2 and LTC_4 levels in the acetic acid model (Table 2). PAF levels in the colonic mucosa of TNB treated rats were significantly decreased one day after damage induction (11 $\pm$ 1.5 pg/10 mg) in the ketotifen protected rats as compared with controls (21 $\pm$ 4.5 pg/10 mg).

172

Table 1. Effect of ketotifen on gastric mucosal damage and mediators after various insults to the rat gastric mucosa

Treatment	No. of rats	Lesions (mm^2/rat)	PAF (pg/10 mg)	LTC_4 (ng/g)	LTB_4 (ng/g)
0.9% Saline	8	0	16.0 ± 1.0	2.8 ± 0.7	1.5 ± 0.3
96% Ethanol	11	$46 \pm 10*$	17.0 ± 2.6	$14.4 \pm 3.6*$	2.6 ± 0.3
96% Ethanol + K	5	$0**$	–	$0**$	$0.8 \pm 0.1**$
96% Ethanol + SP	13	$111 \pm 15*$	$41.0 \pm 5.0*$	$13.1 \pm 2.0*$	$3.6 \pm 0.3*$
96% Ethanol + SP + K	5	$2.4 \pm 1**$	$12.1 \pm 1.0**$	$0.9 \pm 0.4**$	$1.9 \pm 0.3**$
96% Ethanol + VIP	17	$133 \pm 26*$	–	–	$5.5 \pm 0.6*$
96% Ethanol + VIP + K	17	$2.5 \pm 2**$	–	–	$3.5 \pm 1.0**$
25% NaCl	10	$33 \pm 12*$	–	1.4 ± 0.3	$2.4 \pm 0.2*$
25% NaCl + K	12	$4.0 \pm 4**$	–	1.1 ± 0.2	$1.6 \pm 0.2**$
0.6 N HCl	5	$76 \pm 11*$	–	$8.4 \pm 1.3*$	$7.8 \pm 0.5*$
0.6 N HCl + K	5	$6 \pm 2**$	–	$1.9 \pm 0.3**$	$2.5 \pm 0.4**$
Indomethacin	5	$19 \pm 4*$	–	2.1 ± 0.3	1.2 ± 0.1
Indomethacin + K	6	$0**$	–	$0.8 \pm 0.1**$	0.8 ± 0.1

Ketotifen (K) was adminstered i.g. 30 minutes before 1.0 ml ethanol 96% with or without substance P (SP) (1 μmol^{-1} $(100 \ g)^{-1}$) or VIP (0.1 μmol^{-1} $(100 \ g)^{-1}$) i.v. and prior to IG administration of 1.0 ml 25% NaCl, 0.6 N HCl or s.c. indomethacin (30 mg/kg). In the first three sets of experiments rats were killed 10 minutes after damage induction, 1 hour after damage induction with NaCl or HCl and 3 hours after damage induction with indomethacin. The stomachs were washed, lesions were measured and mucosa obtained for PAF, LTC_4 and LTB_4 determination. Results are expressed as mean $\pm$ SE.
* = significantly different from saline treated rats, $p < 0.05$
** = significantly different from the relevant experiment without pretreatment with ketotifen, $p < 0.05$

DISCUSSION

Ketotifen, a drug mainly used for the treatment of asthma and allergic disorders, has proven its effectiveness in preventing mucosal damage in the rat stomach and colon. Ketotifen totally prevented the mucosal damage induced by ethanol and its augmentation by substance P or VIP. The same was true when indomethacin, 0.6 N HCl or 25% NaCl were used as irritants.

Mast cells are thought to be involved in the pathogenesis of ethanol induced gastric damage [4] and there appears to be a correlation between ethanol induced damage and gastric mucosal histamine levels [4]. Mucosal mast cells differ from connective tissue mast cells in their granular content and in their response to drugs [3]. Mucosal mast cells from several species do not respond to disodium cromoglycate. Along these lines, we have shown that ketotifen is one hundred times more potent than sodium cromoglycate in the prevention of gastric mucosal injury [10].

Table 2. Effect of ketotifen on lesion score and mucosal mediators in two experimental models of colitis in the rat

	AA	AA + K	TNB	TNB + K
	24 hours		3 weeks	
n	9	8	3	12
Lesion score	5.8 ± 0.6	$1.8 \pm 0.4^*$	6.2 ± 1.0	$0.8 \pm 0.1^*$
MPO ($\mu g/g$)	3.7 ± 0.7	$1.9 \pm 0.3^*$	3.0 ± 0.7	1.6 ± 0.4
TXB_2 ($\mu g/g$)	0.5 ± 0.02	0.5 ± 0.02	0.8 ± 0.1	$0.4 \pm 0.02^*$
PGE_2 (ng/g)	46.2 ± 4.1	$32.2 \pm 1.4^*$	38.7 ± 5.4	32.6 ± 1.3
LTC_4 (ng/g)	3.6 ± 0.4	$1.9 \pm 0.9^*$	11.9 ± 1.6	$2.8 \pm 0.4^*$

Rats were given ketotifen (100 μg/100 g) i.g. twice daily 48 hours prior to intracolonic administration of 0.25 ml of 50% ethanol containing 30 mg TNB or 2.0 ml of 5% acetic acid and throughout the experiment. Rats were sacrificed 1 and 21 days after induction of injury with TNB and, 24 hours after damage induction with acetic acid, the colon isolated and a 10 cm segment of the distal colon resected. The lumenal region was rinsed with ice cold saline and weighed. The mucosa were scraped and processed for MPO, TXB_2, PGE_2 and LTC_4 determination.
AA = acetic acid
* = significantly different $p < 0.05$ from TNB or acetic acid alone

Ketotifen may act by blocking the production of inflammatory mediators in mast cells and/or other inflammatory cells (e.g. histamine, PAF, eicosanoids, etc) or by blocking their action on target organs. We have shown that the reduction in mucosal damage by ketotifen was accompanied by decrease in the synthesis of these inflammatory mediators. The same is true for experimental models of inflammatory bowel disease. Ketotifen significantly decreased the mucosal damage in the models tested. Both mast cells and eosinophils, two major target cells of ketotifen activity, are found in increased numbers in the active site of inflammatory bowel diseases [6–8,13]. The damage reduction was accompanied here, too, by decreased levels of mediators in the inflamed mucosa.

In summary, we have provided information regarding a new avenue in the use of ketotifen to protect the gastrointestinal mucosa from damage induced by various irritants. The results presented herewith advocate the testing of its efficacy in the protection of the human gut. Other points to be evaluated are whether pretreatment with the drug is needed or whether it can be co-administered and, if pretreatment is needed, for how long and at what dose?

REFERENCES

1. Grant SM, Goa KL, Fitton A, Sorkin EM. Ketotifen. A review of its pharmacodynamic and pharmacokinetic properties, and therapeutic use in asthma and allergic disorders. Drugs. 1990;40:412–448.

2. Gilead L, Livni N, Eliakim R, Ligumsky M, Fich A, Okon E, Rachmilewitz D, Razin E. Human gastric mucosal mast cells are chondroitin sulphate E containing mast cells. Immunology. 1987;62:23–28.

3. Pearce FL, Befus AD, Gauldie J, Beinenstock J. Mucosal mast cells. II. Effects of anti-allergic compounds on histamine secretion by isolated intestinal mast cells. J Immunol. 1982;128:2481–2486.

4. Oates PJ, Hakkinen JP. Studies on the mechanism of ethanol induced gastric damage in rats. Gastroenterology. 1988;94:10–21.

5. Lemanske Jr RF, Atkins FM, Metcalfe DD. Gastrointestinal mast cells in health and disease, part II. J Pediatr. 1983;103:343–351.

6. Kirsner JD, Shorter RG. Recent developments in nonspecific inflammatory bowel disease. N Engl J Med. 1982;306:775–785.

7. Rao SN. Mast cells as a component of the granuloma in Crohn's disease. J Pathol. 1973;109:79–82.

8. Fox CC, Lazenby AJ, Moore WC, Yardley JH, Bayless TM, Lichtenstein LM. Enhancement of human intestinal mast cell mediator release in active ulcerative colitis. Gastroenterology. 1990;99:119–124.

9. Peppercorn MA. Advances in drug therapy for inflammatory bowel disease. Ann Intern Med. 1990;112:50–60.

10. Karmeli F, Eliakim R, Okon E, Rachmilewitz D. Gastric mucosal damage by ethanol is mediated by substance P and prevented by ketotifen, a mast cell stabilizer. Gastroenterology. 1991;100:1206–1216.

11. Eliakim R, Karmeli F, Rachmilewitz D. Ketotifen effectively prevents mucosal damage in two models of experimental colitis (abstract). Gastroenterology. 1991;100:A578.

12. Wallace JL, MacNaughton WK, Morris GP, Beck PL. Inhibition of leukotriene synthesis markedly accelerates healing in a rat model of inflammatory bowel disease. Gastroenterology. 1989;96:29–36.

13. Sarin SK, Malhotra V, Sen Gupta S, Karol A, Gaur SK, Anand BS. Significance of eosinophil and mast cell counts in rectal mucosa in ulcerative colitis. A prospective controlled study. Dig Dis Sci. 1987;32:363–367.

22

The hepatotoxicity of non-steroidal anti-inflammatory drugs

L.F. Prescott

University Department of Clinical Pharmacology, The Royal Infirmary,
Edinburgh, EH3 9YW, Scotland

INTRODUCTION

Serious liver damage is not common with the normal therapeutic use of currently available non-steroidal anti-inflammatory drugs. However, as with virtually all other drugs, liver toxicity has been reported at some time with most, if not all of these agents, and a variety of hepatic reactions have been described. Against this low but variable 'background' incidence, several drugs in this group have emerged with a more obvious profile and these seem able to produce more specific forms of liver damage under certain conditions [1–5]. It should also be remembered that hepatotoxicity was an important factor in the removal of ibufenac, sudoxicam, fenclozic acid and benoxaprofen from the market. The liver is likely to be involved in generalized hypersensitivity reactions to drugs, but this should not be interpreted as evidence that the drug in question necessarily has specific hepatotoxicity. Paradoxically, it is the salicylates and paracetamol which have the greatest potential for hepatotoxicity [2], and both are freely available without prescription in most countries. Although the mechanisms of paracetamol hepatotoxicity following overdosage are well established, very little is known of the way in which the other drugs under consideration cause liver injury.

SALICYLATES

Salicylate hepatitis was described 35 years ago by Manso and his colleagues [6] and it was discovered again in the early 1970s [7,8]. Typically, it presented as a mild dose-dependent hepatitis during the first few weeks of treatment. Most cases were reported in young females with connective tissue disorders taking doses of 50 mg kg^{-1} day^{-1} or more, but this probably reflected the selective use of high dose salicylate therapy at

Side-effects of Anti-inflammatory Drugs 3. Rainsford KD, Velo GP (eds),
Inflammation and Drug Therapy Series, Volume V.

that time [9–12]. Abnormalities of liver function are usually mild and rapidly reversible, and not infrequently the condition is asymptomatic and only discovered incidentally during routine biochemical testing. Salicylate hepatitis is usually associated with sustained plasma salicylate concentrations above 250 mg/L, but it may occur at lower levels [11]. Histological examination of the liver usually shows patchy necrosis with variable portal and parenchymal inflammatory cell infiltration [9,10]. A picture resembling chronic active hepatitis has also been described [13]. The incidence of symptomatic salicylate hepatitis is not known, but abnormal elevation of plasma transaminases has been observed in 50–60% of patients taking full anti-inflammatory doses of aspirin [3,11].

Rarely, liver damage may be more severe with hepatic failure, encephalopathy and a profound metabolic disturbance with acidosis and hypoglycaemia. In such circumstances, the outcome may be fatal and the condition may be indistinguishable from Reye's syndrome [14–19]. Most of these serious reactions have occurred in children but cases have been reported in adults [20–22]. The association between the use of aspirin and Reye's syndrome has been established beyond any reasonable doubt and the incidence of this condition has declined greatly as the indiscriminate and unnecessary use of aspirin in young children has been curtailed [23,24].

PARACETAMOL

Although normally very safe when used properly, paracetamol can cause acute hepatic necrosis when taken in overdosage [25–27]. In many areas, paracetamol has become the most popular non-prescription analgesic, and as a result, it is frequently used for self-poisoning. The usual single adult threshold dose of paracetamol which must be taken to produce severe liver damage (plasma aminotransferase activity 1000 units/L or more) is 150–250 mg/kg and this corresponds to plasma concentrations above 200 mg/L at 4 hours after ingestion. Without specific antidotal therapy, about 10% of adults referred to hospital with paracetamol poisoning develop severe liver damage and 1–2% die several days later with acute liver failure [27]. Paracetamol poisoning is less of a problem in young children. Not only are they less susceptible than adults to the acute toxicity of paracetamol, but they rarely take enough to be at great risk [28].

In patients with moderate to severe liver damage following paracetamol overdosage there is a dramatic increase in plasma aminotransferase activity to 10,000 units/L or greater with a more modest rise in the plasma bilirubin concentration and prothrombin time ratio. Serial estimations of the latter probably provide the best guide to prognosis in patients with severe liver injury [29]. The maximum abnormality of liver function tests is delayed at least until the third day, after which time there is usually rapid recovery in survivors with return of liver function tests to normal in 1–3 weeks. Other biochemical abnormalities include hypophosphataemia with phosphaturia [30] and an initial metabolic acidosis in severely poisoned patients [31]. Delayed haematological abnormalities include thrombocytopenia which in some cases may be due to disseminated intravascular coagulation. Histological examination of the liver shows extensive centrilobular hepatic necrosis with no inflammatory reaction [32].

Paracetamol causes acute liver damage through its conversion by hepatic mixed function oxidase to N-acetylbenzoquinoneimine, a highly reactive intermediate metabolite. Following a therapeutic dose, this metabolite is normally inactivated by conjugation with glutathione and excreted in the urine as cysteine and mercapturic acid conjugates. Following overdosage however, hepatic glutathione is depleted and the reactive metabolite is free to bind covalently to liver cells and this initiates a train of events which results in irreversible injury and necrosis of hepatocytes [33,34]. The critical sites of injury are SH-containing translocases of the cell membrane which control calcium homeostasis [35,36] and intracellular calcium appears to be directly involved in the toxicity of paracetamol [37]. Elucidation of the mechanisms of paracetamol toxicity led to the introduction of N-acetylcysteine and methionine as effective antidotes for paracetamol poisoning [38–40]. Intravenous N-acetylcysteine is the preferred treatment and both agents must be given within 8–10 hours after the paracetamol is taken as efficacy declines rapidly after this time. Recent studies suggest that late treatment up to 24 hours is safe and may confer some benefit [41–42]. N-acetylcysteine protects against paracetamol hepatotoxicity primarily by facilitating glutathione synthesis [43] but it can probably also reverse post-arylation inactivation of the SH-containing enzymes of the plasma membrane [44].

Over the years there have been numerous anecdotal reports claiming that severe and sometimes fatal liver damage may occur during the therapeutic use of paracetamol, particularly in chronic alcoholics. However, a review of these cases reveals that in most, excessive doses were taken while in others there was incidental disease or exposure to other drugs and solvents [2]. Further similar cases have been reported, and again, most have involved chronic alcoholics [45–52]. Chronic alcoholics probably are at increased risk of paracetamol hepatotoxicity but most investigators have uncritically attributed this to increased production of toxic metabolite as a result of microsomal enzyme induction. While chronic administration of ethanol may stimulate the metabolic activation of paracetamol in animals, there is no evidence that it does so in man [53] and the increased susceptibility of alcoholics can be explained rather by their reduced capacity for glutathione synthesis [54]. The maximum single adult therapeutic dose of paracetamol is 1.0 g and this may be repeated 4–6 hourly up to a maximum of 4 g in 24 hours. While a dose of 1.0 g is clearly insufficient to generate enough toxic metabolite to deplete hepatic glutathione and cause liver damage, problems could arise when excessive doses are taken repeatedly.

Hepatitis and jaundice are recognized features of measles in young adults [55], and in a recent study 56% of 118 patients had abnormal liver function tests and 5% were jaundiced. Some 60% of these patients who were treated for pyrexia with paracetamol had elevated plasma aminotransferase activity compared with 15% of those treated with dipyrone [56], and severe hepatotoxicity in children has again been attributed to repeated gross therapeutic overdosing with paracetamol [57].

PHENYLBUTAZONE

Phenylbutazone is the oldest established non-steroidal anti-inflammatory drug and there have been many reports of liver injury associated with its use [1,58]. Phenylbutazone hepatotoxicity usually becomes apparent during the first few weeks of treatment with anorexia, nausea, vomiting, abdominal pain and progressive jaundice. Biochemical abnormalities of liver function include increased plasma aminotransferase and alkaline phosphatase activity and increased bilirubin concentrations. The histological appearances of the liver are usually those of a toxic hepatitis with diffuse or focal hepatic necrosis, a variable inflammatory reaction, prominent cholestasis, and in some cases, granuloma formation [58]. Although recovery is the rule on discontinuation of the drug, fatalities have been recorded [59–61]. Acute hepatic injury with a delayed onset of jaundice is a consistent finding in severe phenylbutazone poisoning [62–64].

Azapropazone is related to phenylbutazone, and a case of reversible liver damage has been reported in association with erythema multiforme after treatment with this drug for 2 weeks. A liver biopsy showed a mild non-specific hepatitis with cholestasis and granulomas [65].

PIROXICAM

There have been several reports of liver damage associated with piroxicam therapy in recent years but this is probably a consequence of its extensive use in some countries. In some cases the liver has been involved in a multisystem reaction [66], while in others the evidence points to more specific hepatotoxicity of piroxicam, although this must be a rare event [67,68]. Liver biopsies have shown subacute hepatitis with cholestasis [68,69]. Fatal submassive hepatic necrosis occurred in a 64-year old woman who developed acute hepatitis after taking 40 mg of piroxicam daily for 3 weeks [70] and piroxicam poisoning in a young child resulted in severe multisystem toxicity with acute liver damage [71].

SULINDAC

There have been many reports of liver damage following the use of sulindac and it seems to have a clear potential for hepatotoxicity [72–82]. The onset usually occurs within a few days or weeks of starting treatment and is characterized by malaise, nausea, vomiting, vague abdominal pain and jaundice with disordered liver function tests. Liver biopsies have shown a variable picture with necrosis of hepatocytes, cholestasis and portal inflammation [1]. Sulindac hepatitis is usually reversible but liver damage may be severe [72,79,82] and a fatal outcome has been reported [78].

CLOMETACIN

This drug is related to indomethacin and it also seems to carry a small but definite risk of liver toxicity. A considerable number of cases, some with fatalities, have been reported from France and these have shown an atypical pattern of toxicity with a syndrome resembling aggressive chronic hepatitis developing after the drug has been taken for a period of months. Liver damage may be persistent with possible progression to cirrhosis [83–92] and the development of primary biliary cirrhosis has been attributed to treatment with clometacin [93]. In a retrospective study of 30 cases of clometacin hepatitis seen over 9 years, most were females and the mean duration of treatment with the drug was 445 days. Clinical features included jaundice, anorexia, weight loss, oedema, ascites, renal impairment and thrombocytopenia. The histological appearances of liver biopsies in 25 patients showed acute hepatitis in 8 and chronic active hepatitis in 17 including 6 with cirrhosis. Hepatitis was directly responsible for the death of 3 patients. Clometacin was proposed as a model for drug-induced autoimmune liver disease [92].

PIRPROFEN

Attention has been drawn previously to the possible hepatotoxicity of pirprofen [2]. There has been a further report of fatal liver injury in a 71-year old man who developed anorexia, confusion and jaundice some 2 months after being given pirprofen 800 mg daily. He died a week after admission to hospital and a post-mortem examination revealed a shrunken, yellow liver with massive necrosis [94].

180

DICLOFENAC

There have been many reports of liver damage following the use of diclofenac, and this drug must be considered to be potentially hepatotoxic. Typically, malaise, anorexia, vomiting, abdominal discomfort and jaundice develop during the first few weeks of treatment and there is considerable disturbance of liver function tests. Examination of liver biopsies and post-mortem specimens has shown hepatocellular damage, portal inflammation and cholestasis [95–104]. In some cases hepatotoxicity has been associated with rashes and nephrotoxicity [102,103], and chronic hepatitis has also been described [104]. In one unit, 5 cases of diclofenac hepatitis were encountered in one year [100].

DIAGNOSIS AND INCIDENCE

The incidence of significant hepatotoxicity caused by non-steroidal anti-inflammatory drugs in unknown. Most reports have involved middle-aged and elderly females, but this is to be expected on the basis of the use of these drugs in the population. There is often considerable difficulty in establishing a cause and effect relationship between hepatic pathology and the use of a drug, and the position is invariably complicated by polypharmacy and underlying or incidental diseases such as systemic lupus erythematosus, infectious hepatitis and alcoholism. In any such assessment, a number of factors must be considered, including dose-toxicity relationships, the time course of the reaction in relation to exposure to the drug and recovery after the drug is discontinued. Diagnosis may be easier if the clinical presentation is typical and the case is strengthened by a plausible mechanism of toxicity and the detection of liver injury during preclinical toxicity studies. Challenge tests are not recommended, but it is not uncommon for an offending drug to be unwittingly (or witlessly) prescribed again with recurrence of the hepatic reaction.

The rank order of the non-steroidal anti-inflammatory drugs for potential hepatotoxicity is unknown and impressions gained from literature reports can be misleading. Some limited information can be obtained from spontaneous reporting of adverse drug reactions to Drug Regulatory Agencies such as the Yellow Card system of the Committee on Safety of Medicines in the United Kingdom. Such data must be assessed with great caution as there are many shortcomings. The number of events should be set against the number of patients at risk but unfortunately the essential information on prescribing rates is not available. In addition, notification is incomplete and subject to bias. Thus reporting rates are very low, especially from hospital medical staff and the rates are much higher for new than for old established drugs, and are increased by publicity.

Many of these problems can be minimised by comparing the number of reports of liver toxicity with the total number of reports for each drug (Figure 1). Although still liable to bias, this shows that hepatotoxicity accounts for only a small fraction of the total reports for most of the non-steroidal anti-inflammatory drugs but that this proportion is apparently substantially increased for phenylbutazone, fenbufen, diclofenac and sulindac (Committee on Safety of Medicines, personal communication). With the exception of fenbufen, this result corresponds exactly with the incidence as indicated by the number of reports of hepatotoxicity in the literature [2,3].

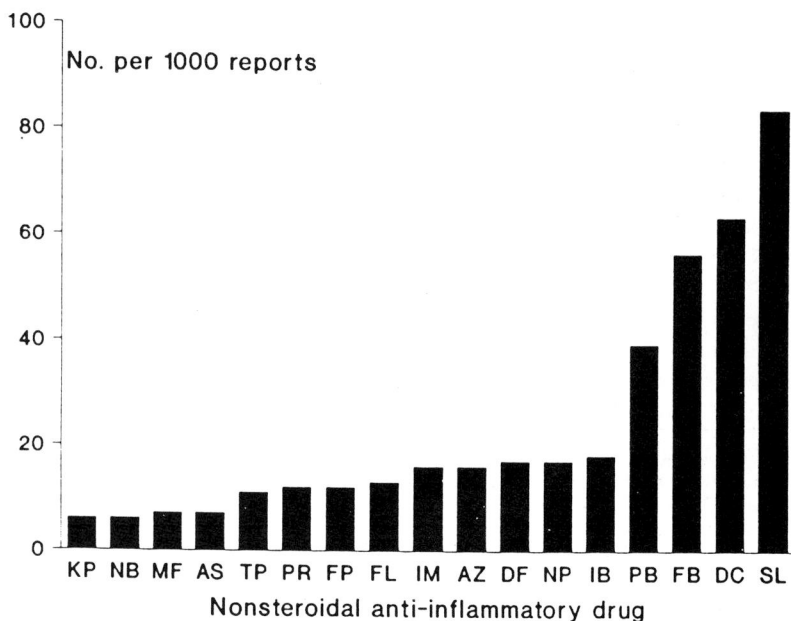

Figure 1. Number of reports relating to hepatotoxicity made to the British Committee on Safety of Medicines for non-steroidal anti-inflammatory drugs from their introduction up to July 1990. The numbers are expressed as a rate per 1000 reports of all reactions involving each drug. The total number of reports is given in brackets after the key for each drug: KP = ketoprofen (1607), NB = nabumetone (1152), MF = mefenamic acid (1574), AS = aspirin (891), TP = tiaprofenic acid (995), PR = piroxicam (3558), FP = fenoprofen (512), FL = flurbiprofen (1318), IM = indomethacin (3842), AZ = azapropazone (621), DF = diflunisal (965), NP = naproxen (2898), IB = ibuprofen (2522), PB = phenylbutazone (1636), FB = fenbufen (720), DC = diclofenac (2777), SL = sulindac (642)

182

CONCLUSION

Hepatotoxicity is not a common problem with the normal use of currently available non-steroidal anti-inflammatory drugs but there are considerable difficulties with diagnosis and confirmation of a causal relationship. The greatest risk appears to be with salicylates and paracetamol. However, there is no indication now for prolonged high dose salicylate therapy and paracetamol is unlikely to cause liver damage unless it is taken in overdosage. Of the other drugs, phenylbutazone, clometacin, pirprofen, diclofenac and sulindac may be identified as carrying an increased risk of hepatotoxicity, but the risk is small and should not be sufficient in itself to restrict their use.

REFERENCES

1. Zimmerman HJ, Lewis JH. Drug-induced cholestasis. Med Toxicol Adverse Drug Experience. 1987;2:112–160.
2. Prescott LF. Liver damage with non-narcotic analgesics. Med Toxicol. 1986;1:44–56.
3. Tolman KG. Hepatotoxicity of antirheumatic drugs. J Rheumatol. 1990;17:(Suppl. 22):6–11.
4. Doube A. Hepatitis and non-steroidal anti-inflammatory drugs. Ann Rheum Dis. 1990;49:489–490.
5. Velo GP, Milanino R. Nongastrointestinal adverse reactions to NSAID. J Rheumatol. 1990;17(Suppl. 20):42–45.
6. Manso C, Taranta A, Mydick I. Effect of aspirin administration on serum glutamic oxaloacetic and glutamic pyruvic transaminases in children. Proc Soc Exper Biol Med. 1956;93:84–88.
7. Russell AS, Sturge RA, Smith MA. Serum transaminases during salicylate therapy. Br Med J. 1971;2:428–429.
8. Rich RR, Johnson JS. Salicylate hepatotoxicity in patients with juvenile rheumatoid arthritis. Arthritis Rheum. 1973;16:1–9.
9. Saltzman DA, Gall EP, Robinson SF. Aspirin-induced hepatic dysfunction in a patient with adult rheumatoid arthritis. Dig Dis Sci. 1976;21:815–820.
10. Wolf JD, Metzger AL, Goldstein RC. Aspirin hepatitis. Arch Intern Med. 1974;80:74–76.
11. Bernstein BH, Singsen BH, King KK, Hanson V. Aspirin-induced hepatotoxicity and its effect on juvenile rheumatoid arthritis. Am J Dis Child. 1977;131:659–663.
12. Hamdan JA, Manasra K, Ahmed M. Salicylate-induced hepatitis in rheumatic fever. Am J Dis Child. 1985;139:453–455.
13. Seaman WE, Ishak KG, Plotz PH. Aspirin-induced hepatotoxicity in patients with systemic lupus erythematosus. Ann Intern Med. 1974;80:1–8.
14. Petty BG, Zahka KG, Bernstein MT. Aspirin hepatitis associated with encephalopathy. J Pediatr. 1978;93:881-882
15. Mäkelä A-L, Lang H, Korpela P. Toxic encephalopathy with hyperammonaemia during high-dose salicylate therapy. Acta Neurol Scand. 1980;61:146–156.
16. Ulshen MH, Grand RJ, Crain JD, Gelfand EW. Hepatotoxicity with encephalopathy associated with aspirin therapy in rheumatoid arthritis. J Pediatr. 1978;93:1034–1037.
17. Christoffersen F, Faarup P, Geertinger P, Krogh P. Reye's syndrome in a child on long-term salicylate medication. Forensic Sci Intern. 1980;15:129–133.
18. Sillanpää M, Mäkelä AL, Koivikko A. Acute liver failure and encephalopathy (Reye's syndrome?) during salicylate therapy. Acta Paediatr Scand. 1975;64:877–880.
19. Young RSK, Torretti D, Williams RH, Hendriksen D, Woods M. Reye's syndrome associated with long-term aspirin therapy. J Am Med Assoc. 1984;251:754–756.

20. Stillman A, Gitter H, Shillington D, Sobonya R, Payne CM, Ettinger D, Lee SM. Reye's syndrome in the adult: case report and review of the literature. Am J Gastroenterol. 1983;78:365–368.
21. Tumiati B, Azzalito C, Veneziani M. Reye's syndrome in an adult following therapy with salicylates in Still's disease. Medicina. 1989;9:64–65.
22. Jolliet P, Widmann J-J. Reye's syndrome in adult with AIDS. Lancet. 1990;335:1467.
23. Pinsky PF, Hurwitz ES, Schonberger LB, Gunn WJ. Reye's syndrome and aspirin. Evidence for a dose-response effect. J Am Med Assoc. 1988;260:657–661.
24. Porter JDH, Robinson PH, Glasgow JFT, Banks JH, Hall SM. Trends in the incidence of Reye's syndrome and the use of aspirin. Arch Dis Child. 1990;65:826–829.
25. Davidson DGD, Eastham WN. Acute liver necrosis following overdose of paracetamol. Br Med J. 1966;2:497–499.
26. Proudfoot AT, Wright N. Acute paracetamol poisoning. Br Med J. 1970;4:557–558.
27. Prescott LF. Paracetamol overdosage: pharmacological considerations and clinical management. Drugs. 1983;25:290–314.
28. Rumack BH. Acetaminophen overdose in children and adolescents. Pediatr Clin N Am. 1986;33:691–701.
29. Harrison PM, O'Grady JG, Keays RT, Alexander GJM, Williams R. Serial prothrombin time as prognostic indicator in paracetamol induced fulminant hepatic failure. Br Med J. 1990;301:964–966.
30. Jones AF, Harvey JM, Vale JA. Hypophosphataemia and phosphaturia in paracetamol poisoning. Lancet. 1989;2:608–609.
31. Flanagan RJ, Mant TGK. Coma and metabolic acidosis early in severe acute paracetamol poisoning. Human Toxicol. 1986;5:256–259.
32. Portmann B, Talbot IC, Day DW, Davidson AR, Murray-Lyon IM, Williams R. Histopathological changes in the liver following a paracetamol overdosage: correlation with clinical and biochemical parameters. J Pathol. 1975;117:169–181.
33. Mitchell JR, Thorgeirsson SS, Potter WZ, Jollow DJ, Keiser H. Acetaminophen-induced hepatic injury: protective role of glutathione in man and rationale for therapy. Clin Pharmacol Ther. 1974;16:676–684.
34. Corcoran GB, Mitchell JR, Vaishnav YN, Horning EC. Evidence that acetaminophen and N-hydroxyacetaminophen form a common arylating intermediate, N-acetyl-p-benzoquino-neimine. Mol Pharmacol. 1980;18:536–542.
35. Mitchell JR. Acetaminophen toxicity. N Engl J Med. 1988;319:1601–1602.
36. Tsokos-Kuhn JO, Hugh H, Smith CV, Mitchell JR. Alkyation of the liver plasma membrane and inhibition of the Ca^{2+}-ATPase by acetaminophen. Biochem Pharmacol. 1988;37:2125–2131.
37. Boobis AR, Seddon CE, Nasseri-Sina P, Davies DS. Evidence for a direct role of intracellular calcium in paracetamol toxicity. Biochem Pharmacol. 1990;39:1277–1281.
38. Prescott LF, Illingworth RN, Critchley JAJH, Stewart MJ, Adam RD, Proudfoot AT. Intravenous N-acetylcysteine: treatment of choice for paracetamol poisoning. Br Med J. 1979;2:1097–1100.
39. Vale JA, Meredith TJ, Goulding R. Treatment of acetaminophen poisoning: the use of oral methionine. Arch Intern Med. 1981;141:394–396.
40. Smilkstein MJ, Knapp GL, Kulig KW, Rumack BH. Efficacy of oral N-acetylcysteine in the treatment of acetaminophen overdose. N Engl J Med. 1988;319:1557–1562.
41. Parker D, White JP, Paton D, Routledge PA. Safety of late acetylcysteine treatment in paracetamol poisoning. Human Exp Toxicol. 1990;9:25–27.
42. Harrison PM, Keays R, Bray GP, Alexander GJM, Williams R. Improved outcome of paracetamol-induced fulminant hepatic failure by late administration of acetylcysteine. Lancet. 1990;335:1572–1573.
43. Lauterburg BH, Corcoran GB, Mitchell JR. Mechanism of action of N-acetylcysteine in the protection against hepatotoxicity of acetaminophen in rats in vivo. J Clin Invest. 1983;71:980–991.
44. Tee LBG, Boobis AR, Huggett AC, Davies DS. Reversal of acetaminophen toxicity in isolated hamster hepatocytes by dithiothreitol. Toxicol Appl Pharmacol. 1986;83:294–314.

45. Wootton FT, Lee WM. Acetaminophen hepatotoxicity in the alcoholics. South Med J. 1990;83:1047–1049.
46. Florén C-H, Thesleff P, Nilsson A. Severe liver damage caused by therapeutic doses of acetaminophen. Acta Med Scand. 1987;222:285–288.
47. Roseau G. Hépatotoxicité du paracétamol chez l'alcoolique par déficit en glutathion. Presse Méd. 1989;18:510.
48. Foust RT, Reddy KR, Jeffers LJ, Schiff ER. Nyquil-associated liver injury. Am J Gastroenterol. 1989;84:422–425.
49. Maddrey WC. Hepatic effects of acetaminophen. Enhanced toxicity in alcoholics. J Clin Gastroenterol. 1987;9:180–185.
50. Denison H, Kaczynski J, Wallerstedt S. Paracetamol medication and alcohol abuse: a dangerous combination for the liver and kidney. Scand J Gastroenterol. 1987;22:701–704.
51. Bell H, Raknerud N. Alvorlig leverskade – etter terapeutisk dose av paracetamol. Tidsskr Nor Laegeforen. 1987;107:1037–1040.
52. Bidault I, Lagier G, Garnier R, Pallot JL, Larrey D. Les hépatites par toxicité subaigu du paracétamol existent-elles? Thérapie. 1987;42:387–388.
53. Prescott LF, Critchley JAJH. Drug interactions affecting analgesic toxicity. Am J Med. 1983;75(5A):113–116.
54. Lauterburg BH, Velez ME. Glutathione deficiency in alcoholics: risk factor for paracetamol hepatotoxicity. Gut. 1988;29:1153–1157.
55. Gavish D, Kleinman Y, Morag A, Chajek-Sharl T. Hepatitis and jaundice associated with measles in young adults. Arch Intern Med. 1983;143:674–677.
56. Ackerman Z, Flugelman MY, Wax Y, Shouval D, Levy M. Hepatitis during measles in young adults: possible role of antipyretic drugs. Hepatology. 1989;10:203–206.
57. Henretig FM, Selbst SM, Forrest C, Kearney TK, Orel H, Werner S, Williams TA. Repeated acetaminophen overdosing causing hepatotoxicity in children. Clin Pediatr. 1989;28:525–528.
58. Benjamin SB, Ishak KG, Zimmerman HJ, Gruska A. Phenylbutazone liver injury: a clinico-pathologic survey of 23 cases and review of the literature. Hepatology. 1981;1:255–263.
59. Catterall RD. Fatal reaction to phenylbutazone in a patient with Reiter's disease. Br J Ven Dis. 1968;44:151–153.
60. Fisher JH. Fatal phenylbutazone hepatitis. Can Med Assoc J. 1960;83:1211–1212.
61. Muscat-Baron JM, Freeman DM. Toxic hepatitis following phenylbutazone therapy. Br J Clin Pract. 1966;20:437–439.
62. Berlinger WG, Spector R, Flanigan MJ, Johnson GF, Groh MR. Hemoperfusion for phenylbutazone poisoning. Ann Intern Med. 1982;96:334–335.
63. Prescott LF, Critchley JAJH, Balali-Mood M. Phenylbutazone overdosage: abnormal metabolism associated with hepatic and renal damage. Br Med J. 1980;281:1106–1107.
64. Strong JE, Wilson J, Douglas JF, Coppel DL. Phenylbutazone self-poisoning treated by charcoal haemoperfusion. Anaesthesia. 1979;34:1038–1040.
65. Lo TCN, Dymock IW. Azapropazone-induced hepatitis. Br Med J. 1988;297:1614.
66. Allier I, Luquel L, Prier A, Offenstadt G. Acute haemolytic anaemia and hepatonephritis due to piroxicam. Thérapie. 1988;48:504.
67. Lee SM, Williams R. Subacute hepatic necrosis induced by piroxicam. Br Med J. 1984;293:540–541.
68. Caballeria E, Masso RM, Arago JV, Sanchis A. Piroxicam hepatotoxicity. Am J Gastroenterol. 1990;85:898–899.
69. Mitnick PD, Klein WJ. Piroxicam-induced renal disease. Arch Intern Med. 1984;144:63–64.
70. Planas R, De Léon R, Quer JC, Barranco C, Bruguera M, Gassull MA. Fatal submassive necrosis of the liver associated with piroxicam. Am J Gastroenterol. 1990;85:468–470.
71. MacDougal LG, Taylor-Smith A, Rothberg AD, Thomson PD. Piroxicam poisoning in a 2-year-old child. S Afr Med J. 1984;66:31–33.
72. Anderson RJ. Severe reaction associated with sulindac administration. N Engl J Med. 1979;300:735–736.
73. Dhand AK, La Breque DR, Metzger J. Sulindac (clinoril) hepatitis. Gastroenterology. 1981;80:585–586.

74. Giroux Y, Moreau M, Kass TG. Cholestatic jaundice caused by sulindac. Can J Surg. 1982;25:334-335.
75. Kaul A, Reddy JC, Fayman E, Smith GF. Hepatitis associated with the use of sulindac in a child. J Pediatr. 1981;99:650–651.
76. Klein SM, Khan MA. Hepatitis, toxic epidermal necrolysis and pancreatitis in association with sulindac therapy. J Rheumatol. 1983;10:512–513.
77. MacIndoe GAJ, Menzies KW, Reddy J. Sulindac (clinoril) and cholestatic jaundice. N Z Med J. 1981;94:430–431.
78. Park GD, Spector R, Headstream T, Goldberg M. Serious adverse reactions associated with sulindac. Arch Intern Med. 1982;142:1292–1294.
79. Smith FE, Lindberg PJ. Life threatening hypersensitivity to sulindac. J Am Med Assoc. 1980;244:269–270.
80. Whittaker SJ, Amar JN, Wanless IR, Heathcote J. Sulindac hepatotoxicity. Gut. 1982;23:875–877.
81. Wolfe PB. Sulindac and jaundice. Arch Intern Med. 1979;91:656.
82. Daniele B, Pignata S, D'Agostino L, Vecchione R, Mazzacca G. Sulindac-induced severe hepatitis. Am J Gastroenterol. 1988;83:1429–1431.
83. Goldfarb G, Pessayre D, Boisseau C, Degott C, Beraud C, Benhamou J-P. Hépatite à la clométacine. Gastroenterol Clin Biol. 1979;3:537–540.
84. Lenoir C, Lababyle D, Buffet C, Lauriat H, Blanchon P, Etienne J-P. Hépatite au clométacine. Nouv Presse Méd. 1978;7:3035–3036.
85. Mamou P, Levy VG. Atteintes hépatiques après clométacine. 6 cas dont 2 mortels. Nouv Presse Méd. 1981;10:2719–2722.
86. Manigand G, Pointud P, Taillandier J, Martin E, Bard H, Benoist J. Hépatite à la clométacine. Nouv Presse Méd. 1979;8:213.
87. Poitrine A, Poynard T, Naveu S, Hilpert G, Chapeut JC. Clometacine-induced hepatitis: a fatal crisis. Gastroenterol Clin Biol. 1983;7:99.
88. Spreux A, Larousse C. Hepatites survenant au cours d'un traitment par la clométacin. Thérapie. 1981;36:293–297.
89. Tassou J-J, Bretagne J-F, Marion J. Hépatite à la clométacine. Concours Méd. 1981;103:679–683.
90. Seigneuric C, Oksman F, Tkaczuk J, Plantavid M, Damoran J, Lala JL. Hépatite et thrombopénie autoimmune au cours d'un traitment par la clométacine. Nouv Presse Méd. 1983;12:106–107.
91. Parini M, Benevent D, Leroux-Robert C. Insuffisance rénale aigue et hépatite lors d'un traitment par clométacine. Nouv Presse Méd. 1982;11:2641.
92. Pariente EA, Hamoud A, Goldfain D, Latrive JP, Gislon J, Cassan P, Morin T, Staub JL, Ramain JP, Bertrand JL. Hépatites a la clométacine (Dupéran). Étude retrospective de 30 cas. Un modele d'hépatite autoimmune médicamenteuse? Gastroenterol Clin Biol. 1989;13:769–774.
93. Andrieu J, Doll J, Gardon JD, Ramaud S. Clometacin-induced hepatitis and primary biliary cirrhosis. Ann Gastroenterol d'Hepatol. 1989;25:259–260.
94. Depla ACTM, Vermeersch PHMJ, Van Gorp LHM, Nadorp JHSM. Fatal acute liver damage associated with pirprofen. Report of a case and review of the literature. Neth J Med. 1990;37:32–36.
95. Babany G, Bernuau J, Danan G, Rueff B, Benhamou J-P. Hépatite fulminante chez une femme prenant de la glafénine et du diclofénac. Gastroenterol Clin Biol. 1985;9:185.
96. Deshayes P, Leloet X, Bercoff E, Fouin-Fortunet H. Hépatite au diclofénac. Nouv Presse Méd. 1984;13:1847.
97. Dunk AA, Walt RP, Jenkins WJ, Sherlock SS. Diclofenac hepatitis. Br Med J. 1982;284:1605–1606.
98. Lascar G, Grippon P, Levy VG. Hépatite aigue mortelle au cours d'un traitment par le diclofénac (Voltarène). Gastroenterol Clin Biol. 1984;8:881–882.
99. Helfgott SM, Sandberg-Cook J, Zakim D, Nestler J. Diclofenac-associated hepatotoxicity. J Am Med Assoc. 1990;264:2660–2662.

100. Iveson TJ, Ryley NG, Kelley PMA, Trowel JM, McGee JO'D, Chapman RW. Diclofenac associated hepatitis. J Hepatol. 1990;10:85–89.
101. Sallie R. Diclofenac hepatitis. J Hepatol. 1990;11:281.
102. Diggory P, Golding RL, Lancaster R. Renal and hepatic impairment in association with diclofenac administration. Postgrad Med J. 1989;65:507–508.
103. Hovette Ph, Touze JE, Debonne JM, Delmare B, Rogier C, Schmoor P, Aubry P. Hépatite cholestatique et insuffisance rénale aigue au cours d'un traitment par diclofénac. Ann Gastroenterol d'Hepatol. 1990;25:257–258.
104. Mazeika PK, Ford MJ. Chronic acute hepatitis associated with diclofenac sodium therapy. Br J Clin Prac. 1989;43:125–126.

23

Paracetamol (acetaminophen) bioactivation by liver microsomes – its role in hepatotoxicity

Chifumi Sato and Fumiaki Marumo
Division of Health Science and Second Department of Internal
Medicine, Faculty of Medicine, Tokyo Medical and Dental University,
Tokyo, Japan

INTRODUCTION

Paracetamol (acetaminophen) produces severe hepatic injury in man [1,2] when taken in large doses mostly for suicidal purposes. In recent years, paracetamol-induced hepatic injury is one of the most frequent causes of fulminant hepatic failure in European countries and has drawn much interest from clinicians. Paracetamol in therapeutic doses is believed to be safe and is frequently prescribed instead of aspirin which causes various adverse effects. Clinical observations, however, have suggested that chronic alcoholics are susceptible to paracetamol hepatotoxicity [3,4] and relatively small doses of paracetamol such as 3 g produce hepatic injury in those patients.

These hepatotoxic effects of paracetamol can be reproduced in experimental animals [5] and mechanisms of the effects have been extensively studied [6,7].

MECHANISMS OF PARACETAMOL HEPATOTOXICITY

Paracetamol is mainly metabolized by glucuronidation and sulphation, and the metabolites are excreted into the urine. A small proportion of the paracetamol is metabolized by the cytochrome P-450-mediated drug oxidizing system (mixed function oxidases) (Figure 1). A reconstituted system containing NADPH-cytochrome P-450 reductase, cytochrome P-450, and phospholipid has been shown to activate paracetamol to a reactive metabolite [8]. A resulting metabolite, supposedly N-acetyl-p-benzoquinoneimine [9], is highly reactive in binding covalently to cellular

Side-effects of Anti-inflammatory Drugs 3. Rainsford KD, Velo GP (eds),
Inflammation and Drug Therapy Series, Volume V.

macromolecules and the amount of the covalent binding correlates well with the hepatotoxicity of paracetamol. In the presence of glutathione, however, the reactive metabolite is detoxified by binding with glutathione. Covalent binding occurs only after depletion of hepatic glutathione. Taking these findings into account, paracetamol hepatotoxicity could be modified in four ways.

Firstly, induction or depression of mixed function oxidases results in the potentiation or attenuation, respectively, of paracetamol hepatotoxicity. For example, 3-methylcholanthrene pretreatment [10] or chronic ethanol administration [11] induces mixed function oxidases and markedly increases paracetamol hepatotoxicity. In fact, recent studies have revealed that ethanol-inducible subspecies of cytochrome P-450 (cytochrome P-450 IIE1) and 3-methylcholanthrene-inducible cytochrome P-450 (cytochrome P-450 IA2) are most active in paracetamol activation [12]. On the other hand, cobaltous chloride pretreatment diminishes mixed function oxidases resulting in the attenuation of paracetamol hepatotoxicity [10].

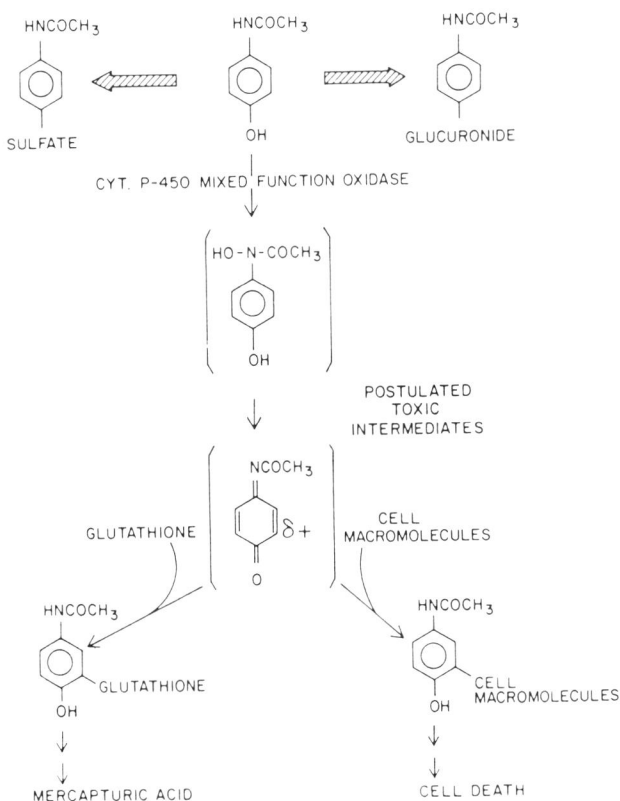

Figure 1. Metabolic disposition of paracetamol (acetaminophen)

Secondly, paracetamol hepatotoxicity could be decreased in the presence of compounds which inhibit mixed function oxidases. This type of inhibition has been reported in piperonyl butoxide [10] and cimetidine [13]. Surprisingly, caffeine potentiates paracetamol hepatotoxicity in the rat [14] although its inhibitory effect has been reported in the mouse [15]. The former effect of caffeine is associated with an increased production of the reactive metabolite.

Thirdly, manoeuvres which decrease hepatic glutathione content potentiate paracetamol hepatotoxicity, and vice versa. For instance, fasting [16] or diethyl maleate pretreatment [17] enhances paracetamol hepatotoxicity by decreasing hepatic glutathione. In contrast, administration of thiol compounds such as *N*-acetylcysteine generally prevents paracetamol hepatotoxicity [18] either by scavenging the reactive metabolite or by enhancing glutathione synthesis. *N*-acetylcysteine has been clinically utilized as a treatment of paracetamol-induced hepatic injury [19]. Inhibition of hepatotoxicity by propylthiouracil may occur through a similar type of mechanism [20]; the production of paracetamol-propylthiouracil conjugate has been reported.

Finally, inhibition of the other two major pathways may theoretically result in the potentiation of paracetamol hepatotoxicity since paracetamol elimination from the plasma is retarded and the substrate for mixed function oxidases is continuously supplied for a longer period.

ASSESSMENT OF PARACETAMOL ACTIVATION

In vivo, glutathione depletion after paracetamol administration has been used as a marker for the production of the reactive metabolite. Renal excretion of mercapturic acid (*N*-acetyl-cysteine conjugate), that reflects the *in vivo* production of paracetamol–glutathione conjugate, has also been utilized to evaluate the production of the reactive metabolite *in vivo*. The amount of covalent binding to cellular proteins, that correlates with the severity of hepatotoxicity, is not a marker for the production of the reactive metabolite but a marker for the net consequences of the production–detoxification balance.

In vitro, however, covalent binding has been believed to indicate the production of the reactive metabolite. To assess the production of the reactive metabolite of paracetamol, the radioactive paracetamol bound covalently to microsomal proteins has been measured. Generally NADPH is used as an electron donor. Addition of glutathione to an *in vitro* system almost completely inhibits covalent binding of the reactive metabolite to microsomal proteins [21]. This is not due to the inhibition of the reactive metabolite production but due to the conjugation of the reactive metabolite with glutathione. A production of paracetamol–glutathione conjugate has been reported in liver microsomes [22] as well as isolated hepatocytes [23]. Those findings suggest that affinity of the reactive metabolite to proteins is by far exceeded by that to glutathione. Thus, we suggest that NADPH-dependent paracetamol–glutathione conjugate production may be a better marker of paracetamol activation than covalent binding.

CHARACTERIZATION OF PARACETAMOL–GLUTATHIONE CONJUGATE PRODUCTION

Characteristics of NADPH-dependent paracetamol–glutathione conjugate production were studied in rat liver microsomes [24]. Briefly, NADPH-dependent production of paracetamol–glutathione conjugate was measured in liver microsomes from male Sprague–Dawley rats, (C57BL/6 × DBA/2)F_1 strain (BDF$_1$) mice, and Japanese white rabbits. The incubation system contained 0.1 mol/L potassium phosphate buffer (pH 7.4), 1 mmol/L glutathione, 8 mmol/L paracetamol, 0.4 mmol/L NADPH, and 1 mg/ml microsomal proteins unless otherwise stated. The conjugate was analyzed by a HPLC system (Shimadzu 9A, Japan) equipped with a reverse-phase column (Shimadzu ODS, Japan) according to Buckpitt et al. [22]. The reaction was glutathione concentration-dependent (Figure 2). When glutathione was present in excess (more than 0.2 mmol/L), this reaction was dependent on time, temperature, pH, and protein concentrations. This reaction required NADPH and oxygen, and was inhibited by CO. Those characteristics of the present reaction were similar to those of mixed function oxidases [24].

There were species differences in paracetamol–glutathione conjugate production. Mouse microsomes were more active than rat and rabbit microsomes [24]. This observation is in accordance with the *in vivo* findings that the mouse is more susceptible to paracetamol hepatotoxicity than the others.

EFFECTS OF VARIOUS DRUGS ON PARACETAMOL ACTIVATION

To study the relation between paracetamol activation and hepatotoxicity, the effects of various compounds which have been shown to affect paracetamol hepatotoxicity were studied (Table 1). Cimetidine at 1 mmol/L inhibited paracetamol activation whereas ranitidine did not (data not shown). The compounds which reportedly attenuate paracetamol hepatotoxicity inhibited this reaction with a few exceptions. L-Ascorbic acid has been shown to inhibit paracetamol hepatotoxicity by decreasing covalent binding of the reactive metabolite *in vivo* and also *in vitro* [25]. In the present study, L-ascorbic acid did not affect the production of paracetamol–glutathione conjugate. L-Ascorbic acid may not inhibit the

191

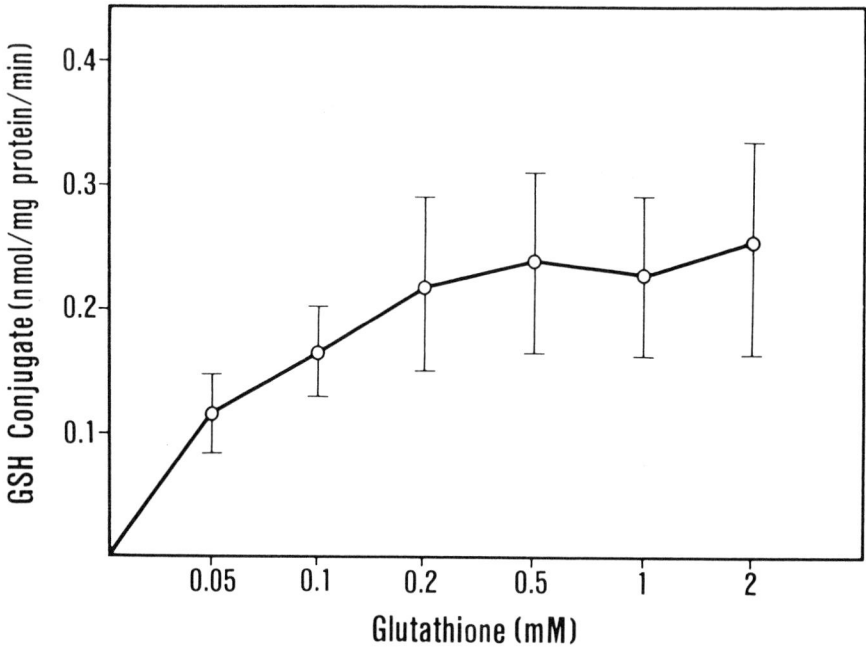

Figure 2. Effect of glutathione concentrations on NADPH-dependent paracetamol–glutathione conjugate production in rat liver microsomes.

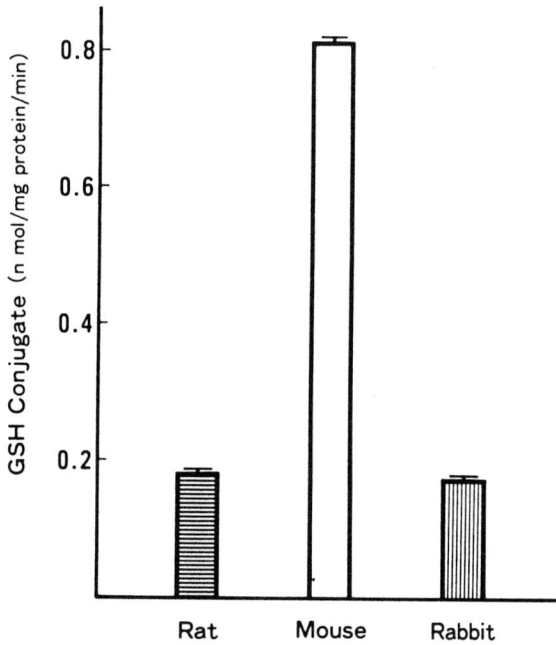

Figure 3. Species differences in paracetamol activation by liver microsomes (from ref. 24)

production of the reactive metabolite but scavenge the reactive metabolite of paracetamol [25] or reduce the reactive metabolite back to paracetamol. If the kinetic constant of glutathione conjugation was exceeded by that of interaction with L-ascorbic acid, this would agree well with existing data. In the case of propylthiouracil, similar mechanisms could be postulated [20].

Interesting is the effects of acetone and caffeine on this reaction. There were species differences in the effects of these two compounds. Acetone enhanced paracetamol–glutathione conjugate production in rat microsomes whereas it inhibited the production in mouse microsomes [24]; the findings are compatible with the existing data that acetone potentiates cell injury in rat hepatocytes but not in mouse hepatocytes [26]. Caffeine enhanced the production of the conjugate in rat microsomes, whereas a minimal effect was observed in mouse microsomes (Table 1), which again is compatible with the *in vivo* observation that caffeine potentiates paracetamol-induced liver injury in the rat [14] but not in the mouse [15].

Table 1. Effects of various compounds on paracetamol–glutathione conjugate production (nmol (mg protein)$^{-1}$ (15 min)$^{-1}$) in rat, mouse and rabbit microsomes

	Rat	*Mouse*	*Rabbit*
Control	3.10 ± 0.28	13.28 ± 1.03	3.58 ± 0.49
Ethanol (10 mmol/L)	2.03 ± 0.09^a	6.74 ± 0.41^a	3.10 ± 0.22
Mannitol (100 mmol/L)	3.48 ± 0.07	13.31 ± 1.91	3.92 ± 0.35
DMSO (100 mmol/L)^b	1.98 ± 0.31^a	5.85 ± 0.47^a	2.27 ± 0.22^a
Cysteine (1 mmol/L)	1.64 ± 0.30^a	8.21 ± 1.02^a	1.45 ± 0.06^a
N-acetylcysteine (1 mmol/L)	2.26 ± 0.27	10.26 ± 0.65^a	3.12 ± 0.67
Aniline (4 mmol/L)	1.31 ± 0.08^a	2.80 ± 0.20^a	1.81 ± 0.18^a
Acetone (100 mmol/L)	4.26 ± 0.21^a	6.56 ± 0.48^a	3.37 ± 0.59
Sodium fluoride (100 mmol/L)	4.56 ± 0.24^a	14.39 ± 1.53	5.96 ± 0.60^a
PTU (0.5 mmol/L)^c	2.98 ± 0.14	12.03 ± 1.31	3.80 ± 0.55
L-ascorbic acid (0.5 mmol/L)	2.69 ± 0.33	12.82 ± 2.15	3.33 ± 0.38
SOD (50 μg/ml)^d	4.15 ± 0.13	ND^e	ND^e
Caffeine (2 mmol/L)	7.51 ± 0.76^a	11.59 ± 0.49	5.08 ± 0.94

Incubation mixtures contained 0.1 mol/L potassium phosphate buffer (pH 7.4), 1 mmol/L glutathione, 0.4 mmol/L NADPH, 8 mmol/L paracetamol, and compounds as indicated. Paracetamol-glutathione conjugate was measured by HPLC as described in the methods. Values are mean $\pm$ SE ($n = 4$)

[a] $= p < 0.05$ compared with respective controls
[b] $=$ dimethyl sulphoxide
[c] $=$ propylthiouracil
[d] $=$ superoxide dismutase
[e] $=$ not determined

EFFECTS OF ETHANOL ON PARACETAMOL ACTIVATION

Clinical and experimental observations have revealed that simultaneous ethanol drinking with paracetamol attenuates paracetamol-induced hepatic injury [27,28]. The postulated mechanisms, however, are controversial. We previously reported that paracetamol activation in rat microsomes was inhibited in the presence of 50 mmol/L ethanol [29]. Tredger et al. reported the inhibitory effect of ethanol on paracetamol hepatotoxicity in the mouse although microsomal activation of paracetamol was not inhibited by ethanol in that model [30]. More recently Thummel et al. reported that ethanol competitively inhibited paracetamol activation in mouse microsomes [31] but not in rat microsomes [32]. These discrepancies may be due to the assay system. In all studies NADPH-dependent covalent binding of the reactive metabolite was measured using radioactive paracetamol. Then we assessed the effect of ethanol on paracetamol–glutathione conjugate production in rat, mouse, and rabbit microsomes. Ethanol at 10 mmol/L apparently inhibited the conjugation reaction in all microsomes (Table 1) but this inhibition was non-competitive in type. A possible mechanism is that acetaldehyde, a reactive metabolite of ethanol, may scavenge the reactive metabolite of paracetamol. In fact, we recently observed that acetaldehyde at concentrations as low as 0.1 mmol/L could inhibit this reaction in rat liver microsomes (unpublished observation). Since a spectrophotometric study showed that ethanol competitively inhibited paracetamol binding to cytochrome P-450 [29], ethanol may inhibit the paracetamol–glutathione conjugation reaction both by inhibiting the production of the metabolite directly and by scavenging the metabolite by acetaldehyde. In any event, the inhibitory effect of ethanol on paracetamol hepatotoxicity could be explained by the decreased availability of the reactive metabolite that binds to cellular proteins. The present observations are different from those reported by Thummel et al. [31,32].

MECHANISMS OF PARACETAMOL ACTIVATION

paracetamol activation is catalysed by cytochrome P-450 mediated mixed function oxidases. A reconstituted system containing NADPH-cytochrome P-450 reductase, cytochrome P-450, and phospholipids has been shown to activate paracetamol [8]. Among many subspecies, cytochrome P-450 IIE1 is most active in paracetamol activation [12]. These findings have clearly shown that paracetamol can be metabolized by cytochrome P-450. Unknown is the role of other electron transport systems in intact microsomes. Superoxide dismutase (50 μg/ml) or mannitol (100 mmol/L), a hydroxyl radical scavenger, did not inhibit this reaction (Table 1) suggesting these two radical species are not involved in paracetamol

194

activation. Recently we observed an enhancement of paracetamol activation by NADH although NADH itself did not initiate this reaction [33]. The second electron in this reaction may be transferred from NADH. Another interesting finding is that this reaction was inhibited in the presence of low concentrations of cyanide [33]. Although cyanide inhibits mixed function oxidases at high concentrations, it generally potentiates the enzyme reaction at low concentrations. The role of cyanide sensitive factor in the present reaction remains to be studied.

ROLE OF LIPID PEROXIDATION

Alternatively, oxygen radicals have been incriminated in paracetamol hepatotoxicity since paracetamol reportedly causes lipid peroxidation [34] and oxygen radical scavengers can inhibit paracetamol hepatotoxicity under some experimental conditions [35]. To investigate whether lipid peroxidation plays an important role in paracetamol hepatotoxicity, the effects of paracetamol on lipid peroxidation *in vivo* and *in vitro* were studied in the rat.

Diene conjugates in liver mitochondria and microsomes were not increased *in vivo* 2 h after paracetamol treatment (1 g/kg, i.p.). Co-administration of ethanol (3 g/kg) that has been shown to inhibit paracetamol hepatotoxicity [28] did not affect *in vivo* lipid peroxidation. These findings clearly contrasted with the findings that carbon tetrachloride (0.5 ml/kg, i.p.) increased diene conjugates in both mitochondria and microsomes and co-administration of ethanol that had been shown to potentiate carbon tetrachloride-induced hepatotoxicity [28] further enhanced lipid peroxidation.

Enzymatic and non-enzymatic production of malondialdehyde was measured as a marker for lipid peroxidation *in vitro* in rat liver microsomes. Paracetamol (2–8 mmol/L) appeared to inhibit lipid peroxidation whereas carbon tetrachloride (1 µl/ml) apparently enhanced lipid peroxidation. Addition of ethanol (50 mmol/L) did not show any significant effect.

Thus, lipid peroxidation measured *in vivo* and *in vitro* did not correlate with the hepatotoxicity of paracetamol.

CONCLUSION

Covalent binding of the reactive metabolite rather than lipid peroxidation appears to be responsible for paracetamol-induced hepatic injury. Although hepatic glutathione status plays an additive role, paracetamol–glutathione conjugate production may be a good marker for paracetamol activation, which correlates well with paracetamol hepatotoxicity. Further investigations are necessary to clarify why covalent binding causes cell injury.

ACKNOWLEDGEMENTS

Part of this study was supported by Grant-in-aid 02304040 and 02670297 from the Japanese Ministry of Education, Science and Culture (Monbusho). We are grateful to Dr J. Liu for his generous assistance during this study.

REFERENCES

1. Davidson DGD, Eastham WN. Liver necrosis following overdose of paracetamol. Br Med J. 1966;2:497–499.
2. Thompson JS, Prescott LF. Liver damage and impaired glucose tolerance after paracetamol overdosage. Br Med J. 1966;2:506–507.
3. Wright N, Prescott LF. Potentiation by previous drug therapy of hepatotoxicity following paracetamol overdosage. Scot Med J. 1973;18:56–58.
4. Emby DJ, Fraser BN. Hepatotoxicity of paracetamol enhanced by ingestion of alcohol: report of two cases. S Afr Med J. 1977;51:208–209.
5. Boyd EM, Bereczky GM. Liver necrosis from paracetamol. Br J Pharmacol. 1966;26:606–614.
6. Mitchell JR, Jollow DJ. Metabolic activation of drugs to toxic substances. Gastroenterology. 1975;68:392–412.
7. Black M. Acetaminophen hepatotoxicity. Annu Rev Med. 1984;35:577–593.
8. Morgan ET, Koop DR, Coon MJ. Comparison of six rabbit liver cytochrome P-450 isozymes in formation of a reactive metabolite of acetaminophen. Biochem Biophys Res Commun. 1983;112:8–13.
9. Dahlin DC, Miwa GT, Lu AYH, Nelson SD. N-Acetyl-p-benzoquinone imine: a cytochrome P-450-mediated oxidation product of acetaminophen. Proc Natl Acad Sci USA. 1984;81:1327–1331.
10. Mitchell JR, Jollow DJ, Potter WZ, Davis DC, Gillette JR, Brodie BB. Acetaminophen-induced hepatic necrosis. I. Role of drug metabolism. J Pharmacol Exp Ther. 1973;187:185–194.
11. Sato C, Matsuda Y, Lieber CS. Increased hepatotoxicity of acetaminophen after chronic ethanol consumption in the rat. Gastroenterology. 1981;80:140–148.
12. Raucy JL, Lasker JM, Lieber CS, Black M. Acetaminophen activation by human liver cytochromes P450IIE1 and P450IA2. Arch Biochem Biophys. 1989;217:270–283.
13. Mitchell MC, Schenker S, Avant GR, Speeg Jr KV. Cimetidine protects against acetaminophen hepatotoxicity in rats. Gastroenterology. 1981;81:1052–1060.
14. Sato C, Izumi N. Mechanism of increased hepatotoxicity of acetaminophen by the simultaneous administration of caffeine in the rat. J Pharmacol Exp Ther. 1989;248:1243–1247.
15. Gale GR, Atkins LM, Smith AB, Lamar Jr C, Walker Jr EM. Acetaminophen-induced hepatotoxicity: antagonistic action of caffeine in mice. Res Commun Chem Pathol Pharmacol. 1987;55:203–225.
16. Pessayre D, Dolder A, Artigou JY, Wandscheer JC, Benhamou JP. Effect of fasting on metabolite-mediated hepatotoxicity in the rat. Gastroenterology. 1979;77:264–271.
17. Mitchell JR, Jollow DJ, Potter WZ, Gillette JR, Bridie BB. Acetaminophen-induced hepatic necrosis. IV. Protective role of glutathione. J Pharmacol Exp Ther. 1973;187:211-217.

18. Lauterburg BH, Corcoran GB, Mitchell JR. Mechanism of action of N-acetylcysteine in the protection against the hepatotoxicity of acetaminophen in rats *in vivo*. J Clin Invest. 1983;71:980–991.

19. Prescott LF. Treatment of severe acetaminophen poisoning with intravenous acetylcysteine. Arch Intern Med. 1981;141:386–389.

20. Yamada T, Ludwig S, Kuhlenkamp J, Kaplowitz. Direct protection against acetaminophen hepatotoxicity by propylthiouracil. *in vivo* and *in vitro* studies in rats and mice. J Clin Invest. 1981;67:688–695.

21. Potter WZ, Davis DC, Mitchell JR, Jollow DJ, Gillette JR, Brodie BB. Acetaminophen-induced hepatic necrosis. III. Cytochrome P-450-mediated covalent binding *in vitro*. J Pharmacol Exp Ther. 1973;187:203–210.

22. Buckpitt AR, Rollins DE, Nelson SD, Franklin RB, Mitchell JR. Quantitative determination of the glutathione, cysteine, and N-acetyl cysteine conjugates of acetaminophen by high-pressure liquid chromatography. Anal Biochem. 1977;83:168–177.

23. Moldeus P. Paracetamol metabolism and toxicity in isolated hepatocytes from rat and mouse. Biochem Pharmacol. 1978;27:2859–2863.

24. Liu J, Sato C, Marumo F. Characterization of acetaminophen–glutathione conjugation reaction by liver microsomes: species difference in the effect of acetone. Toxicol Lett. 1991;56:269–277

25. Lake BG, Harris RA, Phillips JC, Gangolli SD. Studies on the effects of L-ascorbic acid on acetaminophen-induced hepatotoxicity. 1. Inhibition of the covalent binding of acetaminophen metabolites to hepatic microsomes *in vitro*. Toxicol Appl Pharmacol. 1981;60:229–240.

26. Moldeus P, Gergely V. Effect of acetone on the activation of acetaminophen. Toxicol Appl Pharmacol. 1980;53:8–13.

27. Rumack BH. Acetaminophen overdose. Am J Med. 1983;74:104–112

28. Sato C, Nakano M, Lieber CS. Prevention of acetaminophen-induced hepatotoxicity by acute ethanol administration in the rat: comparison with carbon tetrachloride-induced hepatotoxicity. J Pharmacol Exp Ther. 1981;218:805–810.

29. Sato C, Lieber CS. Mechanism of the preventive effect of ethanol on acetaminophen-induced hepatotoxicity. J Pharmacol Exp Ther. 1981;218:811–815.

30. Tredger JM, Smith HM, Read RB, Portmann B, Williams R. Effects of ethanol ingestion on the hepatotoxicity and metabolism of paracetamol in mice. Toxicology. 1985;36:341–352.

31. Thummel KE, Slattery JT, Nelson SD, Lee CA, Pearson PG. Effect of ethanol on hepatotoxicity of acetaminophen in mice and on reactive metabolite formation by mouse and human liver microsomes. Toxicol Appl Pharmacol. 1989;100:391–397.

32. Thummel KE, Slattery JT, Nelson SD. Mechanism by which ethanol diminishes the hepatotoxicity of acetaminophen. J Pharmacol Exp Ther. 1988;245:129–136.

33. Sato C, Marumo F. Synergistic effect of NADH on NADPH-dependent acetaminophen activation in liver microsomes and its inhibition by cyanide. Life Sci. 1991;48:2423–2427.

34. Wendel A, Feuerstein S, Konz KH. Acute paracetamol intoxication of starved mice leads to lipid peroxidation *in vivo*. Biochem Pharmacol. 1979;28:2051–2055.

35. Kyle ME, Miccadei S, Nakae D, Farber JL. Superoxide dismutase and catalase protect cultured hepatocytes from cytotoxicity of acetaminophen. Biochem Biophys Res Commun. 1987;149:889–896.

24

Increased liver toxicity of diclofenac by paracetamol: results and possible mechanisms

K. Brune and J. Lindner

Department of Pharmacology and Toxicology, University of Erlangen-Nürnberg, Universitätsstrasse 22, 8520 Erlangen, Germany

INTRODUCTION

Diclofenac is the most widely-used non-steroidal anti-inflammatory drug (NSAID) in Europe. Almost twenty years of use in humans have shown that this drug is effective, useful and well tolerated in general [1] despite a few drawbacks concerning (a) the variable and incomplete oral bioavailability [2], and (b) the intensive and immediate oxidative metabolization in the liver [2] which is possibly associated with a measurable and clinical relevant hepatotoxicity [5,6,10]. Recent findings revealed that the well-known hepatotoxicity of paracetamol is related to the production of an unstable reactive electrophilic metabolite [8]. We suppose that similar metabolic processes may occur with diclofenac resulting in comparable reactive metabolites. Moreover, recent observations by Sato and his co-workers have indicated that the co-administration of other drugs may enhance the production of hepatotoxic metabolites of paracetamol [9,10] and, thus, enhance this clinically relevant phenomenon. Similar effects appear possible with diclofenac. They may contribute to the putative toxicity of this drug.

The aim of the work presented in a preliminary form was to investigate whether (a) the hepatotoxicity of diclofenac can be enhanced by paracetamol, (b) diclofenac is metabolized via (as yet unknown) reactive intermediates, and (c) diclofenac interacts with paracetamol competing for the same detoxifying mechanisms.

Side-effects of Anti-inflammatory Drugs 3. Rainsford KD, Velo GP (eds), Inflammation and Drug Therapy Series, Volume V.

MATERIALS AND METHODS

The experiments were performed either *in vivo* or *in vitro*. *In vivo* we scored the lethality to mice treated with different doses of (a) paracetamol alone, (b) paracetamol + diclofenac and (c) paracetamol and diclofenac co-administered with *N*-acetylcysteine. The dosages and time schedules are given in Figure 1.

The concentration of liver-related transaminases, SGOT and SGPT were measured according to standard methods. With Tietze's method [11], we measured the depletion of the liver glutathione content elicited by diclofenac and paracetamol alone or in combination. Finally, histological evaluations of the liver of the intoxicated animals were performed.

Using standard methods of synthetic chemistry, we synthesized a highly reactive derivative of diclofenac (quinoneimine of 5-OH-diclofenac, Figure 3) and defined its chemical characteristics in order to measure the occurrence of this intermediate after exposing diclofenac to liver microsomes. Diclofenac was exposed to liver microsomes (see below) in order to determine if this reactive metabolite and its glutathione conjugate were formed. Different S10-liver enzyme preparations of male mice and rats (the animals had been induced by β-naphthoflavone, phenobarbitone, dexamethasone, clofibrate or acetone) were applied for metabolic studies involving diclofenac and its hydroxymetabolites. Using the same system, we investigated the interaction between the oxidative metabolism of diclofenac and paracetamol.

RESULTS

Diclofenac administered alone was almost devoid of hepatotoxicity in mice, but it could enhance the well-known hepatotoxicity of paracetamol considerably at low doses (0.5-1.5 mg/kg bw). It was mandatory that diclofenac was given prior to paracetamol administration (Figure 1). If given together with paracetamol, the toxicity of paracetamol was (slightly) reduced. These drug effects were accompanied by a reduction of liver glutathione (Figure 2).

Also, it could be demonstrated that the hepatotoxicity of diclofenac combined with paracetamol in mice may be reduced by co-administration of *N*-acetylcysteine as has been shown previously for paracetamol alone. The details are not given in this manuscript.

The *in vitro* investigation performed so far has led to the extraction and definition of a so far unknown diclofenac intermediate (Figure 3). This substance was formed by liver microsomes and detoxified via glutathione conjugation in an enzymatic reaction requiring oxygen, NADPH and microsomal enzymes (Table 1).

Surviving Animals (%)

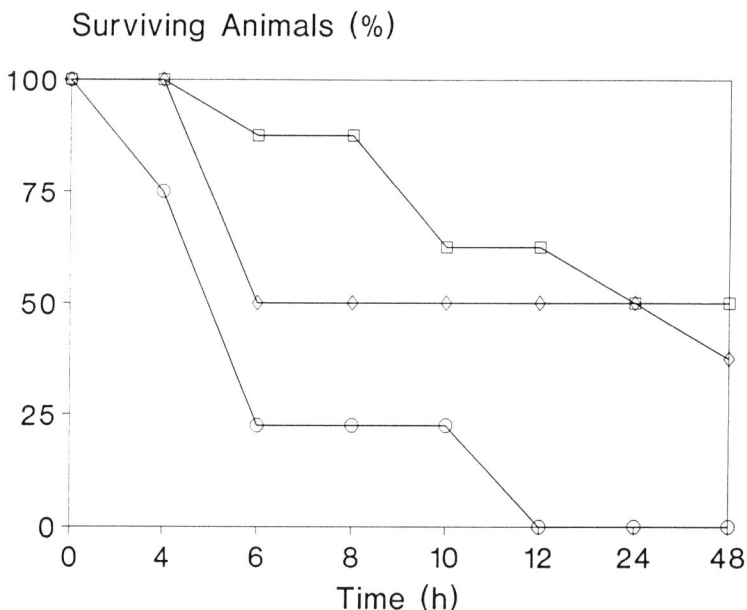

Figure 1. Time course of surviving mice (means of $n = 8$) treated with paracetamol (600 mg/kg body wt, i.p.) alone ($\diamond$) or combined with diclofenac (1 mg/kg body wt, p.o.). Diclofenac was administered either 30 minutes before paracetamol ($\bigcirc$) or simultaneously with paracetamol ($\square$). The differences between the paracetamol group and the diclofenac-plus-paracetamol groups were statistically significant (other groups, not shown)

Table 1. Formation of 5-OH-glutathionyl-diclofenac (5-OH-G-Dic)

	Experimental conditions			
	(1)	(2)	(3)	(4)
Amount 5-OH-G-Dic	2474	436	212	109
(Au/min) formed $\pm$ SD ($n = 3$)	± 313	± 13	± 185	± 95

The results show that 5-OH-glutathionyl-diclofenac is formed by liver enzymes + NADPH + 5-OH-diclofenac (1) but not formed after inhibition of the enzymes by CO (2), lack of NADPH (3), or lack of liver enzymes (4) (S-10-preparation of liver enzymes). This is proof of an enzymatic process leading from diclofenac to 5-OH-glutathionyl-diclofenac as proposed in Figure 1

DISCUSSION

Diclofenac displays comparatively little gastrointestinal toxicity [1]. It is rapidly eliminated by hepatic metabolization and may be handled relatively easily by the treating physician [2]. Other serious side-effects such as CNS effects or overt nephrotoxicity are relatively scarce [1,5]. As with benoxaprofen [12], several cases have been reported showing that diclofenac increased the level of liver related serum transaminases [4–6]. Moreover, diclofenac was occasionally associated with the occurrence of

200

Glutathione [µmol/g Liver]

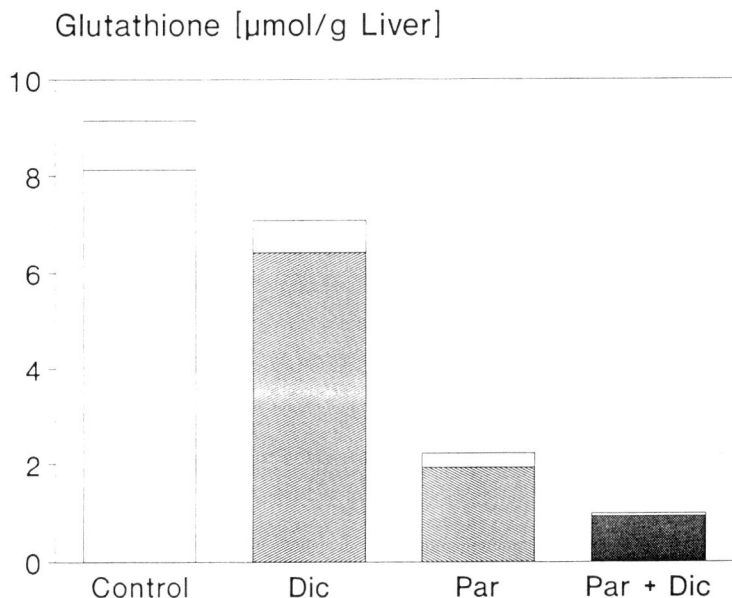

Figure 2. Glutathione concentrations in the livers of a control group and three groups that received paracetamol alone (500 mg/kg body wt, i.p.), diclofenac alone (0.5 mg/kg body wt, p.o.) or both drugs combined. In the co-administered group diclofenac (0.5 mg/kg body wt, p.o.) was given 30 minutes before paracetamol (500 mg/kg body wt, i.p.). The tissue levels of glutathione were measured 2 hours after administration of paracetamol. There was a statistically significant depletion of glutathione levels in the groups treated with diclofenac alone ($p < 0.05$) or in combination with paracetamol ($p < 0.01$) as compared to the control group. Bars show the means (filled) and standard deviations (open) of $n = 10$, respectively.
Abbreviations: Dic = diclofenac, Par = paracetamol

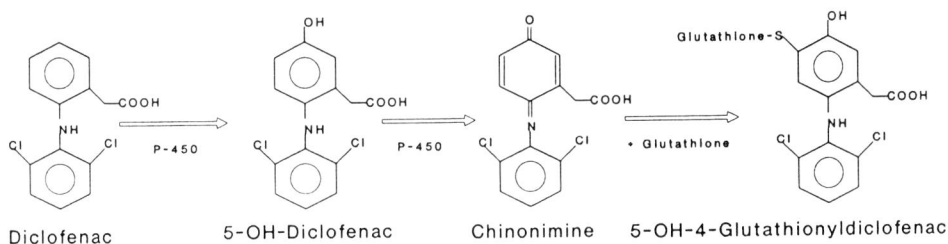

Figure 3. This figure indicates a possible pathway of metabolization of diclofenac via a reactive metabolite: a quinoneimine of 5-OH-diclofenac. The formation of 5-OH-diclofenac and the metabolization to its reactive quinoneimine derivative are P-450 dependent reactions. The reactive metabolite may be detoxified by the formation of a glutathione conjugate (5-OH-glutathionyl-diclofenac)

201

death due to severe liver destruction or damage [7]. Some of this lethal liver damage occurred when diclofenac had been administered with other drugs [6,7]. In two instances, lethal liver damage was reported after administration of diclofenac to patients pretreated with barbiturates or phenytoin. These drugs can induce the production of a sub-group of the P-450 enzyme-system in the liver. Consequently, we believe that some cases of hepatotoxicity related to diclofenac may be caused by the co-administration of other drugs. On the basis of our findings, we suggest that these drugs may either enhance the production of reactive hepatotoxic metabolite(s) of diclofenac via enzyme induction, or compete with the detoxification of the reactive chinonimine metabolite by depleting the glutathione stores.

Our investigations of the hepatotoxic mechanisms of diclofenac in animals, may thus give hints at specific mechanisms of the side effects occasionally observed in man. Further investigations will have to demonstrate the relevance of these *in vivo* and *in vitro* findings. In addition, this research may indicate ways and means to block or prevent the diclofenac-related hepatotoxicity, e.g. by preventing the production of the quinoneimine metabolite or depletion of the glutathione stores.

ACKNOWLEDGEMENTS

This work was supported in part by the German Federal Ministry of Science and Technology (Grant 01VM8917). We thank Dr R. Boecker for helpful discussion and technical support.

REFERENCES

1. Kurowski M, Lanz R, Fenner H, Brune K. Spala, Sicherheitsprofil von Antirheumatika bei Langzeitanwendung. Dtsch Aerztebl. 1990;87:2707–2718.
2. Brune K, Lanz R. Pharmacokinetics of non-steroidal anti-inflammatory drugs. In: Bonta IL, Bray MA, Parnham MJ, eds. Handbook of inflammation. Vol 5. Amsterdam: Elsevier; 1865:413–449.
3. Willis JV, Kenndall MJ, Flinn RM, Thornhill DP, Welling PG. The pharmacokinetics of diclofenac sodium following intravenous administration. Eur J Pharmacol. 1979;16:405–410.
4. Ciccoulunghi SN. Report on a long-term tolerability study of up to two years with diclofenac sodium. Scand J Rheumatol. 1978;22:86–96.
5. Babany G, Bernau J, Danaw G, Rueff B, Benhamou J. Fulminating hepatitis in a woman taking glafenine and diclofenac. Gastroenterol Clin Biol. 1985;9:185.
6. Lasgar G, Grippon P, Levy V. Acute fatal hepatitis during treatment with diclofenac. Gastroenterol Clin Biol. 1984;9:881-882.
7. Helfgott SM, Sandberg-Cook J, Zakim D, Nestler J. Diclofenac-associated hepatotoxicity. JAMA. 1990;264:2660–2662.
8. Albano E, Rundgren M, Harrison PJ, Nelson SD, Moldeus P. Mechanisms of N-acetyl-p-benzoquinoneimine cytotoxicity. Mol Pharmacol. 1985;28:306–311.

9. Sato C, Izumi N. Mechanism of increased hepatotoxicity of acetaminophen by the simultaneous administration of caffeine in the rat. J Pharmacol Exp Ther. 1988;248:1243–1247.

10. Kalhorn TF, Lee CA, Slattery JT, Nelson SD. Effect of methylxanthines on acetaminophen hepatotoxicity in various induction states. J Pharmacol Exp Ther. 1990;252:112–116.

11. Tietze F. Enzymatic method for quantitative determination of nanogram amounts of total and oxidized glutathione. Anal Biochem. 1969;27:502–504.

12. Fowler PD. Major toxic reactions associated with NSAIDs. In: Dudley Hart F, Klinenberg JR, eds. Choosing NSAID therapy. Auckland: ADIS Press; 1985:41–57.

25

Effects of NSAIDs on liver microsomal mono-oxygenase system and products of oxidative metabolism of arachidonic acid

M.E. Fracasso, L. Franco, R. Gasperini and G.P. Velo

Institute of Pharmacology, University of Verona, Verona, Italy

INTRODUCTION

The most common severe adverse reactions to NSAIDs frequently reported in the literature are those affecting the gastrointestinal tract, but substantial numbers of serious reactions affecting the liver (hepatitis, jaundice, hepatic necrosis, hepatic failure) have been seen as well [1]. Recent studies in animals have revealed that acute and/or chronic treatment with NSAIDs may have a toxic effect on hepatic metabolism [2–4]. Pre-clinical studies have been useful both in assessing this toxicity and in sounding an early warning. However, few studies have investigated the mechanism(s) of action of NSAIDs upon the hepatic drug metabolizing P-450 dependent system. *In vitro* data demonstrate that some NSAIDs depress hepatic cytochrome P-450 (cyt. P-450) by converting it to the more labile derivate P-420 [2]. The same group of researchers reported that a concomitant administration of 16,16-dimethyl-$PGF_{2\alpha}$ reversed in part the depressed cytochrome P-450 enzyme system induced by high doses of indomethacin [3]. In the course of studies of side-effects caused by NSAIDs we observed that three drugs with unrelated chemical structures (indomethacin, piroxicam and ibuprofen) inhibited these components of the hepatic microsomal system to a different extent [4]. Therefore, the mechanism by which these drugs induce changes in the hepatic microsomal system may be unique for each class of compounds.

In addition, little attention has been paid to the cyclo-oxygenase inhibitory effect induced by these compounds on the hepatic drug-metabolizing system. The possibility that NSAIDs might destroy cyt. P-450 has increased in importance in view of recent evidence that prostacyclin and thromboxane synthetase resemble P-450 enzymes [5].

Side-effects of Anti-inflammatory Drugs 3. Rainsford KD, Velo GP (eds), Inflammation and Drug Therapy Series, Volume V.

In this study we decided to investigate whether there is a correlation between the hepatic inhibition of arachidonic acid metabolites by NSAIDs and the changes on the mono-oxygenase P-450 system components.

MATERIALS AND METHODS

Male Sprague–Dawley rats (Charles River, Italy) (200–210 g) were treated p.o. with ulcerogenic doses [6–8] of indomethacin (10 mg/kg), piroxicam (50 mg/kg) and ibuprofen (400 mg/kg) for one or three consecutive days. Control rats received the same amount of vehicle (methylcellulose 0.2%). Animals were killed by cervical dislocation 24 hours after the first and third administration. Each liver was immediately removed and homogenized with a cold solution (KCl 0.15 mol/L in phosphate buffer pH = 7.4). The microsomes (105 000 g) were prepared at 4°C by sequential centrifugation [3].

The resulting microsomal pellet was suspended in phosphate buffer (0.1 mol/L, pH 7.4) to a final volume of 1 ml/g of liver weight. Microsomes were maintained at –80°C until use. The amount of microsomal protein was measured by the method of Lowry et al. [9]. The concentrations of cytochrome P-450 and cytochrome b_5 (cyt. b_5) were measured by the technique of Omura and Sato [10]. NADPH cytochrome c reductase (NADPH cyt. c red.) activity was measured by the method of Phillips and Langdon [11], NADH cytochrome b_5 reductase (NADH cyt. b_5 red.) by the method of Minara and Sato [12]. Aminopyrine N-demethylase (AD) activity was determined by the Nash reaction according to Werringloer [13]. PGE_2 levels were measured by radioimmunoassay. PGE_2 was measured in duplicate by radioimmunoassay using a highly sensitive PGE_2 ^{125}I RIA kit (Du-Pont, Nen Division, Germany) and assay standards of 0.25 to 25 pg PGE_2. Cross-reactivity with PGE was 3.7% and with all other prostaglandins less than 0.4%. Lipid peroxidation *in vitro* was carried out by the method of Jordan and Schenkman [14].

RESULTS AND DISCUSSION

After one day treatment indomethacin significantly decreased NADPH-cyt. c reductase with piroxicam decreasing cyt. P-450 content and NADH-cyt. b_5 reductase; ibuprofen had no effect on hepatic mono-oxygenase components (Table 1). Conversely, 24 hours after the third day of treatment indomethacin induced a marked loss of the haemoproteins, cyt. P-450 and cyt. b_5, and a decrease in the enzymatic activities of NADPH-cyt. c reductase, NADH-cyt. b_5 reductase and aminopyrine N-demethylase. Piroxicam significantly reduced all parameters, except cyt. b_5, and ibuprofen caused only a significant decrease in cyt. b_5 (Table 2).

Table 1. Effect of 1 day treatment on hepatic haemoproteins and drug-metabolizing enzyme activities

	Total haem	Cyt. P-450	Cyt.b$_5$	NADPH cyt.c red.	NADH cyt.b$_5$ red.	APD
	(nmol/mg microsomal prot.)			*(nmol/min/mg microsomal prot.)*		
Control (6)	1.248 ±0.153	0.756 ±0.074	0.389 ±0.057	174.83 ±18.10	3.74 ±0.68	3.05 ±0.85
Indomethacin (6) (10 mg/kg)	1.121 ±0.197	0.652 ±0.120	0.380 ±0.058	99.21** ±41.40	3.58 ±0.53	2.89 ±0.53
Ibuprofen (6) (400 mg/kg)	1.169 ±0.207	0.613 ±0.156	0.325 ±0.037	113.89 ±49.52	3.55 ±0.84	3.08 ±0.53
Piroxicam (6) (50 mg/kg)	1.078 ±0.239	0.422** ±0.163	0.368 ±0.079	143.93 ±41.73	2.33** ±0.51	2.09 ±1.09

The values are expressed as mean ± SD (in brackets number of individual rats).
**$p < 0.01$ (Student's t test)
APD = aminopyrine demethylase

Table 2. Effect of 3 days treatment on hepatic haemoproteins and drug-metabolizing enzyme activities

	Total haeme	Cyt. P-450	Cyt.b$_5$	NADPH cyt.c red.	NADH cyt.b$_5$ red.	APD
	(nmol/mg microsomal prot.)			*(nmol/min/mg microsomal prot.)*		
Control (6)	1.267 ±0.225	0.832 ±0.069	0.427 ±0.059	184.53 ±27.64	3.98 ±0.44	3.47 ±0.13
Indomethacin (6) (10 mg/kg)	0.504*** ±0.100	0.188*** ±0.046	0.194*** ±0.041	58.12*** ±12.93	2.33*** ±0.51	1.26*** ±0.22
Ibuprofen (6) (400 mg/kg)	1.189 ±0.133	0.783 ±0.097	0.224** ±0.036	164.28 ±24.00	3.52 ±0.21	2.73 ±0.90
Piroxicam (6) (50 mg/kg)	0.838* ±0.186	0.350* ±0.118	0.374 ±0.092	110.68** ±23.95	2.26** ±0.42	1.60** ±0.30

The values are expressed as mean ± SD (in brackets number of individual rats). *$p < 0.05$,
**$p < 0.01$, ***$p < 0.005$ (Student's t test)

These data indicate that these three drugs administered in ulcerogenic doses induce different depressions on the components of the P-450 mono-oxygenase system.

The mechanisms whereby NSAIDs induce changes in the hepatic drug-metabolizing system may operate in different ways. Each drug studied inhibits the arachidonic acid cascade through cyclo-oxygenase blocking. Little attention has been given to the possible inhibitory effect of this enzyme on the hepatic drug-metabolizing system. In order to understand if the lack and/or low production of the metabolites of arachidonic acid in the liver could cause the cytochrome depression, we measured the *in vivo* levels of prostaglandin E_2 (PGE_2).

Figure 1 shows the hepatic content of PGE_2 in control rats and in treated animals 24 hours after the first and third day of treatment. After indomethacin administration PGE_2 levels in microsomal fractions were significantly lower than controls both after the first and third day; PGE_2 content in piroxicam-microsomes were significantly lower than controls only after three doses. Ibuprofen-microsomes had PGE_2 concentrations similar to those of the control group in both considered times.

These data suggest that when there is a decrease in PGE_2 content there is concomitantly a loss in haemoproteins and/or in reductase activities; however, when PGE_2 production is normal, no modification occurs in the hepatic microsomal parameters. This correlation is evident only after three days of treatment. After one day the components of the microsomal system are not basically affected by indomethacin treatment, even if PGE_2 is significantly lowered; conversely, with piroxicam we noted a decrease in cyt. P-450 without a corresponding significant decrease in PGE_2 levels.

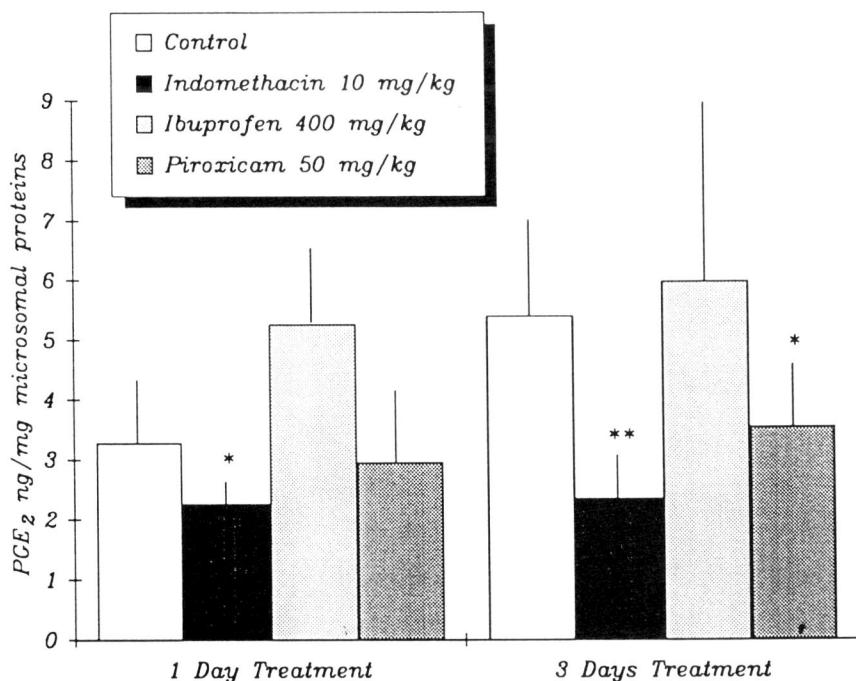

Figure 1. Effect of treatments on hepatic PGE_2 production. The values are expressed as means $\pm$ SD of 5 individual rats. *$p < 0.05$, **$p < 0.01$ (Student's t test)

This might be due to the fact that even if these drugs ultimately block PG synthesis, they exhibit different types of inhibition on the arachidonic acid cascade [15].

To better understand these first steps we assessed the presence of arachidonic acid in the microsomal fractions. It is generally assumed that one of the important sources of malondialdehyde (MDA) is from oxidation of arachidonic acid [14]. Using this method we studied the rate of MDA production after *in vitro* lipid peroxidation in microsomal fractions of control and treated rats (Figure 2).

The rate of MDA production following indomethacin administration was significantly higher than controls after the first dose. After the third dose the rate returned to control values. This suggests a utilization of the arachidonic acid accumulated in the microsomal membranes during drug treatment.

The block of cyclo-oxygenase by indomethacin may initially lead to an increase of arachidonic acid [16], followed after three days of treatment by a decrease through alternative metabolic pathways [17] and this could partially explain the reduction of microsomal parameters.

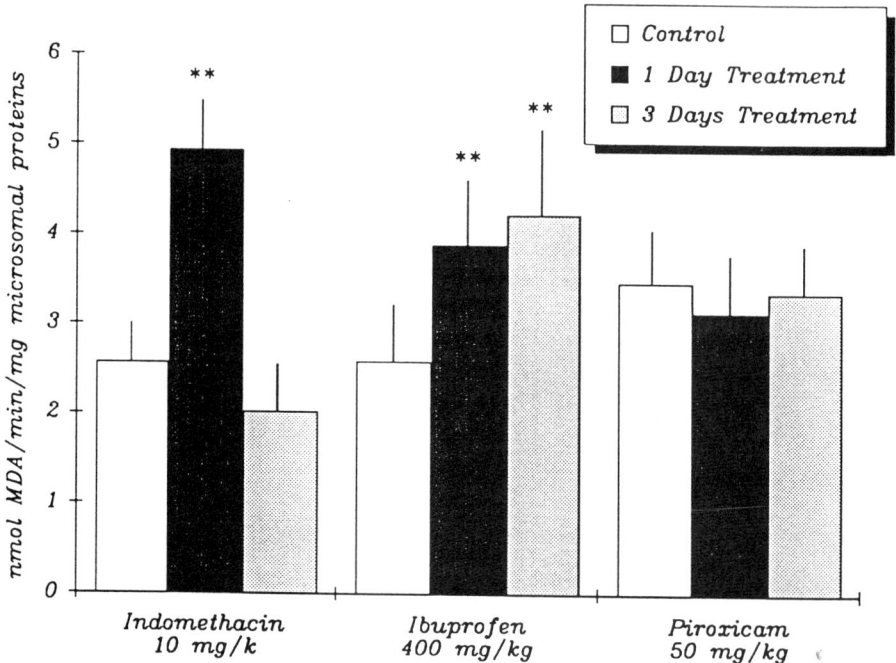

Figure 2. Effect of treatments on production of MDA during 10 min of NADPH-supported lipid peroxidation. The values are expressed as mean $\pm$ SD of 6 individual rats. **$p < 0.01$ (Student's t test)

The rate of MDA production by piroxicam treatment was consistently the same as the control group. This led us to believe that piroxicam might have a different impact upon the utilization of arachidonic acid by blocking its metabolites (i.e. PGE_2). MDA production following ibuprofen treatment significantly increased after the first and third administration. Therefore, there is evidence of fatty acid accumulation (i.e. arachidonic acid). This has been noted by other authors [18] and is also in agreement with our finding of an increase in hepatic weight after the third day of treatment (liver wt. % of body wt.: 5.45 $\pm$ 0.59 vs control 4.12 $\pm$ 0.46).

CONCLUSIONS

Although further evidence is needed to confirm these preliminary data, there is already some evidence suggesting that the varying degrees of hepatic damage may be related to the multiplicity of the metabolites of arachidonic acid. Thus, a lack of the protective effect of PGs (i.e. PGE_2), as described for the gastrointestinal system, might be one of the causes of a loss of hepatic haemoproteins (i.e. cyt. P-450, cyt. b_5) and/or enzymatic activities.

Moreover, it is interesting to note that the three NSAIDs might interfere with the metabolism of arachidonic acid in different ways. In fact, this finding was corroborated evaluating the *in vitro* production of MDA, the principal product of arachidonic acid oxidation [14].

We note that there is an individual mechanism by which each NSAID blocks PG production (PGE_2) and this leads to a different utilization of arachidonic acid. Therefore, we suppose that NSAID inhibiting effect on the hepatic microsomal system is provoked not only by low levels of PGs, but also by the presence of other products of the metabolism of arachidonic acid. Further developments of this research should lead to a better understanding of the mechanisms of these drugs on the hepatic microsomal system.

REFERENCES

1. Del Favero A. Anti-inflammatory analgesics and drugs used in rheumatoid arthritis and gout. In: Dukes MNG, Beeley L, eds. Side effects of drugs annual. Amsterdam: Elsevier Science Publishers; 1988;12:79–100.

2. Falzon M, Nielsch A, Burke MD. Denaturation of cytochrome P-450 by indomethacin and other non-steroidal antiinflammatory drugs: evidence for a surfactant mechanism and a selective effect of a p-chlorophenyl moiety. Biochem Pharmacol. 1986;35:4019–4024.

3. Burke MD, Falzon M, Milton AS. Decreased hepatic microsomal cytochrome P450 due to indomethacin: protective roles of 16,16,-dimethylprostaglandin $F_{2\alpha}$ and inducing agents. Biochem Pharmacol. 1982;389–397.

4. Gasperini R, Leone R, Velo GP, Fracasso ME. The inhibition of hepatic microsomal drugs metabolism in rats by non-steroidal anti-inflammatory drugs. Pharm Res. 1990;22(Suppl. 3):115–116.

5. Ullrich V, Graf H, Haurand M. In: Boobis AR, Caldwell J, De Matteis F, Elcombe CR, eds. Microsomes and drug oxidations. London: Taylor and Francis; 1986:95–104.
6. Weissenborn V, Maedge S, Buettner D, Sewing KF. Indomethacin-induced gastrointestinal lesions in relation to tissue concentration, food intake and bacterial invasion in the rat. Pharmacology. 1985;30:32–39.
7. Wiseman EH, Moguchi Y. Limitations of laboratory models in predicting gastrointestinal toleration of oxicams and other anti-inflammatory drugs. In: Rainsford KD, Velo GP, eds. Side effects of anti-inflammatory drugs (Part II: Studies in major organ systems). Lancaster: MTP Press; 1987:41–54.
8. Reineke C, Klinger W. Influence of ibuprofen on drug metabolizing enzymes in rat liver in vivo and in vitro. Biochem Pharmacol. 1974;24:145–147.
9. Lowry HD, Rosenbrough MJ, Farr AL, Randall R. Protein measurement with the folin phenol reagent. J Biol Chem. 1951;193:265–275.
10. Omura T, Sato R. The carbon monoxide binding pigment of the liver microsomes. J Biol Chem. 1964;239:2370–2378.
11. Phillips AV, Langdon RG. Hepatic triphosphopyridina nucleotide-cytochrome C reductase: isolation, characterization and kinetic studies. J Biol Chem. 1962;237:2652–2660.
12. Minara K, Sato R. Partial purification of NADH-cytochrome b_5 reductase from rabbit liver microsomes with detergents and its properties. J Biochem. 1972;71:725–735.
13. Werringloer J. Assay of formaldehyde generated during microsomal oxidation reactions. In: Fleisher S, Parker L, eds. Methods in enzymology. New York: Academic Press; 1978:297–302.
14. Jordan R, Schenkman JB. Relationship between malondialdehyde production and arachidonic consumption during NADPH-supported microsomal lipid peroxidation. Biochem Pharmacol. 1982;31:1393–1400.
15. Lands WEM. Actions of anti-inflammatory drugs. TIPS. 1981;March:78–80.
16. Vane JR. Inhibition of prostaglandin synthesis as a mechanism of action for aspirin-like drugs. Nature (New Biol). 1971;231:232–235.
17. Taylor GW, Morris HR. Lipoxygenase pathways. Med Bull. 1983;39(3):219–222.
18. Cox JW, Cox SR, Van Giessen G, Ruwart MJ. Ibuprofen stereoisomer clearance and distribution in normal and fatty in situ perfused rat liver. J Pharmacol Exp Ther. 1985;232:636–643.

26

Hepatitis due to non-steroidal anti-inflammatory drugs (NSAIDs)

William M. O'Brien

Professor of Internal Medicine Emeritus, The University of Virginia, Charlottesville, VA, USA

INTRODUCTION

Very rare adverse drug reactions can have devastating effects on the future use of the drug. Such rare but potentially lethal reactions often result in withdrawal or restricted use of a drug. The worst such reactions are aplastic annaemia, anaphylaxis, erythema multiforme and hepatitis.

Since non-steroidal anti-inflammatory drugs (NSAIDs) are the most widely used drugs in the world, such an immense population exposure makes hepatitis a major concern. There are three possible relationships of hepatitis to NSAIDs:

1. The offending drug is excreted in the liver, is insoluble, and precipitates in the liver. This results in direct liver damage.

2. An idiosyncrasy occurs. The patient has signs of allergy: skin rash, fever, eosinophilia and an enlarged tender liver.

3. The presence of hepatitis is coincidental. Non-A/non-B hepatitis is common, as is alcohol abuse, and NSAIDs are in wide use, so the appearance of hepatitis could be a phenomenon due solely to chance.

We must clearly distinguish between *hepatitis* and *transaminitis*. *Hepatitis* is a disease: the patient is clinically ill; he is jaundiced, febrile, sick, and has abnormal laboratory values etc. *Transaminitis* is the result from an abnormal laboratory test, and the patient is healthy. The *ascertainment* is totally different: hepatitis is an illness, the transaminase is a laboratory report.

Side-effects of Anti-inflammatory Drugs 3. Rainsford KD, Velo GP (eds), Inflammation and Drug Therapy Series, Volume V.

INSOLUBILITY

Benoxaprofen had linear pharmacokinetics and formed crystalline bodies in the urine. Its precipitation in liver and kidney may explain its propensity to cause hepatic and renal failure.

Sulindac is also very insoluble and does occasionally produce an unusual granulomatous hepatitis. Surveys in Denmark [1], Sweden [2] and France [3] have shown this drug does have the highest rate of hepatotoxicity of any NSAID. Two years ago the United States Food and Drug Administration knew of 437 cases, and four deaths. Sulindac is excreted in the liver; the drug does cause gall stones, renal stones, and acute pancreatitis [4,5]. The liver reaction is probably due to precipitation of sulindac in the liver parenchyma, rather than an idiosyncratic reaction, although definite idiosyncrasy has been reported. The occurrence of transaminitis with sulindac may be dose related [6]. The frequency of the phenomena is emphasized by reports of two or more cases from a single institution [7,8].

IDIOSYNCRASY

Hepatitis due to NSAIDs is a rare event. In 1984, I reviewed the world's literature and found 16 cases due to NSAIDs in now common use in the United States (this excludes indomethacin and phenylbutazone) [9]. No patient died and eleven had evidence of hypersensitivity. From 1986 to 1990, I found 12 further cases, with three deaths. Over a fifteen-year period there was an average of 2 reports per year, with a death reported every other year. These cases are so rare that this is *less* than would be expected in the 2% of the population of western countries receiving NSAIDs who are exposed to hepatotoxic viruses and consume excessive amounts of alcohol.

True idiosyncrasy (as defined by eosinophilia, fever, skin rash, and an AST/ALT ratio of less than 1) does occur.

Perhaps the most striking case was a female receiving naproxen [10]. On rechallenge with fenoprofen, these events recurred. Striking eosinophilia occurred in a naproxen case with colitis [11]. Renal and hepatic biopsy revealed eosinophils in a diclofenac case [12], while another had renal insufficiency [13]. The case from Israel had a skin biopsy which demonstrated vasculitis. The piroxicam case cleared over one month [15]. All cases were remarkably benign.

This accounts for only one half of cases reported in the past 15 years, and none of the three fatalities. Many of the reports do not have sufficient detail to be certain of the cause. Were any of these cases coincidental – due to background noise?

212

Table 1. Hepatitis due to sulindac (Clinoril)

Insolubility
      Gall stones
      Renal stones
      Acute pancreatitis
      Transaminitis at high doses
      Granulomatous hepatitis
Hypersensitivity
Prevalence
      USA 437 cases known to FDA
      Highest rate of NSAID induced hepatitis
            Sweden
            Denmark
            France

Table 2. Idiosyncratic liver disease due to NSAIDs

Ref.	Drug	Eosinophils	Fever	AST/ALT	Remarks
10	Naproxen	+		0.73	
10	Fenoprofen	+	+	0.93	Rechallenge
11	Naproxen	+ + +		0.42	Colitis
12	Diclofenac	+ + +		?	Acute nephritis
13	Diclofenac	−	−	0.75	Acute nephritis
14	Diclofenac	+ + +	+	?	Skin vasculitis
14	Diclofenac	+	−	?	Rash
15	Piroxicam	+	−	0.48	

Two diclofenac cases developed chronic active hepatitis [16,17], suggesting that they were actually due to non-A/non-B hepatitis. All seven cases in one report of 'hepatotoxicity' had elevated AST/ALT ratios [18]. One died, the other six had mild transaminitis. Another series included two cases of mild transaminitis, without information on AST/ALT ratios, MCV or serum iron levels [17].

The three deaths are all suspicious. The naproxen case [19] had received only 5 naproxen suppositories one month before she became ill – the AST/ALT ratio was 1.73. One Irish case attributed to diclofenac had received indomethacin for two weeks, and had received diclofenac for five weeks [20], while a Spanish case had received indomethacin for 6 weeks, and then piroxicam for 5 days; her death was blamed on piroxicam [21]. No history of falls or aspiration pneumonia is mentioned in the Boston case reported to be due to diclofenac [18]; the AST/ALT ratio was 1.55.

From the small number of case reports, it is obvious that true idiosyncrasy does occur. The remaining case reports suggest viral infection and alcoholism might be the cause of hepatic dysfunction rather than drug

213

induced illness. Jick [22] pointed out that when an illness is rarely induced by a drug, and this same illness is common in the absence of drug therapy, that the discovery of drug-induced disease is extremely difficult or impossible.

Can we trust these individual case reports? In a population the size of the United States (250 000 000), about 2% of the population take NSAIDs (5 000 000). Of these arthritics, 10% abuse alcohol (500 000), idiopathic non-A/non-B hepatitis without needle exposure or transfusion can occur (325). Each year in the world, 2 cases are reported, with a death every other year. Assume only 1 in 100 cases is reported, we would have 400 cases and 50 deaths. But 500 325 arthritis patients have other causes of hepatic dysfunction.

VIRAL INFECTION

In the past we had markers only for hepatitis A and B. The transaminase was a surrogate test for all other viral causes of hepatitis. In the United States in 1987, there were 5949 reports of non-A/non-B hepatitis with 168 deaths in patients with no exposure to blood products or illicit drugs [23]. By sheer change, about 120 of these patients would be on NSAIDs, and 3 would die. The rate of idiopathic non-A/non-B hepatitis would be 2 per 100 000. The careful studies in five countries, suggest this rate may be as high as 6.5 per 100 000 [24]. Multiple hospitalization without transfusion or use of blood products was a major risk in this study.

The older data on hepatitis associated with NSAIDs can be confused because a test for hepatitis C was only recently available, and because viral hepatitis is a true allergic hepatitis, with the AST/ALT ratio less than 1. It is estimated that 40–60% of the 150 000 new cases of hepatitis C are idiopathic [25], with multiple sexual partners being the only risk factor indentified.

ALCOHOLISM

The transaminase is the best surrogate test for alcoholism, since it is easier to interpret than an elevated MCV or the serum iron or transferritin.

Transaminases are protein enzymes, and are much less stable than a metallic ion such as sodium. In normal individuals, transaminase levels fluctuate widely. The National Institutes of Health [26] conducted a detailed study of the variation of duplicate determinations of the blood constituents of 68 normal individuals for 12 consecutive weeks. Thus, they could precisely estimate the individual variation, group variation, and analytical variation over time [27]. After removing all of these sources of variation, the authors could estimate how much of a change in the laboratory test was necessary to reach medical significance.

On duplicate serum specimens, the coefficient of variation was lowest for the sodium: 0.6%. It was highest for the transaminase (AST, SGOT): 10.4%, 17 times greater than the sodium. For the sodium, with a mean of 139.4 mmol/L, a change of 2.0 was considered medically significant. For the transaminase, the duplicate, weekly, and analytical variations were so great that the magnitude of a medically significant change could not be estimated [28].

Age and obesity both raise the level of the aminotransferases [29]. About 3% of the blood collected in the United States is discarded because of transaminitis. Studies of otherwise healthy blood donors with unexplained elevations of aminotransferases reveal that many are alcoholic, some abuse paracetamol (acetaminophen), and some are obese. Liver biopsy in these obese donors often reveal fatty infiltration of the liver [30]. The variability of this test is emphasized by the observation that 4 of 891 patients receiving placebo in rheumatic disease trials were forced to withdraw because of significant hepatotoxicity [31].

The AST/ALT ratio is particularly helpful. Workers in New Zealand [32] have carefully studied liver function during acute alcohol detoxification, and note the AST (ASpartate aminoTransferase or 'SGOT') is characteristically more strikingly elevated than the ALT (ALanine aminoTransferase, or 'SGPT'). The reverse is true in hepatitis B, liver cancer, and obstructive jaundice. For alcoholic hepatitis the ratio of AST/ALT is 1.50, in hepatitis B it is 0.51.

The reason for the high AST/ALT ratio in alcoholics is that these patients often have a poor diet, and are deficient in pyridoxine. ALT has pyridoxine as a coenzyme. Thus the alcoholic patient has difficulty in making ALT, but still can make AST. These effects are well demonstrated by adding pyridoxal 5' phosphate to liver biopsies taken from alcoholic patients, and by changes in the AST/ALT ratios when pyridoxine is added to the diet of chronic alcoholics [33].

Table 3. Alcoholics and pyridoxal-5'-phosphate deficiency

		Liver		Biopsy	
	AST/ALT	AST	ALT	AST	ALT
Before treatment	5.3	524	99		
% change on adding pyridoxal-5'-phosphate				+8.6	+38.2
One month on pyridoxine	2.9	601	207		

215

Careful studies of the AST/ALT ratio have not been published for transaminitis secondary to NSAIDs but data from the arthritis patients in the ARAMIS data base [34] suggest the ratio may be less than 1. For naproxen, 2.46% of 325 AST determinations were elevated, while 4.92% of 183 ALT tests were above normal. Similar trends were seen for salicylates, sulindac and piroxicam.

Alcohol abuse is a far greater problem than viral infection. Eleven percent of the caloric consumption of Americans is alcohol. The Kaiser Permanente health plan estimates that 14% of its male patients and 6% of its female patients abuse alcohol. Six drinks a day doubles the mortality rate, and 3 to 5 drinks increases the rate by 50%. Based on the widespread use of NSAIDs each year in the United States one would expect 1650 deaths due to alcoholism and its complications in patients incidentally receiving NSAIDs.

In the United States the death rate from cirrhosis of the liver is 14.3 per 100 000 for males, and 7.6 for females [36]. Each year about 550 patients with arthritis receiving NSAIDs would be expected to die of alcoholic liver disease.

In any arthritic patient with hepatic abnormalities, a careful search should be made for a high AST/ALT ratio, elevations of the γ-glutamyl transpeptide (GGT), large red cells best detected by an elevated MCV, and a high serum iron or desialylated transferrin. A search for these markers must be carefully made before assuming the damage is due to an NSAID. Further, a careful history of the other sequelae of alcoholism (accidents, falls, aspiration pneumonia) should be sought by history before the episode of abnormal liver function is attributed to the NSAID.

BIASES IN CASE REPORTS

Can we trust individual case reports? In a population the size of the United States (250 000 000), about 2% of the population take NSAIDs (5 000 000). Of these arthritics, 10% abuse alcohol (500 000), and idiopathic non-A/non-B hepatitis without needle exposure or transfusion can occur (1000). Each year in the world, 2 cases are reported with a death every other year. Assume only 1 in 100 cases is reported. We would have 400 cases and 50 deaths. But 501 000 arthritis patients would have other causes of hepatic dysfunction.

To demonstrate these biases, we can study the report of seven cases of 'hepatotoxicity' reported by Helfgott and his associates [18]. The case did not come from a single institution; there being four institutions involved. These cases are 'collected', and the method of collection may be severely biased.

216

Differential referral rates – Berkson's fallacy

Berkson [37] long ago pointed out the fallacy of differential referral rates in retrospective studies: patients with several serious conditions, such as arthritis and abnormal liver function tests are more likely to be referred to major hospital centres. Pseudo-associations may occur. An example of this fallacy follows:

Assume a major medical centre draws on a population of	10 000 000
Serious arthritis requiring NSAID therapy is present in 10% of this population	1 000 000
Non-A/non-B hepatitis not due to transfusion or drug abuse is present in 0.02% of this population	2000

Public Health officials know this rate is 20 cases per 100 000!

Our population looks like this:

	No arthritis	Arthritis	Totals
No hepatitis	8 998 200	999 800	9 998 000
Hepatitis	1 800	200	2 000
Totals	9 000 000	1 000 000	10 000 000

If we did a *prospective* study of this population, we would find that the hepatitis rate was the same in the NSAID users as the rest of the population.

Now assume that 1% of this population is referred to our regional medical centre. Some go because of cancer, some to have small cysts removed, some because of arthritis or hepatitis. The population at the referral centre looks like this:

	No arthritis	Arthritis	Totals
No hepatitis	89 982	9 998	99 980
Hepatitis	18	2	20
Totals	90 000	20 000	100 000

It is extremely naive to assume that all diseases would have the same referral rate! Almost every cancer case would appear at our regional centre, while most cysts would be removed locally without referral to a major centre. There are **differential referral rates** depending on the severity of the disease.

217

Hepatitis is a serious illness, as is arthritis. Assume that the referral rates are:

2% of arthritic patients (**4 have hepatitis**)

50% of hepatitis patients (**100 have arthritis**)

Our hospital population now looks like this:

	No arthritis	Arthritis	Totals
No hepatitis	89982	19996	109978
Hepatitis	900	104	1004
Totals	90882	20100	110982

We do a **retrospective** study of our arthritis clinic records and discover that we have **517 cases of hepatitis per 100 000 arthritic patients!** A quick consultation with Public Health Authorities tells us that the rate should be **20** per hundred thousand. We have found a strong association between taking NSAIDs and hepatitis! Should we rush into print?

Perhaps not! There is **no** true association in the population. This is **Berkson's Fallacy**, a pseudo-association due to differential referral rates. This is why we cannot believe Helfgott's [18] collection of cases; it may well be an artifact of differential hospital referral rates!

Further, these cases were collected from several institutions who wished to report their adverse experiences with diclofenac. This raises the question of the 'volunteer effect'.

The volunteer effect

In the National Halothane Study [38] many hospitals who had bad experiences 'volunteered', and demonstrated that halothane was the most dangerous anaesthetic. When hospitals who failed to volunteer were studied, halothane was found to be quite safe. When the volunteer and non-volunteer hospitals were pooled, halothane was exactly in the middle of all anaesthetics in its hepatotoxicity.

This again demonstrates the need for examining a total population, rather than a report from a few selected hospitals.

Deliberate over-reporting for commercial purposes

Voluntary reporting of adverse drug reactions has always resulted in under-reporting. In 1989 a pharmaceutical firm made a grant to the American Liver Foundation which sent a letter to every American physician warning of hepatotoxicity to diclofenac [39]. Many physicians thought that this was an FDA warning.

Helfgott's paper received wide attention and shortly after its publication the FDA has required a 'Dear Doctor' letter to be sent to all American physicians. Immediately after the JAMA report, large numbers of reprints of the Helfgott paper were distributed to physicians in Virginia by pharmaceutical firms which compete against diclofenac. Often FDA form 1639 was left with the report from the Brigham [18] so that further reports of diclofenac hepatotoxicity could be submitted. Surprisingly, when the Brigham and Women's Hospital earlier reported two similar cases with hepatitis in which patients received NSAIDs [40], the liver dysfunction was attributed to underlying rheumatoid disease, and no reprints were distributed by pharmaceutical representatives in this area.

I am concerned that we may see a new era in adverse drug reporting. Whenever a new drug is widely used, a rival drug firm can search through large referral centres, and can find transaminitis and submit reports of 'hepatotoxicity' to a leading journal. The lucrative sale of reprints might offer an inducement to both the author and the journal to generate such reports, when, in fact the transaminitis is because of nothing more than background 'noise' and Berkson's fallacy.

NATIONAL REGISTRIES

National registries for adverse drug reactions provide the best and most unbiased data on hepatitis caused by NSAIDs. The best registries are in Scandinavia. Since Danish and Swedish physicians are required by law to report all adverse effects, these countries have given a highly accurate evaluation of the relative toxicities of various NSAIDs. It is well to remember that Denmark was the first country to recognize the unusual toxicity of benoxaprofen [41].

A careful recent survey of the Danish data [1] did reveal a high reaction rate for sulindac, but failed to demonstrate any unusual reaction rates for other NSAIDs. Wilholm and his associates from the Department of Drugs of the National Board of Health and Welfare of Sweden, also found the highest rate of reactions with sulindac [2], without any unusual rates for other NSAIDs.

Mason and his associates [42] studied all reports made to the United States Food and Drug Administration for an 18 month period after the marketing of diclofenac, and in spite of the considerable commercial stimulus for over-reporting, diclofenac's rates were exactly in the middle of the five most frequently used NSAIDs.

The French data deserves special comment. The consumption of alcohol in France is 13.5 litres of pure alcohol per person per year (in the USA, 8.0). The death rate from liver disease is 18.3 per 100 000 in France (in the USA, 10.2). In all France in 1985, there were about 1 000 000

Table 4. Hepatitis due to NSAIDs in France (Centre de Pharmacovigilance)

NSAID	Incidence of hepatitis per month of treatment	Years of treatment for one case
Sulindac Ibuprofen Indomethacin	1/50 000 to 1/100 000	6 000
Ketoprofen Diclofenac	1/100 000 to 1/300 000	17 000
Piroxicam Flurbiprofen	1/300 000 to 1/500 000	33 000
Naproxen	1/500 000	42 000
Idiopathic non A/non B hepatitis		13 000 to 40 000

patients receiving NSAIDs, with 56 cases of hepatitis due to NSAIDs, and 3 deaths. Of NSAIDs in use in the United States, there were 44 cases and no deaths [3]. These rates reported from France are shown in Table 4.

The data from these national registries clearly indicate that hepatitis due to NSAIDs is a rare event. True allergic hepatitis does occur, but it seems likely that other cases of transaminitis and hepatitis are probably due to natural variation in the serum transaminase and hepatic damage due to viruses and alcohol.

ACKNOWLEDGEMENT

Jane Chapman O'Brien provided expert assistance in typing this manuscript.

REFERENCES

1. Kromann-Anderson H, Pedersen A. Reported adverse reactions to and consumption of nonsteroidal anti-inflammatory drugs in Denmark over a 17-year period. Dan Med Bull. 1988;35:187–192.
2. Wiholm BE, Myrhed M, Ekman E. Trends and patterns in adverse drug reactions to non-steroidal anti-inflammatory drugs reported in Sweden. In: Rainsford KD, Velo GP (eds.), Side-effects of anti-inflammatory drugs, Vol. 1. Lancaster: MTP Press:1987:55–72.
3. Castot A, Netter P, Larrey D, Carlier P, Gaire M, Bannwarth B. Hepatites aux anti-inflammatories non-steroidiens. Bilan cooperatif des centres regionaux de pharmacovigilance pour l'annee 1985. Therapie. 1988;43:229–233.
4. Zimmerman H. Update on hepatotoxicity due to classes of drugs in common clinical use: non-steroidal drugs, anti-inflammatory drugs, antibiotics, antihypertensives, and cardiac and psychotropic drugs. Sem Liv Dis. 1990;10:322–338.
5. U.S. Food and Drug Administration. Meeting of the Arthritis Advisory Committee May 28, 1988.

6. Atkinson M, Germain G, Lee P. The efficacy and safety of sulindac (400 mg vs 600 mg daily) in rheumatoid arthritis. A Canadian multicentre study. J Rheumatol. 1988;15:1001–1004.

7. Whittaker SJ, Amar JN, Wanless IR et al. Sulindac hepatotoxicity. Gut. 1982;23:875–877.

8. Wood LJ, Searle J, Mundo F et al. Sulindac hepatotoxicity: effects of acute and chronic exposure. Aust NZ J Med. 1985;15:397–401.

9. O'Brien WM, Bagby GF. Rare adverse reactions to nonsteroidal anti-inflammatory drugs. J Rheumatol. 1985;12:13–20, 347–353, 562–567, 785–790.

10. Andrejak M, Davion T, Gineston JL, Capron JP. Cross hepatotoxicity between non-steroidal anti-inflammatory drugs. Br Med J. 1987;295:180–181.

11. Bridges AJ, Marshall JB, Diaz-Arias AA. Acute eosinophilic colitis and hypersensitivity reaction associated with naproxen therapy. Am J Med. 1990;89:526–527.

12. Diggory P, Golding RL, Lancaster R. Renal and hepatic impairment in association with diclofenac administration. Postgrad Med J. 1989;65:507–508.

13. Hovette P, Touze JE, Debonne B et al. Hepatite cholestatique et insuffisance renale aigue au cours d'un traitement par diclofenac. Ann Gastroenterol Hepatol. 1989;25:257–258.

14. Schapira D, Bassan L, Nahir AM, Scharf Y. Diclofenac-induced hepatotoxicity. Postgrad Med J. 1986;62:63–65.

15. Caballeria E, Masso RM, Arago JV, Sanchis. Piroxicam hepatotoxicity. Am J Gastroenterol. 1990;85:898–899.

16. Mazeika PK, Ford MJ. Chronic active hepatitis associated with diclofenac sodium therapy. Br J Clin Pract. 1989;43:125–126.

17. Iveson TJ, Ryley NG, Kelly PM, McGee JO, Chapman RW. Diclofenac associated hepatitis. J Hepatol. 1990;10:85–89.

18. Helfgott SM, Sandberg-Cook J, Zakin D, Nestler J. Diclofenac-associated hepatotoxicity. JAMA. 1990;264:2660–2662.

19. Giarelli L, Falconieri G, Delendi M. Fulminant hepatitis following naproxen administration. Hum Pathol. 1986;11:1019.

20. Breen EG, McNicholl J, Cosgrove E et al. Fatal hepatitis associated with diclofenac. Gut. 1986;27:1390–1393.

21. Planas R, De Leon R, Quer JC et al. Fatal submassive necrosis of the liver associated with piroxicam. Am J Gastroenterol. 1990;85:468–470.

22. Jick H. The discovery of drug-induced illness. N Engl J Med. 1977;296:481–485.

23. Centre for Disease Control. Non-A/non-B hepatitis rates. MMWR. 1988;36:840.

24. Francis DP, Hadler SC, Prendergast TJ et al. Occurrence of hepatitis A,B and Non-A/Non-B in the United States. Am J Med. 1984;76:69–74.

25. Alter MJ, Coleman PJ, Alexander WJ et al. Importance of heterosexual activity in the transmission of hepatitis B and non-A, non-B hepatitis. JAMA. 1989;262:1201–1205.

26. Williams GZ, Young DS, Stein MR, Cotlove E. Biological and analytic components of variation in long-term studies of serum constituents in normal subjects. I. Objectives, subject selection, laboratory procedures and estimation of analytic deviation. Clin Chem. 1970;16:1016–1021.

27 Harris EK, Kanofsky P, Shakarji G, Cotlove E. Biological and analytical components of variation in long-term studies of serum constituents in normal subjects. II. Estimating biological components of variation. Clin Chem. 1970;16:1022–1027.

28. Cotlove E, Harris EK, Williams GZ. Biological and analytical components of variation in long-term studies of serum constituents in normal subjects. III. Physiological and medical implications. Clin Chem. 1970;16:1028–1321.

29. Siest G, Schiele F, Galteau M et al. Aspartate aminotransferase and alanine aminotransferase activities in plasma: statistical distributions, individual variations, and reference values. Clin Chem. 1975;21:1077–1087.

30. Hultcrantz R, Glaumann H, Lindberg G, Nilsson HS. Liver investigation in 149 asymptomatic patients with moderately elevated activities of serum aminotransferase. Scand J Gastroenterol. 1986;21:109–113.

31. Felson DT, Anderson JJ, Meenan RF. The comparative efficacy and toxicity of second-line drugs in rheumatoid arthritis. Arthritis Rheum. 1990;33:1449–1461.

32. Kawachi I, Robinson GM, Stace NH. A combination of raised serum AST:ALT ratio and erythrocyte mean cell volume level detects excessive alcohol consumption. NZ Med J. 1990;103:145–148.

33. Diehl AM, Potter J, Boitnott J, van Duyn MA, Herlong HF, Mezey E. Relationship between pyridoxal 5-phosphate deficiency and aminotransferase levels in alcoholic hepatitis. Gastroenterology. 1984;86:632–636.

34. Fries JF, Singh G, Lenert L, Furst DE. Aspirin, hydroxychloroquine, and hepatic enzyme abnormalities with methotrexate in rheumatoid arthritis. Arthritis Rheum. 1990;33:1611–1619.

35. Klatsky AL, Friedman GD, Siegelaub AB. Alcohol and mortality. Ann Intern Med. 1981;95:139–145.

36. Center for Disease Control. Deaths from chronic liver disease – United States, 1986. MMWR. 1989;38:46–49.

37. Berkson J. Limitations of the application of fourfold table analysis to hospital data. Biometrics Bull. 1946;2:47–55.

38. The National Halothane Study. Possible associations between halothane anesthesia and postoperative hepatic necrosis. JAMA. 1966;197:775–788.

39. American Liver Foundation. Hepatotoxicity Update. Considerations when selecting a nonsteroidal anti-inflammatory drug. San Francisco: Professional Health Care Communications [updated].

40. Roberts WN, Coblyn JS. Rheumatoid arthritis and granulomatous hepatitis: a new association. J Rheumatol. 1983;10:969–972.

41. Pedersen A. More light on the side effects of benoxaprofen (Translation from Danish). Ugeskr Laeger. 1982;144:2236–2237.

42. Mason DH, Bernstein J, Bortnichak EA, Ehrlich GE. Spontaneous reporting of adverse drug reactions: diclofenac sodium and four other leading NSAIDs. Intern Med Specialist. 1990;11:1–8.

27

Current status of nephrotoxicity caused by non-steroidal anti-inflammatory drugs

L.F. Prescott and U. Martin

University Department of Clinical Pharmacology, The Royal Infirmary, Edinburgh, EH3 9YW, Scotland

INTRODUCTION

The potential of the non-narcotic analgesics to cause renal damage has long been recognized. Thus the salicylates and pyrazolone analgesics such as amidopyrine were known to cause fluid retention and impairment of renal function at the beginning of the century and similar problems were encountered with phenylbutazone soon after its introduction some 40 years ago [1,2]. In the 1950s an association was noted between chronic excessive consumption of combination analgesics and a form of chronic interstitial nephritis [3] and subsequently analgesic nephropathy became established as a major problem in many countries [4]. Papillary necrosis was recognized as the primary renal lesion, and at the time, phenacetin was universally incriminated as the causal agent on the basis of the common denominator theory. It has since become obvious that phenacetin itself played only a minor aetiological role, and that the typical changes of analgesic nephropathy can be produced more readily in experimental animals and man by salicylates and the non-steroidal anti-inflammatory drugs [5,6].

The more recent discovery that many of the actions of aspirin and other non-steroidal anti-inflammatory analgesics are mediated by inhibition of prostaglandin synthesis [7] has led to renewed interest in their effects on the kidney, and in particular, their role in the control of the renal circulation [8–10]. The potential of these drugs to cause serious nephrotoxicity is now widely accepted and many cases have been reported in recent years. Several different mechanisms may be involved, and as a result the clinical presentations and pathological features vary.

Side-effects of Anti-inflammatory Drugs 3. Rainsford KD, Velo GP (eds),
Inflammation and Drug Therapy Series, Volume V.

PROSTAGLANDIN-DEPENDENT ACUTE IMPAIRMENT OF RENAL FUNCTION

Although renal blood flow, glomerular filtration and the tubular reabsorption of water and electrolytes may all be influenced by the action of renal prostaglandins, the non-steroidal anti-inflammatory drugs have no significant effect on renal function in healthy adults under normal conditions because the actions of powerful vasodilator prostaglandins (PGs) such as PGE_2 and I_2 (prostacyclin) are not necessary for the maintenance of renal blood flow. However, non-steroidal anti-inflammatory agents can cause major impairment of renal function in predisposed individuals in whom renal blood flow is already compromised because of conditions such as underlying renal disease, systemic lupus erythematosus, cardiac failure, hypertension, renal artery stenosis, patent ductus arteriosus, diabetes, gout, hepatic cirrhosis, myeloma, infection, dehydration, hypovolaemia, sodium depletion, other drug therapy (especially with diuretics), surgery, relief of urinary retention and the extremes of age. In many of these conditions the production of vasoconstrictors such as angiotensin II, noradrenaline and antidiuretic hormone is increased to support blood pressure and these effects may be balanced by a corresponding increase in the synthesis of vasodilator prostaglandins which then play a vital role in maintaining renal perfusion [e.g. refs. 11–29]. Deterioration in renal function secondary to decreased prostaglandin synthesis is probably the commonest adverse effect of the non-steroidal anti-inflammatory drugs on the kidney. The onset is rapid, and within limits, the decline in renal function is dose-dependent [20,30]. The changes are usually reversible on withdrawal of the offending drug and are often reassuringly described as 'functional'. However, this 'functional' impairment can progress to ischaemic tubular necrosis with acute irreversible renal failure and fatalities have been recorded [31–33].

FLUID RETENTION, HYPONATRAEMIA AND HYPERKALAEMIA

These adverse effects are also thought to be mediated by the actions of non-steroidal anti-inflammatory drugs on the renal prostaglandins which are involved in water and sodium balance [10,24,34]. Fluid retention with weight gain and oedema is a common complication of the use of these drugs and overt cardiac failure with pulmonary oedema may be precipitated even in patients with previously normal cardiac function. Haemodilution contributes to the hyponatraemia which is more likely to occur in the presence of predisposing factors such as underlying renal disease and concomitant therapy with diuretics. These abnormalities of fluid and sodium balance are of particular importance in the elderly and in patients with cardiovascular, hepatic and renal disease [35,36]. It is not surprising that many clinically significant adverse interactions have been described between the non-steroidal anti-inflammatory agents and cardiovascular drugs (see below).

The non-steroidal anti-inflammatory drugs can also cause severe life-threatening hyperkalaemia in a setting of hyporeninaemic hypoaldosteronism, and repeated episodes have been described in some patients [17,37]. It can occur in patients with normal renal function, but renal disease, old age and concomitant intake of potassium supplements or potassium-retaining diuretics are important predisposing factors [13,38,39]. It has been suggested that non-steroidal anti-inflammatory drugs are a risk factor for sudden death in marathon runners because they may potentiate hyperkalaemia induced by strenuous exercise and dehydration [40].

ACUTE INTERSTITIAL NEPHRITIS

This condition is characterized by progressive renal failure during the first few weeks after starting treatment with a non-steroidal anti-inflammatory drug. In some cases there are no obvious predisposing factors and interstitial nephritis may appear to follow on from the early acute deterioration in renal function described above. There is often oliguria and in some patients there is proteinuria in the range associated with the nephrotic syndrome [41]. Less often, multisystem involvement or eosinophilia may point to an allergic or immunological mechanism [42]. Renal function usually improves when the drug is discontinued but recovery can be slow and incomplete [29,39,43–45]. Irreversible fatal renal failure has been described [31,33]. Drug-induced interstitial nephritis may be superimposed on the changes caused by other conditions in which the kidney is involved, such as systemic lupus erythematosus [21].

The histological appearances in acute interstitial nephritis caused by non-steroidal anti-inflammatory drugs include a dense inflammatory infiltrate of lymphocytes, plasma cells and in some cases, eosinophils, with diffuse interstitial oedema and tubular degeneration and atrophy [41,42]. These changes may be associated with glomerulosclerosis [41,46,47] and granulomas have been described [48]. In patients with long standing renal impairment the picture is likely to be complicated further by the development of interstitial fibrosis [11].

NEPHROTIC SYNDROME

The nephrotic syndrome is a less common manifestation of non-steroidal inflammatory nephrotoxicity and it usually has a delayed insidious onset after treatment for several months. It seems most likely to occur in patients with pre-existing renal disease, those taking diuretics and the elderly, but it has also been described in the young [49]. The heavy proteinuria usually disappears on withdrawal of the drug concerned, but may return if it is reintroduced [50]. Histological abnormalities include minimal change glomerulopathy, mild mesangial prominence and glomerulosclerosis together with variable tubular damage, interstitial infiltration and oedema [33,49,51,52]. In some cases the appearances resemble those of acute interstitial nephritis and the appearance of large numbers of T lymphocytes in interstitial infiltrates may suggest an immunologically mediated cytotoxic reaction [41,53,54]. The drugs implicated as a cause of the nephrotic syndrome include fenoprofen, ibuprofen, naproxen, indomethacin, phenylbutazone, alclofenac* and tolmetin [55,56].

ANALGESIC NEPHROPATHY (RENAL PAPILLARY NECROSIS AND CHRONIC INTERSTITIAL NEPHRITIS)

The syndrome of analgesic nephropathy was originally described in patients who had abused analgesic combinations containing phenacetin [3]. It is characterized by insidious, slowly progressive renal failure which may be discovered incidentally. In other cases, attention may be drawn to the kidney by episodes of recurrent loin pain and haematuria caused by necrosis of papillae, or by pyelonephritis, urinary obstruction, hypertension or the development of uroepithelial tumours or end-stage renal failure. The primary renal lesion of analgesic nephropathy is papillary necrosis, but secondary changes in the corresponding cortex progress to give a picture which resembles chronic interstitial nephritis. Over a period of years further changes result in the generalized non-specific fibrosis and destruction of end-stage renal disease [6].

In the early reports, the combination analgesics abused by these patients invariably contained phenacetin and it is not surprising that it was quickly singled out for blame. However, this drug was never taken alone and it has subsequently been shown that both phenacetin and paracetamol (its major metabolite) are probably the safest non-narcotic analgesics as far as the kidney is concerned. Thus renal papillary necrosis is more readily produced by the other drugs with which the phenacetin was necessarily taken although the latter agent had central nervous system effects which may have resulted in abuse [5]. The long-term use of non-steroidal anti-inflammatory drugs in the treatment of arthritis is clearly associated with the risk of development of chronic renal failure, and most, if not all of these drugs can cause renal papillary necrosis with all the predisposing factors and typical features of analgesic nephropathy [6,11,57–67]. The mechanism

---

*discontinued

is probably related to chronic damage to tubular structures in the renal papilla and inner medulla caused by ischaemia secondary to inhibition of prostaglandin synthesis.

Recent studies have again confirmed the association between heavy chronic consumption of combination analgesics and chronic renal disease [68,69]. However, these findings certainly do not imply that phenacetin (or paracetamol) necessarily played an exclusive aetiological role. Studies have consistently shown a very high incidence of papillary necrosis in patients with rheumatoid arthritis [6], and chronic renal failure due to the long-term use of non-steroidal anti-inflammatory drugs cannot be distinguished on clinical or pathological grounds from the condition which was formerly known as analgesic nephropathy [70].

OBSTRUCTIVE UROPATHY

Most non-steroidal anti-inflammatory drugs and their active metabolites are weak organic acids and as such they are potential substrates for active tubular transport. They may compete with other anions for active tubular secretion and reabsorption, and on this basis, drugs such as phenylbutazone may have a potent uricosuric action. Under conditions of low urine flow rate and low pH, uric acid may precipitate in the renal tubules and collecting system resulting in crystalluria, acute loin pain, and haematuria followed by oliguria and anuria [71]. There have been recent reports of a similar syndrome following the use of suprofen. It occurred most often in young men and was associated with the use of other analgesics (especially ibuprofen), physical activity and exposure to sun [72,73]. Multiple ureteric strictures and retroperitoneal fibrosis are rare complications of analgesic nephropathy [5].

RENAL DRUG INTERACTIONS

Many important interactions between non-steroidal anti-inflammatory agents and other drugs have been recognized, and most have been obvious in retrospect. Reversal of the blood pressure-lowering effects of hydrochlorothiazide and guanethidine by phenylbutazone and related drugs in hypertensive patients was reported nearly 25 years ago [74], and in recent years there have been numerous further reports of similar antagonism of the action of diuretics and other drugs used in the treatment of hypertension and cardiac failure [75–81 and many others]. These important interactions are common and the mechansims are presumably related to the fluid and sodium retention induced by non-steroidal anti-inflammatory drugs. Severe life-threatening hyponatraemia and water intoxication was reported in a 68-year-old man with myeloma who was given low-dose cyclophosphamide in combination with indomethacin [82]. The basis for this interaction, if real, is obscure. It can also be predicted that hyperkalaemia associated with the latter drugs could be potentiated to a dangerous degree in patients who are also prescribed angiotensin converting enzyme (ACE) inhibitors, potassium-retaining diuretics and potassium supplements.

Another important group of non-steroidal anti-inflammatory drug interactions involves the potentiation of toxicity of drugs which have a low therapeutic ratio and which depend primarily on renal excretion for elimination from the body. In these circumstances it is obvious that drug accumulation and toxicity may occur if the renal clearance of such drugs is reduced by the non-steroidal anti-inflammatory agents. The possible mechanisms of renal interactions with these drugs include reduction in glomerular filtration rate and renal blood flow, competition for active renal tubular secretion, and in some cases, mutual potentiation of nephrotoxicity. Examples of drugs which might be involved in such interactions include lithium [83–85], cyclosporin [86–88], methotrexate [89–91], cisplatin [92], cadmium [93], ACE inhibitors [94] and digoxin [95]. Triamterene causes disastrous potentiation of the nephrotoxicity of indomethacin to the extent that the combination can induce acute renal failure even in healthy young adults [96]. The mechanism is unknown. Probenicid can compete with drugs such as indomethacin, naproxen, diflunisal and ketoprofen for biliary or renal excretion [79] but any such interaction is unlikely to be of great clinical significance. Finally, there have been two recent reports in which it has been suggested that the nephrotoxicity of glafenine and floctafenine may be potentiated by ethanol [97,98].

ARE ALL NON-STEROIDAL ANTI-INFLAMMATORY DRUGS NEPHROTOXIC?

All non-steroidal anti-inflammatory drugs seem able to cause the acute adverse renal effects mediated by inhibition of prostaglandin synthesis. Sulindac is said to have less effect on renal prostaglandins than the other drugs, but reports have been inconsistent in this respect [19,99–101]. However, sulindac can cause significant impairment of renal function [20,28] and hyponatraemia [102] and it antagonizes the actions of drugs such as frusemide [75] and labetolol [81]. The renal effects of the non-steroidal anti-inflammatory drugs which are mediated by prostaglandins are probably dose-dependent [30] and in keeping with this, acute renal failure is a recognized complication of gross overdosage with these drugs [103]. The non-steroidal anti-inflammatory drugs all seem able to produce renal papillary necrosis and the typical lesions of analgesic nephropathy [5,6].

Not all non-steroidal anti-inflammatory drugs have been reported to cause the other syndromes of renal toxicity. Thus reports of obstructive uropathy caused by uric acid crystalluria have been limited to phenylbutazone and suprofen, and so far, relatively few drugs have been implicated as a cause of the nephrotic syndrome (see above).

Paracetamol differs from the non-steroidal anti-inflammatory drugs in a number of respects and it is not normally considered to share their adverse effects on the kidney or to have important effects on prostaglandins. Paracetamol seems not to antagonize the action of antihypertensive drugs [76] but variable effects on inhibition of renal prostaglandin synthesis have been reported. In one study in healthy young women, paracetamol had no significant effect on urinary prostaglandin E_2 excretion [104] and similar findings were reported by Berg et al. [105] in young subjects. The latter investigators observed moderate depression of urinary prostaglandin E_2 in healthy elderly subjects and patients with chronic renal failure but sodium excretion was reduced only in the elderly. In contrast, the administration of 4.0 g of paracetamol daily for 3 days under conditions of controlled fluid and sodium intake in healthy female volunteers resulted in a highly significant reduction in urinary prostaglandin E_2 and sodium output which was similar to that produced by indomethacin. Paracetamol also delayed the onset of diuresis after an acute water load [106]. There was no effect on glomerular filtration rate or renal blood flow in any of these studies. In another study, paracetamol significantly reduced the transient increase in urinary prostaglandin E_2 excretion and plasma renin activity induced by frusemide in healthy females, but it had no effect on natriuresis and diuresis [107].

Despite these findings, and the demonstration that paracetamol can be converted to the same highly reactive potentially cytotoxic metabolite in the kidney as is responsible for hepatic necrosis following overdosage [108], there is very little evidence of serious nephrotoxicity with normal clinical use of the drug. However, acute tubular necrosis is a recognized complication of overdosage [109]. Paracetamol is clearly not a major cause of analgesic nephropathy even though there is widespread deep suspicion on the grounds that it is the major metabolite of phenacetin [5]. In spite of the enormous scale of its use in many countries, there have been very few reports of analgesic nephropathy caused by paracetamol alone [110] or acute impairment of renal function following its normal use [111].

INCIDENCE

The true incidence of serious adverse renal effects caused by nonnarcotic analgesics is unknown, but overall it is probably low in relation to their extensive use. In a controlled longitudinal study of the use of mixed non-prescription analgesics containing phenacetin over 20 years in a group of

Swiss working women, the absolute incidence of impaired renal function was very low, but there was a highly significant increase in the risk of death not only from renal disease, but also from cancer and cardiovascular disease [69]. The incidence of nephrotoxicity is much higher in the elderly and susceptible individuals taking non-steroidal anti-inflammatory drugs. Thus, in a retrospective survey in a large medical practice, impairment of renal function was observed in 343 of 1908 (18%) of patients given ibuprofen [112], while in 15 of 114 elderly institutionalized subjects, the blood urea nitrogen concentration increased by a mean of 89% within 5 to 7 days of starting treatment with ibuprofen, sulindac, piroxicam or naproxen [20]. A similar very high incidence of renal impairment was observed in a comparative study of ibuprofen, sulindac and piroxicam given for 11 days to 12 patients with mild stable chronic renal failure [28].

The rank order of the nephrotoxic potential of different non-steroidal anti-inflammatory drugs is unknown. The relative number of cases reported in the literature is no indication, and the data obtained from the spontaneous adverse reaction reporting systems of Drug Regulatory Authorities must be interpreted with great caution. The number of reports is obviously dependent on the scale of use of the different drugs, and this vital prescribing information is not available. Reporting rates are much higher for recently introduced than for old established drugs, and the rate can be greatly influenced by publicity in both the medical and lay press. Only a very small fraction of the total number of events is notified, and reporting rates for hospital doctors in the United Kingdom are even lower than those for general practitioners. There is no proof that a reaction was caused by a particular drug, and interpretation is made more difficult by the presence of underlying disease and polypharmacy.

Despite all these problems, the data from spontaneous reporting systems can have limited utility, and one approach is to express the number of reports of a particular event as a fraction of the total number of reports attributed to that drug. Such data is clearly still subject to major bias, but limited comparisons can be made between drugs. The number of cases which could be interpreted as adverse renal effects to currently available non-steroidal anti-inflammatory drugs which were reported to the Committee on Safety of Medicines up to July 1990 are shown in Figure 1 [Committee on Safety of Medicines, personal communication]. The data are expressed as a fraction of the total number of reactions reported for each drug. It is obvious that adverse renal reactions account for only a small proportion of the total number of reports for most of these drugs, and that the relative rates are somewhat higher for diclofenac, naproxen, fenoprofen, azapropazone, fenbufen, and notably much higher for mefenamic acid. It is not known whether these different rates represent true differences in the incidence of nephrotoxicity caused by these drugs.

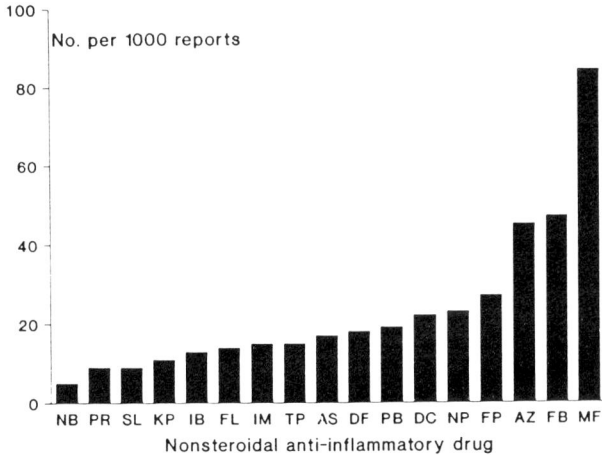

Figure 1. Number of reports relating to nephrotoxicity made to the British Committee on Safety of Medicines for non-steroidal anti-inflammatory drugs up to July 1990. The numbers are expressed as a rate per 1000 reports of all reactions involving each drug. The total number of reports is given in brackets after the key for each drug: NB = nabumetone (1152), PR = piroxicam (3558), SL = sulindac (642), KP = ketoprofen (1607), IB = ibuprofen (2522), FL = flurbiprofen (1318), IM = indomethacin (3842), TP = tiaprofenic acid (995), AS = aspirin (891), DF = diflunisal (965), PB = phenylbutazone (1746), DC = diclofenac (2777), NP = naproxen (2898), FP = fenoprofen (512), AZ = azapropazone (621), FB = fenbufen (720), MF = mefenamic acid (1574)

REFERENCES

1. Hanzlik PJ, Scott RW, Reycraft JL. The salicylates. VIII. Salicyl edema. Arch Intern Med. 1917;20:329–340.
2. Burns JJ, Rose RK, Chenkin T, Goldman A, Schulert A, Brodie BB. The physiological disposition of phenylbutazone in man and a method for its estimation in biological material. J Pharmacol Exp Ther. 1953;109:346–357.
3. Spühler O, Zollinger HU. Die chronische interstitielle Nephritis. Z Klin Med. 1953;151:1–50.
4. Kincaid-Smith P. Analgesic nephropathy: a common form of renal disease in Australia. Med J Aust. 1969;2:1131–1135.
5. Prescott LF. Analgesic nephropathy: a reassessment of the role of phenacetin and other analgesics. Drugs. 1982;23:75–149.
6. Kincaid-Smith P. Renal toxicity of non-narcotic analgesics: at-risk patients and prescribing applications. Med Toxicol Adverse Drug Exp. 1986;1(Suppl. 1):14–22.
7. Ferreira SH, Moncada S, Vane JR. Indomethacin and aspirin abolish prostaglandin release from the spleen. Nature. 1971;231:237–239.
8. Kimberly RP, Sherman RL, Mouradian J, Lockshin MD. Apparent acute renal failure associated with therapeutic aspirin and ibuprofen administration. Arth Rheum. 1979;22:281–285.
9. Dunn MJ, Zambraski EJ. Renal effects of drugs that inhibit prostaglandin synthesis. Kidney Int. 1980;18:609–622.
10. Clive DM, Stoff JS. Renal syndromes associated with non-steroidal anti-inflammatory drugs. N Engl J Med. 1984;310:563–572.

11. Adams DH, Howie AJ, Michael J, McConkey B, Bacon PA, Adu D. Non-steroidal anti-inflammatory drugs and renal failure. Lancet. 1986;1:57–60.
12. Atkinson LK, Goodship THJ, Ward MK. Acute renal failure associated with acute pyelonephritis and consumption of non-steroidal anti-inflammatory drugs. Br Med J. 1986;292:97–98.
13. Andrejak M, Makdassi R, Fievet P, Coevoet B, Lambrey G, Bataille P, Sebert JL, Fournier A. Toxicité rénale des anti-inflammatoires non-stéroïdiens et de la clométacine. Thérapie. 1986;41:331-337.
14. Blackshear JL, Napier JS, Davidman M, Stillman MT. Renal complications of non-steroidal anti-inflammatory drugs: identification and monitoring of those at risk. Sem Arth Rheum. 1985;14:163–175.
15. Brater DC. Adverse effects of non-steroidal anti-inflammatory drugs on renal function. Ann Int Med. 1990;112:559–560.
16. Carmichael J, Shankel SW. Effects of non-steroidal anti-inflammatory drugs on prostaglandins and renal function. Am J Med. 1985;78:992–1000.
17. Corwin HL, Bonventre JV. Renal insufficiency associated with non-steroidal anti-inflammatory agents. Am J Kid Dis. 1984;4:147–152.
18. Demandt E, Legius E, Devlieger H, Lemmens F, Proesmans W, Eggermont E. Prenatal indomethacin toxicity in one member of monozygous twins: a case report. Eur J Obst Gynecol Reprod Biol. 1990;35:267–269.
19. Eriksson L-O, Sturfelt G, Thysell H, Wollheim FA. Effects of sulindac and naproxen on prostaglandin excretion in patients with impaired renal function and rheumatoid arthritis. Am J Med. 1990;89:313–321.
20. Gurwitz JH, Avorn J, Ross-Degnan O, Lipsitz LA. Nonsteroidal anti-inflammatory drug-associated azotemia in the very old. JAMA. 1990;264:471–475.
21. Ling BN, Bourke E, Campbell WH, Delaney VB. Naproxen-induced nephropathy in systemic lupus erythematosus. Nephron. 1990;54:249–255.
22. Loeffler M, Hanson G, Philp T. Piroxicam-induced renal failure following relief of chronic retention. Br J Urol. 1989;63:438–439.
23. Menkes CJ. Renal and hepatic effects of NSAIDs in the elderly. Scand J Rheumatol. 1989;18(Suppl. 83-1):11–14.
24. Seyberth HW. Die Bedeutung der renalen Prostaglandine für die Nierenfunktion im frühen Kindesalter. Monatsschr Kinderheilkd. 1987;135:178–184.
25. Shpilberg O, Douer D, Ehrenfeld M, Engelberg S, Ramot B. Naproxen-associated fatal acute renal failure in multiple myeloma. Nephron. 1990;55:448–449.
26. Stillman MT. Interaction and selection of therapeutic agents in the elderly. NSAIDs and the ageing kidney. Scand J Rheumatol. 1989;18(Suppl. 82):33–38.
27. ter Borg EJ, De Jong PE, Meijer S, Kallenberg CGM. Renal effects of indomethacin in patients with systemic lupus erythematosus. Nephron. 1989;53:238–243.
28. Whelton A, Stout RL, Spilman PS, Klassen DK. Renal effects of ibuprofen, piroxicam and sulindac in patients with asymptomatic renal failure. A prospective, randomized, crossover comparison. Ann Intern Med. 1990;112:568–576.
29. Velo GP, Milanino R. Nongastrointestinal adverse reactions to NSAIDs. J Rheumatol. 1990;17(Suppl. 20):42–45.
30. Muther RS, Potter DM, Bennett WM. Aspirin-induced depression of glomerular filtration rate in normal humans: role of sodium balance. Ann Intern Med. 1981;94:317–321.
31. Boletis J, Williams RJ, Shortland JR, Brown CB. Irreversible renal failure following mefenamic acid. Nephron. 1989;51:575–576.
32. Itami N. Progressive renal failure despite discontinuation of mefenamic acid. Nephron. 1990;54:281–282.
33. Sarma PSA. Fatal acute renal failure after piroxicam. Clin Nephrol. 1989;31:54.
34. Dunn MJ. Nonsteroidal anti-inflammatory drugs and renal function. Ann Rev Med. 1984;35:411–428.
35. Goodenough GK, Lutz LJ. Hyponatremic hypervolaemia caused by a drug-drug interaction mistaken for a syndrome of inappropriate ADH. J Am Geriat Soc. 1988;36:285–286.

36. Van Den Ouweland FA, Gribnau FWJ, Meyboom RHB. Congestive heart failure due to non-steroidal anti-inflammatory drugs in the elderly. Age Ageing. 1988;17:8–16.
37. Ohguchi Y, Ajifu K, Yoshida K. Repeated episodes of hyperkalaemia induced by non-steroidal anti-inflammatory drugs in a patient with rheumatoid arthritis. Rinsho Seijinbyo. 1988;18:115.
38. Goldszer RC, Coodley EL, Rosner MJ, Simons WM, Schwartz AB. Hyperkalemia associated with indomethacin. Arch Intern Med. 1981;141:802–804.
39. Reeves WB, Foley RJ, Weinman EJ. Nephrotoxicity from non-steroidal anti-inflammatory drugs. South Med J. 1985;78:318–322.
40. Johnson RB. Use of NSAIDs in long distance runners: a risk factor for sudden death? South Med J. 1989;82:95.
41. Bender WL, Whelton A, Beschorner WE, Darwish MO, Hall-Craggs M, Solez K. Interstitial nephritis, proteinuria, and renal failure caused by non-steroidal anti-inflammatory drugs. Am J Med. 1984;76:1006-1012.
42. Ray PE, Rigolizzo D, Wara DR, Piel CF. Naproxen nephrotoxicity in a 2-year old child. Am J Dis Child. 1988;142:524–525.
43. Buysen JGM, Houthoff HJ, Krediet RT, Arisz L. Acute interstitial nephritis: a clinical and morphological study in 27 patients. Nephrol Dial Transplant. 1990;5:94–99.
44. Levin ML. Patterns of tubulo-interstitial damage associated with non-steroidal anti-inflammatory drugs. Sem Nephrol. 1988;8:55–61.
45. Toto RD. Acute tubulointerstitial nephritis. Am J Med Sci. 1990;299:392–410.
46. Abraham PA, Keane WF. Glomerular and interstitial disease induced by non-steroidal anti-inflammatory drugs. Am J Nephrol. 1984;4:1–6.
47. Porile JL, Bakris GL, Garella S. Acute interstitial nephritis with glomerulopathy due to non-steroidal anti-inflammatory agents. J Clin Pharmacol. 1990;30:468–475.
48. Schwarz A, Krause PH, Keller F, Offerman G, Mihatsch MJ. Granulomatous interstitial nephritis after non-steroidal anti-inflammatory drugs. Am J Nephrol. 1988;8:410–416.
49. Robinson J, Malleson P, Lirenman D, Carter J. Nephrotic syndrome associated with non-steroidal anti-inflammatory drug use in two children. Pediatrics. 1990;85:844–847.
50. Tietjem DP. Recurrence and specificity of nephrotic syndrome due to tolmetin. Am J Med. 1989;87:354–355.
51. Warren GV, Korbet SM, Schwarz MM, Lewis EJ. Minimal change glomerulopathy associated with non-steroidal anti-inflammatory drugs. Am J Kid Dis. 1989;13:127–130.
52. Bander SJ. Reversible renal failure and nephrotic syndrome without interstitial nephritis from zomepirac. Am J Kid Dis. 1985;6:233–236.
53. Finkelstein A, Fraley DS, Stachura I, Feldman HA, Gandy DR, Bourke E. Fenoprofen nephropathy: lipoid nephrosis and interstitial nephritis. A possible T-lymphocyte disorder. Am J Med. 1982;72:81–87.
54. Feinfeld DA, Olesnicky L, Pirani CL, Appel GB. Nephrotic syndrome associated with use of the non-steroidal anti-inflammatory drugs. Nephron. 1984;37:174–179.
55. Kamiya Y, Nakabayashi K, Suzuki M, Motohashi S, Maemura C. A case of concurrent occurrence of acute renal failure and nephrotic syndrome induced by alclofenac. Nippon Naika Gakki Zasshi. 1989;78:60–65.
56. Hoitsma AJ, Wetzels JFM, Koene AP. Drug-induced nephrotoxicity: aetiology, clinical features and management. Drug Safety. 1991;6:131–147.
57. Prescott LF. Renal papillary necrosis and aspirin. Scot Med J. 1969;14:82–85.
58. Gokal R, Matthews DR. Renal papillary necrosis after aspirin and alclofenac. Br Med J. 1977;2:1517–1518.
59. Jackson B, Lawrence JR. Renal papillary necrosis associated with indomethacin and phenylbutazone treated rheumatoid arthritis. Aust N Z J Med. 1978;48:165–167.
60. Husserl FE, Lange RK, Kantrow CM. Renal papillary necrosis and pyelonephritis accompanying fenoprofen therapy. JAMA. 1979;242:1896–1898.
61. Robertson CE, Ford MJ, Van Someren V, Dlugolecka M, Prescott LF. Mefenamic acid nephropathy. Lancet. 1980;2:232–233.
62. Wortmann DW, Kelsch RC, Kuhns L, Sullivan DB, Cassidy JT. Renal papillary necrosis in juvenile rheumatoid arthritis. J Pediatr. 1980;97:37–40.

63. Lourie SH, Denman SJ, Schroeder ET. Association of renal papillary necrosis and ankylosing spondylitis. Arthritis Rheum. 1977;20:917–921.
64. Shah GM, Muhalwas KK, Winer RL. Renal papillary necrosis due to ibuprofen. Arthritis Rheum. 1981;24:1208–1210.
65. Munn E, Lynn KL, Bailey RR. Renal papillary necrosis following regular consumption of non-steroidal anti-inflammatory drugs. N Z Med J. 1982;95:213–214.
66. Erwin L, Jones JMB. Benoxaprofen and papillary necrosis. Br Med J. 1982;285:694.
67. Baillie MD. Renal papillary necrosis in children with chronic arthritis. Am J Dis Child. 1986;140:16–17.
68. Sandler DP, Smith JC, Weinberg CR, Buckalew VM, Dennis VW, Blyth WB, Burgess WP. Analgesic use and chronic renal disease. N Engl J Med. 1989;320:1238–1243.
69. Dubach UC, Rosner B, Sturmer T. An epidemiologic study of abuse of analgesic drugs. Effects of phenacetin and salicylate on mortality and cardiovascular morbidity (1968 to 1987). N Engl J Med. 1991;324:155–160.
70. Rossi E, Menta R, Cambi V. Partially reversible chronic renal failure due to long-term use of non-steroidal anti-inflammatory drugs. Nephrol. Dial Transplant. 1988;3:469–470.
71. Lipsett MB, Goldman R. Phenylbutazone toxicity: report of a case of acute renal failure. Ann Intern Med. 1954;41:1075–1079
72. Hart D, Ward M, Lifschitz MD. Suprofen-related nephrotoxicity: a distinct clinical syndrome. Ann Intern Med. 1987;106:235–238.
73. Strom BL, West SL, Sim E, Carson JL. The epidemiology of the acute flank pain syndrome from suprofen. Clin Pharmacol Ther. 1989;46:693–699.
74. Polak F. Die hemmende Wirkung von Phenylbutazon auf die durch einige Antihypertonica hervorgerufene Blutdrucksenkung bei Hypertonikern. Z Gesamte Inn Med Grenzgeb. 1967;22:375–376.
75. Brater DC, Anderson S, Baird B, Campbell WB. Effects of ibuprofen, naproxen and sulindac on prostaglandins in men. Kidney Int. 1985;27:66–73.
76. Radack KL, Deck CC, Bloomfield SS. Ibuprofen interferes with the efficacy of antihypertensive drugs. Ann Intern Med. 1987;107:628–635.
77. Oates J. Antagonism of antihypertensive drug therapy by non-steroidal anti-inflammatory drugs. Hypertension. 1988;11(Suppl. II):II4–II6.
78. Schoenfeld A, Freedman S, Hod M, Ovadia Y. Antagonism of antihypertensive drug therapy in pregnancy by indomethacin? Am J Obst Gynecol. 1989;161:1204–1205.
79. Weinblatt ME. Drug interactions with non-steroidal anti-inflammatory drugs (NSAIDs). Scand J Rheumatol. 1989;18(Suppl. 83-1):7–10.
80. Sahloul MZ. al-Kick R, Ivanovich P, Mujais SK. Nonsteroidal anti-inflammatory drugs and antihypertensives. Cooperative malfeasance. Nephron. 1990;56:345–352.
81. Abate MA, Neely JL, Layne RD, D'Alessandri R. Interaction of indomethacin and sulindac with labetolol. Br J Clin Pharmacol. 1991;31:363–366.
82. Webberley MJ, Murray JA. Life-threatening acute hyponatraemia induced by low dose cyclophosphamide and indomethacin. Postgrad Med J. 1989;65:950–952.
83. Bailey CE, Stewart JT, McElroy RA. Ibuprofen-induced lithium toxicity. South Med J. 1989;82:1197.
84. Stein G, Robertson M, Nadarajah J. Toxic interactions between lithium and non-steroidal anti-inflammatory drugs. Psychol Med. 1989;18:535–543.
85. Ragheb M. The clinical significance of lithium–non-steroidal anti-inflammatory drug interactions. J Clin Psychopharmacol. 1990;10:350–354.
86. Harris KP, Jenkins D, Walls J. Nonsteroidal anti-inflammatory drugs and cyclosporine a potentially serious adverse interaction. Transplantation. 1988;46:598–599.
87. Sesin GP, O'Keefe E, Roberto P. Sulindac-induced elevation of serum cyclosporine concentration. Clin Pharm. 1989;8:445-446.
88. Branthwaite JP, Nicholls A. Cyclosporin and diclofenac interaction in rheumatoid arthritis. Lancet. 1991;337:252.
89. Thyss A, Milano G, Kubar J, Namer M, Schneider M. Clinical and pharmacokinetic evidence of a life-threatening interaction between methotrexate and ketoprofen. Lancet. 1986;1:256–258.

90. Cassano WF. Serious methotrexate toxicity caused by interaction with ibuprofen. Am J Pediat Hematol Oncol. 1989;11:481–482.
91. Dupius LL, Koren G, Shore A, Silverman ED, Laxer RM. Methotrexate–non-steroidal anti-inflammatory drug interaction in children with arthritis. J Rheumatol. 1990;17:1469–1473.
92. de Gislain C, Dumas M, d'Athis P, Chapuis T, Mayer F, Fargeot P, Guerrin J, Escousse A. Evolution de la creatininemie lors d'injections repétees de cisplatine. Influence des associations médicamenteuses. Thérapie. 1990;45:423–427.
93. Bernard AM, de Russis R, Amor AO, Lauwerys RR. Potentiation of cadmium nephrotoxicity by acetaminophen. Arch Toxicol. 1988;62:291–294.
94. Seelig CB, Maloley PA, Campbell JR. Nephrotoxicity associated with concomitant ACE inhibitor and NSAID therapy. South Med J. 1990;83:1144–1148.
95. Jorgensen HS, Christensen HR, Kampmann JP. Interaction between digoxin and indomethacin or ibuprofen. Br J Clin Pharmacol. 1991;31:108–110.
96. Favre L, Glasson P, Vallotton MB. Reversible acute renal failure from combined triamterene and indomethacin: a study in healthy subjects. Ann Intern Med. 1982;96:317–322.
97. Cledes J, Kermanach P, Guillodo MP, Herve JP. Acute renal insufficiency after the prescription of glafenine: role of concomitant alcohol ingestion. Presse Méd. 1989;18:333.
98. Verdier D. Acute renal failure after ingestion of floctafenine. Possible role of concomitant alcohol absorption. Presse Méd. 1990;19:1463.
99. Patrono C. The role of prostaglandin synthesis inhibition in the renal syndromes associated with non-narcotic analgesics. Med Toxicol Adverse Drug Exp. 1986;1(Suppl. 1):23–33.
100. Swainson CP, Griffiths P, Watson ML. Chronic effects of oral sulindac on renal haemodynamics and hormones in subjects with chronic renal disease. Clin Sci. 1986;70:243–247.
101. Ciabattoni G, Cinotti GA, Pierucci A, Simonetti BM, Manzi M et al. Effects of sulindac and ibuprofen in patients with chronic glomerular disease: evidence for the dependence of renal function on prostacyclin. N Engl J Med. 1984;310:279–283.
102. Chamontin B, Fille A, Salva P, Salvador M. Does selective inhibition of prostaglandins exist? Concerning a case of hyponatraemia with sulindac. Presse Méd. 1988;17:2140–2141.
103. Vale JA, Meredith TJ. Acute poisoning due to non-steroidal anti-inflammatory drugs: clinical features and management. Med Toxicol Adverse Drug Exp. 1986;1:12–31.
104. Bippi H, Frölich JC. Effects of acetylsalicylic acid and paracetamol alone and in combination on prostanoid synthesis in man. Br J Clin Pharmacol. 1990;29:305–310.
105. Berg KJ, Djøseland O, Gjellan A, Hundal Ø, Knudsen ER, Rugstad HE, Rønneberg E. Acute effects of paracetamol on prostaglandin synthesis and renal function in normal man and in patients with renal failure. Clin Nephrol. 1990;34:255–262.
106. Prescott LF, Mattison P, Menzies DG, Manson LM. The comparative effects of paracetamol and indomethacin on renal function in healthy female volunteers. Br J Clin Pharmacol. 1990;29:403–412.
107. Martin U, Prescott LF. Interaction of paracetamol with frusemide. Fund Clin Pharmacol. 1991;5:411
108. McMurray RJ, Snodgrass WR, Mitchell JR. Renal necrosis, glutathione depletion and covalent binding after acetaminophen. Toxicol Appl Pharmacol. 1978;46:87–100.
109. Prescott LF. Paracetamol overdosage: pharmacological considerations and clinical management. Drugs. 1983;25:290–314.
110. Segasothy M, Sulieman AB, Puvaneswary M, Rohana A. Paracetamol: a cause for analgesic nephropathy and end-stage renal disease. Nephron. 1988;50:50–54.
111. Gabriel R, Caldwell J, Hartley RB. Acute tubular necrosis caused by therapeutic doses of paracetamol? Clin Nephrol. 1982;18:269–271.
112. Murray MD, Brater DC, Tierney WM, Hui SL, McDonald CJ. Ibuprofen-associated renal impairment in a large general internal medicine practice. Am J Med Sci. 1990;299:222–229.

28

Are oral prostaglandins effective in preventing nephrotoxicity from NSAIDs and cyclosporin?

Fabio Cominelli

Department of Medicine, Division of Gastrointestinal and Liver Diseases, University of Southern California, School of Medicine, Los Angeles, CA 90033, USA

INTRODUCTION

Prostaglandins are modulators of renal excretory function via alterations of intrarenal perfusion pressures and the distribution of blood flow. The predominant renal prostaglandins are prostacyclin (PGI_2), prostaglandin E_2 (PGE_2) and $PGF_{2\alpha}$. Medullary synthesis exceeds cortical synthesis five to ten fold, although PGI_2 appears to be maximally produced in the cortex [1–3]. The regulation of basal prostaglandin production is still poorly understood, but renal injury readily augments output. This appears to be true independent of the mechanism of injury, whether by ischaemia, obstructive uropathy, toxic exposure or immunological disturbance [4,5]. Renal vasoconstriction markedly accelerates prostaglandin synthesis and release, and chronic renal damage is usually characterized by an elevation in renal vascular resistance. In addition, the infusion of exogenous vasoconstrictors such as angiotensin II or norepinephrine elicits release of the vasodilator PGE_2 [4]. Under normal volume replete conditions renal function is to a very limited, if any extent dependent on endogenous prostaglandin synthesis. When maintenance of renal circulation is stressed by vasoconstricting hormones or by diminished circulating volume, then endogenous prostaglandin production becomes critically important in the maintenance of a normal renal blood flow (RBF) and glomerular filtration rate (GFR).

Side-effects of Anti-inflammatory Drugs 3. Rainsford KD, Velo GP (eds), Inflammation and Drug Therapy Series, Volume V.

MISOPROSTOL AND NSAID-INDUCED NEPHROTOXICITY IN PATIENTS WITH CIRRHOSIS AND ASCITES

Renal hemodynamics are frequently abnormal or unstable in patients with cirrhosis and ascites [6,7]. Renal function may deteriorate abruptly if plasma volume is reduced by bleeding, diuresis or paracentesis [6,7]. Vasodilatory prostaglandins oppose the renal effects of vasoconstrictors, such as angiotensin II and norepinephrine, in order to maintain renal perfusion and sodium excretion. Administration of NSAIDs to these patients inhibits renal PGs allowing the unopposed vasoconstrictor activity to reduce the GFR [8–10]. Cessation of NSAID therapy is usually followed by rapid recovery of function suggesting pharmacological rather than structural renal injury [11]. Recently oral prostaglandin analogues, such as misoprostol and enisoprost have become available for clinical studies. These compounds are well absorbed and have a number of measurable systemic effects.

We have recently examined the effects of simultaneous administration of misoprostol with indomethacin in cirrhotic patients with ascites to determine if it can prevent NSAID-induced renal dysfunction [12]. We have performed a randomized double-blind, cross-over study in 10 patients with alcoholic cirrhosis and ascites. Indomethacin (50 mg) was administered orally together with placebo or misoprostol (800 μg). Patients were maintained on constant sodium diet (10 mEq). The efficacy parameters evaluated were urine flow, sodium excretion rate, functional excretion of sodium and potassium, and creatinine clearance. Within 8 hours following a single 50 mg dose of indomethacin there was a fall in prostaglandin excretion in both groups (PGE_2 –69% vs –80%; 6-keto $PGF_{1\alpha}$, –69% vs 80%). However, in the initial 4 hours after receiving the test drugs misoprostol appeared to blunt the indomethacin-induced renal impairment compared to placebo. Urine flow rate was similarly decreased by 43 and 48%; urinary sodium excretion was increased by 31% in the misoprostol group and decreased by 65% in the placebo group; fractional excretion of sodium was +88% vs –33%; fractional excretion of potassium, +1% vs –19%; creatinine clearance, –34% vs 49%, respectively.

Although none of these results reached statistical significance, there was a consistent tendency of reducing the nephrotoxic effects of indomethacin by misoprostol. Our initial observation has been recently confirmed by Wong et al. in a group of patients with well compensated cirrhosis [13]. These data have provided the rationale for a larger study in patients with cirrhosis and ascites. A multicentre trial on the efficacy of misoprostol in reducing ibuprofen-induced renal dysfunction in alcoholic liver disease with ascites is in progress.

CYCLOSPORIN NEPHROTOXICITY

Cyclosporin (Cs) nephrotoxicity is related in part to dose-dependent decreases in RBF and GFR associated with parallel increases in renal vascular resistance. Evidence suggests a major role of cyclo-oxygenase metabolites including PGE_2, PGI_2 and TxB_2 [14]. Rats given Cs show stimulation of the renin-angiotensin system together with an increase in glomerular synthesis and urinary excretion of TxA_2 [15]. Rat vascular smooth muscle cells incubated with Cs demonstrate impaired PGE_2 secretion in response to vasoconstrictor stimuli and decreased sensitivity to angiotensin II and arginine vasopressin [16]. When incubated with Cs, endothelial cells in culture demonstrate a dose-dependent decrease in PGI_2 synthesis [17,18]. Finally, inhibition of prostaglandin synthesis exacerbates Cs-induced renal vasoconstriction. Thus, an increased production of vasoconstrictor metabolites, such as TxB_2 or decreased production of vasodilatory PGs, such as PGE_2 may represent a key factor in the pathogenesis of Cs nephrotoxicity.

THERAPEUTIC USE OF PROSTAGLANDIN ANALOGUES IN PREVENTING CYCLOSPORIN NEPHROTOXICITY

In animal models of Cs nephrotoxicity the prostaglandin analogue 16,16-dimethyl PGE_2 demonstrated protective effects [19]. In addition, misoprostol is capable of reversing acute Cs nephrotoxicity in rats [20]. Cs in a dose of 10 mg/kg caused a decrease in renal function and renal haemodynamics. Conversely, misoprostol caused only little changes in renal haemodynamics or renal function when administered to normal rats. When misoprostol was administered to Cs-treated animals there was a significant reversal of these effects.

A recent study by Moran et al. has described the ability of misoprostol (800 mg/day) to prevent acute graft rejection in renal transplant recipients treated with Cs and prednisone [21]. In the group given placebo there were 62 episodes of acute renal dysfunction in 33 subjects. By contrast, in the group given misoprostol there were 42 episodes in 29 subjects. The number of patients who had acute graft rejection was significant lower in the misoprostol-treated group (10 of 38 (26%) vs 20 of 39 (51%)). Interestingly the incidence of acute nephrotoxicity due to Cs was higher in the misoprostol group. Graft rejection adversely affected renal function in both groups. Treatment with misoprostol, however, was associated with improved renal function whether or not rejection had occurred suggesting that misoprostol treatment may have a beneficial effect on chronic Cs nephrotoxicity.

In a prospective, randomized, double-blind trial Neuberger et al. (unpublished observations) have recently compared the effects of enisoprost, a new orally active PG analogue, versus placebo after orthotopic liver transplantation. Patients were immunosuppressed with Cs, azathioprine and glucocorticoids. The first dose of Cs was given post-transplantation after haemodynamic stability was achieved. Prophylactic dosing with enisoprost or placebo was begun simultaneously and continued for 12 weeks. Sixty-three patients (EP = 32, P = 31) were enrolled, of whom 40 had fully completed the study. The incidence of acute Cs nephrotoxicity was not different (EP = 6 vs P = 6). In this study the PG analogue enisoprost did not reduce the incidence of acute rejection after orthotopic liver transplantation nor the incidence of acute nephrotoxicity. Renal function was improved by prophylactic administration of the drug.

In another study, Adams et al. (unpublished observations) examined the effects of enisoprost in a prospective double-blinded study of 374 patients undergoing renal transplantation at 39 centres. Patients were randomized to receive EP 50 mg q.i.d., EP 100 mg q.i.d. or placebo. There was no significant difference between the treatment groups in regard to graft rejection or renal function. One more time enisoprost had no effect on either the incidence of acute rejection or renal function at two months following renal transplantation.

Finally, Pollak et al. (unpublished observations) have studied the effects of enisoprost in improving renal function in renal transplant recipients chronically exposed to Cs. In this study there was no evidence of concurrent acute renal injury, including that of acute rejection. Therefore, this study represented the best model to study the effects of oral prostaglandins in preventing Cs nephrotoxicity. However, two weeks of therapy with EP did not improve renal function in Cs-treated renal transplant patients.

CONCLUSION

Despite the promising results of animal studies there is not definitive evidence of a protective renal action of prostaglandin analogues, such as misoprostol and enisoprost in man. Further studies are in progress to determine the efficacy of these compounds in preventing cyclosporin and NSAID-induced nephrotoxicity.

REFERENCES

1. Carmichael J, Shankel SW. Effects of non-steroidal anti-inflammatory drugs on prostaglandins and renal function. Am J Med. 1985;992–1000.
2. Ciabattoni G, Cinotti G, Pierucci A, Simonetti BM, Manzi M, Pugliese F, Barsotti P, Pecci G, Taggi F, Patrono C. Effects of sulindac and ibuprofen in patients with chronic glomerular diseases. Evidence for the dependence of renal function on prostacyclin. N Engl J Med. 1984;310:279–283.
3. Hassid A, Dunn MJ. Microsomal prostaglandin biosynthesis of human kidney. J Biol Chem. 1980;55:2472–2475.
4. McGiff JC, Crowshaw K, Terragno NA, Lonigro AJ. Renal prostaglandins: possible regulators of the renal action of pressor hormones. Nature. 1970;227:1255–1257.
5. Dunn MJ, Zambraski EJ. Renal effects of drugs that inhibit prostaglandin synthesis. Kidney Int. 1980;18:609–622.
6. Epstein M, ed. The kidney in liver disease, 2nd ed. New York: Elsevier; 1983.
7. Papper S. Hepatorenal syndrome. Contrib Nephrol. 1980;23:55–70.
8. Zipser RD. Role of renal prostaglandins and the effects of non-steroidal anti-inflammatory drugs in patients with liver disease. Am J Med. 1986;81(Suppl. 2B):95–103.
9. Arroyo V, Gines P, Rimola A, Gaya J. Renal function abnormalities, prostaglandins, and effects of non-steroidal anti-inflammatory drugs in cirrhosis with ascites: an overview with emphasis on pathogenesis. Am J Med. 1986;81(Suppl. 2B):104–122.
10. Zipser RD, Kerlin P, Hoefs JC, Zia P, Barg A. Renal kallikrein excretion in cirrhosis. Relationship to other vasoactive systems. Am J Gastroenterol. 1981;75:183–187.
11. Zipser RD, Hoefs JC, Speckart PF, Zia PK, Horton R. Prostaglandins: modulators of renal function and pressor resistance in chronic liver disease. J Clin Endocrinol Metab. 1979;48:894–900.
12. Antillon M, Cominelli F, Lo S, Moran M, Sonberg K, Reynolds TB, Zipser RD. Effects of oral prostaglandins on indomethacin-induced renal dysfunction in patients with cirrhosis with ascites. J Rheumatol. 1990;17:46–49.
13. Wong F, Massie D, Hsu P, Dudley F. Effect of an oral prostaglandin E1 analogue on indomethacin induced renal dysfunction in alcoholic cirrhosis. Hepatology. [in press]
14. Bennet WM, Elzinga L, Kelley V. Pathophysiology of cyclosporine nephrotoxicity: role of eicosanoids. Transplant Proc. 1988;3(Suppl. 3):628–633.
15. Kawaguchi A, Goldman MH, Shapiro R, Foegh ML, Ranwell PW, Lower RR. Transplantation. 1985;40:214–216.
16. Kurtz A, Pfeilschifter J, Kuhn K, Koch KM. Cyclosporin A inhibits PGE2 release from vascular smooth muscle cells. Biochem Biophys Res Commun. 1987;147:542–549.
17. Lau DC, Wong KL, Hwang WS. Cyclosporine toxicity on cultured rat microvascular endothelial cells. Kidney Int. 1989;35:604–613.
18. Zoja C, Furci L, Ghilardi F, Zilio P, Benigni A, Remuzzi G. Cyclosporin-induced endothelial cell injury. Lab Invest. 1986;55:455–462.
19. Ryffel B, Donatsch P, Hiestand P, Mihatsh MJ. PGE2 reduces nephrotoxicity and immunosuppression of cyclosporine in rats. Clin Nephrol. 1986;25(Suppl. 1):S95–S99.
20. Paller MS. The prostaglandin E1 analog misoprostol reverses acute cyclosporine nephrotoxicity. Transplant Proc. 1988;3(Suppl. 3):634–637.
21. Moran M, Mozes MF, Maddux MS, Veremis S, Bartkus C, Ketel B, Pollak R, Wallermark C, Jonasson O. Prevention of acute graft rejection by the prostaglandin E1 analogue misoprostol in renal-transplant recipients treated with cyclosporine and prednisone. N Engl J Med. 1990;322:1183–1188.

29
Aspirin and Reye's syndrome

Brian L. Strom

Clinical Epidemiology Unit, Section of General Internal Medicine,
Department of Medicine, University of Pennsylvania School of
Medicine, Philadelphia, Pennsylvania, USA

INITIAL STUDIES

Arizona study

The first such study was a case–control study performed in Arizona in December 1978 [1]. Seven school-aged children with Reye's syndrome were compared to 16 classmates, matched for sex and suffering from an illness during the same month as the cases. The parents of patients were interviewed, exploring exposures during the time prior to the vomiting in the cases and during the entire illness in the controls. It was found that fever was more common in the cases ($p = 0.05$) and that cases took more medications ($p = 0.05$). In particular, of the seven cases, all took aspirin. Of the 16 controls, only 8 did. This gave an odds ratio which was indefinite ($p < 0.05$). There was a relationship between dose of aspirin and the severity of the disease which was statistically significant. Finally, analysing only those who had suffered from fever, there still remained a relationship between aspirin and development of Reye's syndrome ($p < 0.01$).

Ohio study

The second study was performed in the state of Ohio and was a case–control study performed between December 1978 and March 1980 [2]. Ninety-seven stage I cases who had been detected using active surveillance were compared to 156 controls matched for age, race, sex and recent illnesses of the same type. Personal interviews were conducted of their parents. Of the 97 cases, 94 were exposed to aspirin. In contrast, of the 156 controls, only 71 were exposed to aspirin. This gave an odds ratio of 37.5 ($p < 0.01$). Controlling for the level of fever, headache, and sore throat yielded an odds ration of 11.5 ($p < 0.001$). A positive dose–response

Side-effects of Anti-inflammatory Drugs 3. Rainsford KD, Velo GP (eds),
Inflammation and Drug Therapy Series, Volume V.

relationship was seen. In contrast, of the 97 cases, only 16 were exposed to paracetamol (acetaminophen). Of the 156 controls, 51 were exposed to paracetamol. This gave an odds ratio of 0.4 ($p < 0.01$).

Michigan study

The third of the initial studies was performed in the state of Michigan [3]. In fact, two such studies were performed and reported together. The first Michigan study collected data from March and April 1980. Twenty-five cases were included, including patients who were reported to the Michigan Department of Health plus others identified by regular contacts with paediatric intensive care units. These were compared to 46 controls matched for school, grade, age, race and absence from school at the same time for the same illness. A subgroup of the controls were matched for the level of fever. An open-ended interview was conducted of the parents, assisted by trade names and asking to see the bottles of medications.

Of the 25 cases, 24 had documented histories of aspirin ingestion. Of the 46 controls, 30 had such histories. In a matched analysis, this gave an odds ratio which was indefinite ($p < 0.002$). Matching on level of fever, of the 14 cases, all 14 were exposed to aspirin. Of the 17 controls, 12 were exposed to aspirin. Again this gave an odds ratio which was indefinite ($p < 0.02$). In contrast, of the 25 cases, four were exposed to paracetamol. Of the 46 controls, 19 were exposed to this drug. This gave an odds ratio of 0.3 ($p < 0.05$). In those matched on level of fever, of the 14 cases, only one was exposed to paracetamol. Of the 19 controls, six were exposed to this drug. This gave an odds ratio of 0.2 ($p > 0.05$).

The second Michigan study collected data during October 1980 through April 1981. The cases were 12 children who were reported to the Michigan Department of Health or identified based on regular contacts with paediatric intensive care units. These cases were compared to 29 controls matched for school, grade, age, race, absence from school at the same time for the same illness, and peak temperature. A more focused interview was conducted of the patients. The cases were interviewed in the hospital and the controls at home. A supplementary questionnaire later asked about whether the subjects knew of the reported link between aspirin and Reye's syndrome and whether this made them change their use of the medications.

Of the 12 cases, all 12 had used aspirin. Of the 29 controls, only 13 did. They gave an odds ratio which was indefinite ($p < 0.002$). Of the 12 cases, none had received paracetamol. Of the 29 controls, 16 did. This gave an odds ratio of zero ($p < 0.005$). No dose- or duration-response relationship was apparent. The controls were more likely to know the link between aspirin and Reye's syndrome than the cases.

242

Synthesis

Based on these initial studies, it appeared very likely that use of aspirin in susceptible individuals during particular viral illnesses was indeed associated with the subsequent development of Reye's syndrome. However, the studies were criticized for a number of valid reasons. First, there may have been inequality between the case group and the control group in the severity of the viral prodromal illness. As such, one could not differentiate whether it was aspirin or, alternatively, the more severe viral infection which was the cause, as it is possible that aspirin had been used more often in those whose viral infection was more severe. Second, sometimes the studies controlled for the presence of fever, but often they did not, nor did they control for the severity or duration of the fever. Third, there was a great potential for recall bias, especially with the open-ended questions, as mothers of children with Reye's syndrome might have remembered the drugs their children received more completely. However, it is important to note the inverse finding with paracetamol, which makes this less likely. Fourth, there was either no control of potential confounding variables or limited control of such variables. Fifth, there was a variable location of the interview, with cases sometimes interviewed in the hospital and controls at home. Sixth, in the later studies there was the possibility of publicity bias, i.e. patients with Reye's syndrome might have been more likely to report use of salicylates, because of their knowledge of this possible link from the lay press. In addition, the presence of aspirin exposure may have made it more likely that physicians would diagnose a case of Reye's syndrome – a diagnosis bias.

Because of these criticisms, the conclusions made in late 1981 were that more studies were needed. However, in the meantime it was recommended that parents reduce the use of aspirin in children with chicken pox and influenza, as these initial studies were felt to be sufficiently convincing to recommend public health action, despite their limitations.

FOLLOW-UP STUDIES

Public Health Service pilot study

In response to the previous recommendations, the Public Health Service undertook to perform the 'definitive' study of aspirin and Reye's syndrome [4]. They first performed a pilot study, the results of which were sufficiently dramatic that they chose to publish them, so much so that they were accepted for publication in the New England Journal of Medicine [4] – highly unusual for a pilot study. The Public Health Service pilot study was performed between February and May 1984. A total of 30 cases with Stage II Reye's syndrome were studied. It was felt that, by including patients who were more severe, the diagnosis would be less ambiguous, and less subject to a diagnosis bias. The cases were reviewed by a panel of experts to validate whether or not they truly had Reye's syndrome. Four different groups comprising 145 controls were included. Each of these was matched to the cases by age, race and antecedent illness. One group of controls came from the same emergency room to which the cases had presented. A second group of controls were inpatients in the same hospitals. The third group of controls were matched for school. The fourth group of controls were chosen by random digit telephone dialling. A structured interview was conducted of all care providers as soon as possible after the disease had been diagnosed. It included detailed medication histories using brand names, calendars of events, and included requests for identification of the bottles or pictures of the medication actually taken. The onset of the illness was timed precisely, and many potential confounders were measured and controlled for.

Of the 30 cases, 28 had received aspirin during their prodromal illness. Of the 145 controls, only 67 had. This gave an odds ratio of 16.1 ($p < 0.01$). Importantly, the severity of the prodromal illness was less in the cases than in the controls. In contrast to these findings, of the 30 cases, only 8 had received paracetamol. Of the 145 controls, 97 had. This gave an odds ratio of 0.22 ($p < 0.01$).

Public Health Service main study

The Public Health Service proceeded in performing its main study [5,6]. This study was designed in a similar way to that in the pilot study. It was conducted between January 1985 and May 1986. Twenty-seven cases were included, stage II or greater. Again, the cases were reviewed by a panel of experts blinded as to their antecedent aspirin exposure. A total of 140 controls were chosen, using a method similar to that used in the pilot study. The remainder of the design was also similar to that used in the pilot study.

Overall, an odds ratio of 40 was observed with a lower limit of the 95% confidence interval of 5.8 [5]. In the four separate control groups the odds ratio ranged from 33 (matched for school) to 66 (matched for hospital). In all cases, the results were statistically significant. Twenty-six of the 27 cases had been exposed to aspirin. In contrast, the odds ratio for paracetamol was 0.22. Again, the severity of the prodromal illness was less in cases than in controls. Adjusting for the severity of prodromal illness, the odds ratio for aspirin use was 142! A positive dose–response relationship was also seen [6].

Yale study

Finally, an additional study was performed at Yale, funded by aspirin manufacturers [7]. This study was performed during winter 1986–1987. Twenty-four cases stage I or greater were included. These, too, were reviewed by a panel of experts. Forty-eight controls were included, matched for geographical area, specialty of the physicians' practice, race, age, time of onset of the prodromal illness, type of prodromal illness, and cluster and severity of the symptoms. A structured interview of the parents was conducted and identification of the bottles or pictures was sought, plus review of the hospital records, to attempt to optimize drug history. The onset of the illness was timed precisely and, again, many confounders were measured and appropriately controlled.

Of the 24 cases, 22 were exposed to aspirin. Of the 48 controls, only 8 were thus exposed. This gave an odds ratio (95% confidence interval) of 35 (4.2–2.8). A clear dose–response relationship was seen, and the link between aspirin and Reye's syndrome was known more in controls than in the Reye's cases. In contrast to the results with aspirin, of the 24 cases, only 9 had been exposed to paracetamol. Of the 48 controls, 34 had been exposed to paracetamol. This gave an odds ratio of 0.09 (0.02–0.43). Again, this represented a dramatic confirmation of the previous findings, in a study supported by the aspirin industry.

COMMENTS

Thus, after six different studies conducted during seven time periods, a very consistent dramatic association was seen, including a dose–response relationship. A series of criticisms still remained, but each had a reasonable response.

First, the critics stated that Reye's syndrome is a new disease, but aspirin is an old drug. If aspirin is the cause of Reye's syndrome, how can this be? First, it is possible that there was some change in the manufacturing process of aspirin which related to the development of this 'new' disease. However, more likely, Reye's syndrome is in fact not a new disease. It is probably the same illness that previously had been called 'post-infectious metabolic encephalopathy'.

Second, the critics stated that Reye's syndrome was uncommon outside the US and, in particular, the link between Reye's syndrome and aspirin is not as apparent in data outside the US. However, only in the US was aspirin used in children so commonly. In addition, Reye's syndrome, as described elsewhere, seems to be a different illness than that described in the US being present, for example, in younger children.

Third, the critics claim that Reye's original case did not have aspirin exposure. While there were no notations about aspirin exposure in Reye's original paper, unpublished data indicate that 11 of those 21 cases in fact did have aspirin exposure, despite the infrequent use of aspirin at that time in Australia.

Fourth, the critics responded that the pathophysiology of Reye's syndrome is not known. This is true. Reye's syndrome clinically presents similarly to salicylate toxicity, and much is being learned about possible pathophysiological mechanisms, e.g. mitochondrial damage present in Reye's syndrome. However, we also cannot explain the precise pathophysiology of the link between cigarettes and lung cancer, cholesterol and heart disease, diethylstilboestrol and vaginal cancer, etc. The fact that the pathophysiology has not been worked out does not mean the association is not real.

Fifth, critics complain that 'Reye's syndrome' cases are in fact misdiagnosed inborn errors of metabolism, as they present similarly. First, this is not likely to be the case in children of school age, who were the subjects of most of these studies. Second, this is not likely to be related to aspirin use.

Finally, the critics point to a new Australian study which does not demonstrate a link between aspirin and Reye's syndrome [8]. However, drug use in this study was based on chart reviews only, the cases were very young (remaining more likely to be misdiagnosed cases with inborn errors of metabolism), and the use of aspirin is very uncommon in the study [9].

CONCLUSION

Thus, in conclusion, it appears clear that Reye's syndrome is indeed caused by aspirin exposure during an acute viral illness in children. The exact pathophysiology of how this occurs remains to be worked out. Based on these conclusions, use of aspirin in children in the US has dropped dramatically and the occurrence of Reye's syndrome has virtually disappeared in this country. Thus, as final evidence of the correctness of the link, we now have a natural experiment which, fortunately, also represents a major successful public health intervention.

REFERENCES

1. Starko KM, Ray CG, Dominguez LB, Stromberg WL, Woodall DF. Reye's syndrome and salicylate use. Pediatrics. 1980;66:859–864.
2. Halpin TJ, Holtzhauer FJ, Campbell RJ, Hall LJ, Correa-Villasenor A, Lanese R, Rice J, Hurwitz ES. Reye's syndrome and medication use. JAMA. 1982;248:687–691.
3. Waldman RJ, Hall WN, McGee H, Van Amburg G. Aspirin as a risk factor in Reye's syndrome. JAMA. 1982;247:3089–3094.

4. Hurwitz ES, Barrett MJ, Bregman D, Gunn WJ, Schonberger LB, Fairweather WR, Drage JS, LaMontagne JR, Kaslow RA, Burlington DB, Quinnan GV, Parker RA, Phillips K, Pinsky P, Dayton D, Dowdle WR. Public Health Service study on Reye's syndrome and medications. Report of the pilot phase. N Engl Med J. 1985;313:849–857.
5. Hurwitz ES, Barrett MJ, Bregman D, Gunn WJ, Pinsky P, Schonberger LB, Drage JS, Kaslow RA, Burlington B, Quinnan GV, LaMontagne JR, Fairweather WR, Dayton D, Dowdle WR. Public Health Service study of Reye's syndrome and medications. Report of the main study. JAMA. 1987;257:1905–1911.
6. Pinsky PF, Hurwitz ES, Schonberger LB, Gunn WJ. Reye's syndrome and aspirin. Evidence for a dose–response effect. JAMA. 1988;260:657–661.
7. Forsyth BW, Horwitz RI, Acampora D, Shapiro ED, Viscoli CM, Feinstein AR, Henner R, Holabird NB, Jones BA, Karabelas ADE, Kramer MS, Miclette M, Wells JA. New epidemiologic evidence confirming that bias does not explain the aspirin/Reye's syndrome association. JAMA. 1989;261:2517–2524.
8. Orlowski JP, Campbell P, Goldstein S. Reye's syndrome: a case–control study of medication use and associated viruses in Australia. Cleve Clin J Med. 1990;57:323–329.
9. A catch in the Reye is awry. Editorial. Cleve Clin J Med. 1990;57:318–320.

30

Antirheumatic drug therapy in the elderly

W. Watson Buchanan and Walter F. Kean

Rheumatology Unit, Department of Medicine, McMaster University
Faculty of Health Sciences, 1200 Main Street West, Hamilton, Ontario,
L8N 3Z5, Canada

INTRODUCTION

In developed nations about 10 percent of the population are elderly, defined as 65 years or older [1]. Predictions forecast a doubling of this percentage by the year 2030 [2]. At present the elderly use approximately 75 percent of doctors' time and require 20–40 prescriptions per person annually [3]. In the United Kingdom the elderly occupy more than 50 percent of all hospital beds, and some 40 percent of acute speciality beds [4]. Chronic illness, particularly rheumatic disease, is common, and it is therefore not surprising that so many non-steroidal anti-inflammatory analgesics and other antirheumatic drugs are prescribed for the elderly. There is growing evidence that adverse reactions to antirheumatic drugs, especially non-steroidal anti-inflammatory analgesics, may be more common in the elderly, especially women [5]. This can be explained, with respect to elderly patients in general, by three factors: elderly patients receive an increased number of medications, the physiological changes which occur with ageing may affect pharmacokinetic drug distribution, and the elderly patient may be more sensitive to the pharmacodynamic effects of drugs.

DEFINITION OF THE ELDERLY

Since Otto von Bismarck (1815–1898) ordered compulsory retirement of Prussian officers on their 65th birthday [1] this age has been widely accepted as the chronological definition of the elderly. However, a chronological definition is not entirely satisfactory, since many elderly persons maintain good health until at least the age of 75 [6]. Furthermore, healthy elderly subjects differ little from healthy young persons. Ageing should not be considered a pathological process, but a physiological

Side-effects of Anti-inflammatory Drugs 3. Rainsford KD, Velo GP (eds),
Inflammation and Drug Therapy Series, Volume V.

transition. Ideally, drug studies should be performed in patients with hepatic and renal failure or both, irrespective of their age [7]. If such studies are conducted in elderly subjects it is essential that clinical and laboratory details be accompanied by a list of coexisting diseases, smoking habits, alcohol intake, and current medication. Until such methodology is consistently instituted conclusions regarding drug studies in the elderly that do not differentiate subjects according to such characteristics will remain difficult to interpret, especially if there is disagreement in the results. A system for assessment of organ failure in elderly subjects is long overdue.

PHYSIOLOGICAL CHANGES

The physiological changes which occur with ageing and which might influence the pharmacokinetic disposition of a drug [8] are summarized in Table 1.

Table 1. Physiological changes which occur with ageing which may affect drug pharmacokinetics (after Ouslander [8])

Pharmacokinetics	Physiological changes
Absorption	Decreased oesophageal peristalsis
	Atrophy of gastric and small intestinal mucosa
	Decreased gastric and mesenteric blood flow
	Increased gastric pH
	Decrease in gastric emptying
	Decreased active mucosal transport
Distribution	Decrease in lean body mass (total body water)
	Increase in fat
	Decrease in plasma volume
	Decrease in plasma albumin concentration
Hepatic	Decrease in liver mass
biotransformation	Decreased function of microsomal cytochrome P-450 enzymes
	Decrease in enzyme induction
	Decrease in hepatic blood flow as a result of decreased cardiac output
Renal clearance	Decrease in thirst appreciation
	Decreased functioning nephrons
	Decreased cardiac output results in decreased renal blood flow and thus glomerular filtration rate declines
	Decreased creatinine clearance*

*Corrected for lean body mass using the formula of Crockhoff and Gault

$$\text{Creatinine clearance (ml/min)} = \frac{(140 - \text{age}) \times \text{body weight (kg)}}{814 \times \text{serum creatinine (mmol/L)}}$$

The formula should be adjusted in females by multiplying by 0.85

Absorption

Non-steroidal anti-inflammatory analgesics are weak acids which are lipid-soluble, with a pKa of approximately 3–5, i.e. the pH at which ionization occurs. Oral bioavailability of non-steroidal anti-inflammatory analgesics is not impaired in the elderly, since these drugs are passively absorbed [10]. Substances which are absorbed by active transport mechanisms, such as calcium, galactose, iron and thiamine may have a reduced rate of absorption in the elderly [11]. Whether antirheumatic drugs, which are absorbed by active transport mechanisms, e.g. methotrexate, have delayed absorption in the elderly is not known. Only one drug to date, prazosin, has been proven to have diminished absorption in elderly subjects [12]. The rate of many of the non-steroidal anti-inflammatory analgesics is slower when taken with meals or alkalis [13], but this is of no practical importance in the treatment of chronic arthritis. Many elderly subjects, especially women, have diminished oesophageal motility [8] and reduced salivary flow [14]. It has been estimated that normal salivary output is of the order of 500–1500 mL per day. Saliva not only contains mucin and bicarbonate, but also epithelial growth factor, produced by the submandibular glands [15]. Whether a diminished salivary flow plays a role in protecting the gastric mucosa from non-steroidal anti-inflammatory analgesic injury is not known. Epithelial growth factor is known, however, to be protective in rats [16].

Distribution

The extent to which a drug is distributed and the relative distribution to various organs and tissues depends on its chemical characteristics. Drugs which are preferentially bound to plasma proteins, such as the non-steroidal anti-inflammatory analgesics, are confined to extracellular fluids. On the other hand drugs which are water soluble or preferentially bound to tissues have a greater volume of distribution. Changes in body composition, such as reduction in lean body mass, might be expected to increase drug toxicity in the elderly [8]. Elderly patients, especially those who are confined to bed, have low serum albumin concentrations as well as a decreased ability to bind certain drugs [17–19]. Thus, elderly patients may have a disproportionately high level of free non-steroidal anti-inflammatory drugs. This may account for the cognitive changes seen in elderly subjects when treated with these drugs [21].

250

Biotransformation

Although the plasma half-life of a drug may be altered by changes in volume of distribution and clearance it remains a useful pharmacokinetic parameter. Non-steroidal anti-inflammatory analgesics can be broadly classified into two groups according to their half-lives [22] (Table 2). Those with long half-lives e.g. piroxicam, are prescribed on a once daily basis. Exceptions include phenylbutazone and oxyphenbutazone which continue needlessly to be prescribed three times a day. Aspirin (acetylsalicylic acid) has a very short half-life of some 10–15 minutes. Salicylic acid, however, is prolonged, especially when administered in anti-inflammatory dosage of 3 g or more daily. It is therefore unnecessary to prescribe salicylates for inflammatory joint disease more than twice a day [23]. Some of the hepatic enzymes involved in the biotransformation of salicylates are governed by Michaelis-Menten kinetics, so that the plasma half-life increases with the dose of the drug [24]. Non-steroidal anti-inflammatory analgesics with short plasma half-lives can be given on a twice-daily basis and still be effective, due to the fact that the biological duration of action exceeds the rate of drug elimination, as well as persistence in synovial fluid [25]. Patient compliance is improved when fewer tablets have to be taken [26].

The liver has been aptly described as the great 'poison trap', since hepatocytes carry out biotransformation reactions that contribute to the removal of drugs and other foreign chemicals. A useful scheme categorizes these reactions as either 'preparative' (Phase I) or 'synthetic' (Phase II). Phase I reactions include the oxidations (hydroxylation, N-dealkylation, and sulphoxidation), the reductions, and the hydrolyses. These

Table 2. Half-lives ($t_{1/2}$) of some NSAIDs currently available (values represent means in hours)

Short $t_{1/2}$ (<6 hours)		Long $t_{1/2}$ (>6 hours)	
Acetylsalicyclic acid	0.25	Diflunisal	13
Diclofenac	<1	Fenbufen	11
Fenoprofen	2.5	Naproxen	14
Flufenamic acid	1.4	Oxyphenylbutazone	70
Flurbiprofen	3	Phenylbutazone	70
Ibuprofen	2.5	Piroxicam	40
Ketoprofen	1–2	Salicylate[a]	15
Mefenamic acid	2–4	Sulindac[b]	8
Meclofenamate	2–4	(active metabolite)	18
Tiaprofenic acid	2		
Tolmetin[c]	1 & 7		

[a]Salicylate metabolism follows mixed phase kinetics, whereby the $t_{1/2}$ increases in parallel with the plasma level. This $t_{1/2}$ applies to therapeutic doses of 3 g or more daily. With small doses, the $t_{1/2}$ is of the order of 2 hours
[b]The active metabolite of sulindac has a long $t_{1/2}$
[c]Elimination is biphasic

'preparative' reactions generally constitute relatively minor molecular modifications, making drugs more water-soluble (polar) and often retaining the pharmacological action of the parent compound. Phase II reactions involve conjugation of a drug to molecules such as a glucuronide, acetate or sulphate. The resultant conjugates are usually more water-soluble than the parent compounds and are excreted in the urine. Generally the products of Phase II reactions are inactive [27]. As demonstrated for antipyrine [28] oxidative biotransformation, carried out by the cytochrome P-450 mixed function oxidases, may be diminished in the elderly. The plasma half-lives of phenylbutazone [29], piroxicam [30] and ibuprofen [31] have been reported to be prolonged; but has not been confirmed in all studies [32,33]. No prolongation of plasma half-life of isoxicam was observed in elderly versus young patients with rheumatoid arthritis [34]. The ill-fated benoxaprofen had a marked prolongation of plasma half-life in elderly patients, which may explain its toxicity in these subjects [35]. There is evidence that aplastic anaemia in elderly patients receiving phenylbutazone may be related to slower biotransformation, resulting in increased plasma concentration [36]. Whether non-steroidal anti-inflammatory analgesics with long plasma half-lives are more likely to cause gastric complications remains debatable [37].

Synthetic Phase II processes, such as glucuronidation, are not affected by ageing. Salicylates are largely biotransformed by such processes, and their plasma half-lives are not prolonged in elderly patients [38]. Two of the enzyme processes in the biotransformation of salicylates are, however, saturable, so that a sudden increase in plasma concentration can occur causing acute salicylate intoxication [39].

Renal clearance

The glomerular filtration rate declines predictably in old age, with a mean reduction of 35 percent compared with the young [40]. Thus, for drugs whose clearance is accomplished partly or entirely by renal excretion of the intact drug, the total clearance can be expected to decline in elderly subjects. Of the non-steroidal anti-inflammatory analgesics only azapropazone is largely excreted unchanged in the urine, and so may require the dose to be reduced in the elderly or in patients with renal failure [41]. Since non-steroidal anti-inflammatory analgesics are weak acids, their renal clearance is increased as the urinary pH rises. This is of little clinical significance, however, except for salicylates, for which there may be a substantial fall in plasma concentration even with small changes in urinary pH above 6.5 [42].

There is also some evidence that drugs undergoing biotransformation by Phase II reactions are more slowly eliminated in the elderly, as may be the case with ketoprofen and naproxen [43,44]. This is because their acylglucuronides are readily hydrolyzed back to the parent drug in a so-called 'futile cycle' [45]. Many of these drugs are racemic, consisting of R (rectus) and S (sinister) enantiomers. Naproxen is marketed as the S which is active as an anti-inflammatory agent [46], whereas all other proprionic acid derivatives are a mixture of R and S enantiomers. The R enantiomer can be considered somewhat of a pro-drug, since stereo-inversion occurs in the body, converting it to the S enantiomer. In renal failure, not only are the acyl glucuronides capable of being hydrolyzed to the parent drug, but the R enantiomer is converted to an S enantiomer which is more slowly excreted and has therefore potential for toxicity in the elderly [47]. This may have contributed to toxicity of benoxaprofen in elderly patients who had renal failure.

The serum creatinine concentration is an unreliable indicator of renal function in the elderly. There is reduction in muscle and lean body mass in elderly subjects [8] (Table 1), so that there may not be a meaningful rise in serum creatinine in renal failure. The creatinine clearance is a more reliable indicator, but requires correction for age and sex [9].

Receptors

Animal studies have shown that there are fewer corticosteroid binding sites in the adipocytes and leucocytes of elderly animals compared to younger ones [48,49]; no comparable data exists for humans. There is, however, a decreased number of isoprenaline receptors on the lymphocytes of elderly patients [50]. It remains to be determined whether such altered receptor function has relevance to the toxicity of antirheumatic drug therapy.

ADVERSE REACTIONS

Pharmacokinetic disposition plays a surprisingly small part in predicting toxic effects, most of which are idiosyncratic. Measurement of blood levels of antirheumatic drugs is of little value in predicting toxic effects or monitoring clinical response [51–55]. Dose response relationships have only been demonstrated with the three non-steroidal anti-inflammatory analgesics, carprofen [56], fenclofenac [57], and naproxen [58,59]. Measurement of blood levels of salicylates is no longer recommended [60,61], because of their five-fold variations. Serum concentrations of indomethacin do, however, correlate with headache [62]. Tinnitus is not a good sign of salicylate toxicity in elderly patients, since many are intrinsically deaf [63]. Toxic effects, however, with salicylates in the elderly occur with lower doses [64]. Blood levels of gold have not been found to relate to toxicity [65]. Measurement of free drug levels, both for salicylates [66] and gold [67] have been of no more value than measurement of total drug level [68]. It remains to be proven whether measurement of methotrexate polyglutamates in the liver might be helpful in predicting methotrexate hepatotoxicity [69].

A high incidence of adverse drug reactions has been reported in elderly patients [70]. However, elderly patients have multiple drug therapy, and the relationship between the number of drugs and adverse reactions is not linear, but exponential [70]. Also adverse reactions increase with severity of illness [71]. When these factors are taken into account elderly patients are probably no more prone than younger patients to develop drug reactions [72]. As previously mentioned the elderly are not homogenous. The study of Sheldrake et al. [73] with flurbiprofen in patients with rheumatoid arthritis is a case in point: elderly patients had less adverse effects than younger patients, the elderly patients were, however, 'squeaky clean'!

Possession of the HLA-DR3 phenotype predisposes to toxicity with gold and D-penicillamine [74]. Slow acetylators have more nausea and vomiting with sulphasalazine [75]. Poor sulphoxation has been associated with increase in gold toxicity [76]. Drug interactions account for 5–10 percent of adverse reactions [77], but are in general mild [78]. Since elderly patients tend to receive a large number of medications, drug interactions become extremely important. The clinically important interactions have all been well documented [79–82]. Non-compliance is another major factor in drug toxicity in the elderly [83] who are notoriously forgetful in taking medication, especially of salicylates [84]. Perhaps the one drug where prediction of toxicity is more certain in the elderly is allopurinol. The metabolite, oxypurinol has normally a plasma half-life of 15 hours, but this is much prolonged in renal failure. Oxypurinol is potentially very toxic and severe fatal reactions can be avoided if renal function is first assessed before allopurinol is prescribed for elderly patients with gout [85].

Of the major toxicities encountered in the elderly those affecting the gastrointestinal tract and kidneys are the most frequent [86,87]. Although there is little argument whether non-steroidal anti-inflammatory analgesics cause gastric and duodenal mucosal injury [88], there is still controversy regarding their role in acute gastrointestinal haemorrhage [89]. The incidence of major gastrointestinal haemorrhage is low in comparison with the number of prescriptions issued [90]. There is, however, a large corpus of evidence to suggest that the elderly, especially females, may be particularly prone to both acute gastrointestinal haemorrhage and perforation with non-steroidal anti-inflammatory analgesic therapy [5,87]. It should be noted, however, that not all authors have found age to be a factor with non-steroidal anti-inflammatory analgesic toxicity [87]. Again the problem is defining the elderly: there is a considerable difference between a healthy man or woman in their early seventies, and a frail old woman in a long-care institution. There seems little difference in the incidence of acute gastrointestinal haemorrhage among the different non-steroidal anti-inflammatory analgesics, but all seem less toxic than acetyl-salicylic acid [91]. Since non-acetylated salicylates appear less injurious to the gastric mucosa than acetylsalicylic acid [92], and since both are equipotent as anti-inflammatory analgesics [93], there seems little reason why acetylsalicylic acid should be used in rheumatological practice [94]. There is no evidence, at present, that cytoprotective agents, such as misoprostol, will prevent acute gastrointestinal bleeding.

In addition to side effects in the stomach and duodenum other sites of the gastrointestinal tract may be affected with non-steroidal anti-inflammatory analgesics, especially in the elderly. Thus tablets lodging in the oesophagus may cause haemorrhage and stricture. Small and large bowel haemorrhage, perforation and stricture formation have been reported [95,96]. It has been suggested that drugs which have appreciable enterohepatic re-circulation, such as indomethacin and piroxicam, may be more likely to cause lower bowel complications [97], but this awaits confirmation.

Frequently omitted in epidemiological studies of gastrointestinal side effects on non-steroidal anti-inflammatory analgesics are other drugs which are potentially injurious to the gastric and duodenal mucosa, such as potassium. It is uncertain whether oral corticosteroids cause acute gastrointestinal haemorrhage and perforation, at least in the low doses prescribed for patients with rheumatoid arthritis [89]. Whether patients with pre-existing gastric and duodenal ulcers are more prone to bleed when prescribed non-steroidal anti-inflammatory analgesics, and whether the gastric mucosa is more susceptible to injury from these drugs in patients with rheumatoid arthritis, are not known [87]. The effects of smoking on non-steroidal anti-inflammatory analgesic-induced gastric and duodenal ulceration are unclear, but there is evidence that alcohol is a major risk factor [98]. Patients on anticoagulant therapy are clearly more likely to bleed when prescribed non-steroidal anti-inflammatory analgesic therapy, as are patients with oesophageal varices.

Salicylates are well known to cause a 'transaminitis' (a misnomer since there is no inflammation of the enzymes!) and a few patients have developed acute hepatitis as a result of non-steroidal anti-inflammatory analgesic therapy [87]. The latter complication appears to be more common in the elderly, especially women on multiple medications [99]. There is no evidence that hepatic damage from azathioprine or methotrexate is more common in elderly patients. Paracetamol (acetaminophen) may result in liver damage even at recommended daily dosage [87]. Paracetamol should always be considered a potential cause of unexplained liver dysfunction in elderly patients [100].

At least six renal syndromes have been identified with non-steroidal anti-inflammatory analgesic therapy [87] including the flank pain syndrome resulting from suprofen [101]. Three of the syndromes – haemodynamic or

255

functional acute renal failure, hyponatraemia, and hyperkalaemia, are related to inhibition of renal prostaglandin production. These are most commonly seen in elderly patients who are receiving treatment for congestive cardiac failure and have renal insufficiency, or who are hypovolemic owing to diminished fluid intake or excessive loss [87]. Interstitial nephritis is rare and unpredictable, but again tends to occur in older patients. High dose corticosteroid therapy and dialysis may be necessary to assist recovery [87]. Analgesic nephropathy remains despite the removal of phenacetin. Gold and D-penicillamine produce a membranous glomerulonephropathy which responds to discontinuation of therapy. There is no evidence that this complication is more common in the elderly, although it should be noted that these drugs are contra-indicated in patients with renal failure, which excludes many elderly patients. There is evidence, however, that cyclosporin renal toxicity may be more common in those over 60 years of age.

CONCLUSION

It is surprising that although we have recommended drug doses in relation to body size for paediatric use, we have none for geriatric practice. It is important to know the pharmacokinetic behaviour of drugs prescribed for the elderly, and how this may be influenced by physiological changes and concurrent diseases. It is also important for the practising physician to appreciate that new antirheumatic drugs are evaluated in 'squeaky clean' healthy elderly patients without the complicating factors of diseases, such as hypertension, congestive cardiac failure, and renal insufficiency – the 'stuff' of real world, everyday clinical practice. Care must be exercised at all times with all drugs prescribed for the elderly. It is prudent to adhere to the policy of 'go low, go slow' when commencing both non-steroidal anti-inflammatory analgesics and second-line drugs, monitoring for side effects as the clinically effective dose is gradually reached. In this way, it may be possible to avoid or lessen the potential adverse effects of antirheumatic drug therapy in the elderly.

REFERENCES

1. Aiken LR. Later life. New York; Holt, Rinehart and Winston; 1982:201.
2. Carty MA, Everitt DE. Basic principles of prescribing for geriatric outpatients. Geriatrics. 1989;44:85–98.
3. Buchanan WW, Preston SJL & Arnold MH. Antirheumatic drug therapy in the elderly. Resident Staff Physician. 1990;36:31–39.
4. Dall JLC. Introduction of Symposium on the Elderly. Curr Med Res Opin. 1982;7:3.
5. Fries JF, Miller SR, Spitz PW et al. Toward an epidemiology of gastropathy associated with non-steroidal anti-inflammatory drug use. Gastroenterology. 1989;96:647–655.
6. MacLennan WJ. Old age in Scotland. Proc R Coll Physician Edin. 1988;18:252–258.

7. Kean WF, Buchanan WW. Antirheumatic drug therapy in the elderly: a case of failure to identify the correct issues. J Am Geriatr Soc. 1987;35:363–364.
8. Ouslander JG. Drug therapy in the elderly. Ann Intern Med. 1981;95:711–722.
9. Cockcroft DW, Gault MH. Prediction of creatinine clearance from serum creatinine. Nephron. 1976;16:31–41.
10. Kean WF, Buchanan WW. Variables affecting the absorption of non-steroidal anti-inflammatory drugs from the gastrointestinal tract. Jpn J Rheumatol. 1987;1:159–170.
11. Bender AD. Effect of age on intestinal absorption: implications of drug absorption in the elderly. J Am Geriatr Soc. 1968;16:1331–1339.
12. Rubin PC, Scott PJW, McLean K et al. Prazosin disposition in young and elderly subjects. Br J Clin Pharmacol. 1981;12:401–404.
13. Buchanan WW, Kean WF. An overview of current non-steroidal anti-inflammatory drug therapy in rheumatoid arthritis, with emphasis on the use in the elderly. In: Lewis AJ, Furst DF, eds. Nonsteroidal anti-inflammatory drugs, mechanisms and clinical use. New York: Marcel Dekker; 1987:9–29.
14. Whaley K, Williamson J, Chisholm DM et al. Sjögren's syndrome 1. Sicca components Q J Med. 1973;42:279–304.
15. Cohen S. Isolation of a mouse submaxillary gland protein accelerating incisor eruption and eyelid opening of newborn animals. J Biol Chem. 1986;237:1155.
16. Konturek SJ, Dembinski A, Warzecha Z et al. Epidermal growth factor (EGF) in the gastroprotective and ulcer healing actions of colloidal bismuth subcitrate (De Nol) in rats. Gut. 1988;29:894–902.
17. Wallace S, Whiting B. Factors affecting drug binding in plasma of elderly patients. Br J Clin Pharmacol. 1976;3:327–330.
18. Greenblatt DJ. Reduced serum albumin concentration in the elderly: a report from the Boston Collaborative Drug Surveillance Program. J Am Geriatr Soc. 1979;27:20–22.
19. Greenblatt DJ, Sellers EM, Shader RI. Drug disposition in old age. N Engl J Med. 1982;306:1081–1088.
20. Buchanan WW, Kean WF. Implications of antirheumatic drug therapy in elderly patients with osteoarthritis. J Rheumatol. 1987;4:98–100.
21. Goodwin JS, Regan M. Cognitive dysfunction association with naproxen and ibuprofen in the elderly. Arthritis Rheum. 1982;25:1013–1015.
22. Graham GG, Day RO, Champion GD et al. Aspects of the clinical pharmacology of non-steroidal anti-inflammatory drugs. Clin Rheum Dis. 1984;10:229–249.
23. Benson WG, Laskin CA, Parton TW et al. Twice daily dosing of enteric coated aspirin in patients with rheumatoid diseases. J Rheumatol. 1976;6:351–356.
24. Levy G, Tsuchiya T, Amsell LP. Limited capacity for salicylphenolic glucuronide formation and its effect on the kinetics of salicylate elimination in man. Clin Pharmacol Ther. 1972;13:258–268.
25. Dromgoole SH, Furst DE, Desiraju RK et al. Tolmetin kinetics and synovial fluid prostaglandin E levels in rheumatoid arthritis. Clin Pharmacol Ther. 1982;32:371–372.
26. Blackwell B. Patient compliance. N Engl J Med. 1973;289:249–252.
27. Preston S, Arnold M, Buchanan WW. Hepatic biotransformation of antirheumatic drugs. Clinical and theoretical implications. Hung Rheumatol. 1989(Suppl):11–28.
28. Swift CG, Triggs EJ. Clinical pharmacokinetics in the elderly. In: Swift CG, ed. Clinical pharmacology in the elderly. New York: Marcel Dekker; 1987:31–82.
29. O'Malley K, Crooks J, Duke E, Stevenson IH. Effect of age and sex on human drug metabolism. Br Med J. 1971;3:607–609.
30. Richardson CJ, Blocka KLN, Ross SG, Verbeeck RK. Effects of age and sex on piroxicam disposition. Clin Pharmacol Ther. 1985;37:13–18.
31. Greenblatt DJ, Abernethy DR, Matlis R, Hermatz JS, Shader RI. Absorption and disposition of ibuprofen in the elderly. Arthritis Rheum. 1984;27:1066–1069.
32. Triggs EJ, Nation RL. Pharmacokinetics in the aged: a review. J Pharmacokinet Biopharm. 1975;3:387–418.

33. Darragh A, Gordon AJ, O'Bryne H, Hobbs D, Casey E. Single-dose and steady-state pharmacokinetics of piroxicam in elderly vs young adults. Eur J Clin Pharmacol. 1985;28:305–309.
34. Grace EM, Rosenfeld JM, Sweeney GD, Buchanan WW. The pharmacokinetics of isoxicam in elderly patients with rheumatoid arthritis. Curr Med Res Opin. 1987;10:580–591.
35. Taggart H, Alderdice JM. Fatal cholestatic jaundice in elderly patients taking benoxaprofen. Br Med J. 1982;284:1372.
36. Cunningham JL, Leyland MJ, Delamore IW, Price-Evans DA. Acetanilide oxidation in phenyl-butazone-associated hypoplastic anaemia. Br Med J. 1974;3:313–317.
37. Buchanan WW. Anti-rheumatic drug therapy. London: Medi-Copne Communications;1984:29–38.
38. Roberts MS, Rumble RH, Wanwimolruk S, Thoma D, Brooks PM. Pharmacokinetics of aspirin and salicylates in elderly subjects and in patients with alcoholic liver disease. Eur J Clin Pharmacol. 1983;25:253–261.
39. Needs CJ, Brooks PM. Clinical pharmacokinetics of the salicylates. Clin Pharmacokinet. 1985;10:164–177.
40. Rowe JW, Andres R, Tobin JD et al. The effects of age on creatinine clearance in man: a cross-sectional and longitudinal study. J Gerontol. 1976;31:155–163.
41. Ritch AES, Perera WR, Jones CH. Pharmacokinetics of azapropazone in the elderly. Br J Clin Pharmacol. 1982;14:116–119.
42. Graham GG, Champion GD, Day RO, Paull PD. Patterns of plasma concentrations and urinary excretion of salicylate in rheumatoid arthritis. Clin Pharmacokinet. 1977;22:410–420.
43. Advenier C, Roux A, Gobert C et al. Pharmacokinetics of ketoprofen in the elderly. Br J Clin Pharmacol. 1983;16:65–70.
44. Upton RA, Williams RL, Kelly J et al. Naproxen pharmacokinetics in the elderly. Br J Clin Pharmacol. 1984;18:207–214.
45. Verbeeck RK, Wallace SM, Loewen GR. Reduced elimination of ketoprofen in the elderly is not necessarily due to impaired glucoronidation. Br J Clin Pharmacol. 1984;17:783–784.
46. Kean WF, Lock CJL, Rischke J et al. Effect of R and S enantiomers of naproxen on aggregation and thromboxane production in human platelets. J Pharm Sci. 1989;78:324–327.
47. Lee EJ, Williams KM, Graham GG et al. Liquid chromatographic determination and plasma profile of optical isomers of ibuprofen in humans. J Pharm Sci. 1984;73:1542–1544.
48. Roth GS, Livingstone JN. Reductions in glucocorticoid inhibition of glucose oxidation and presumptive glucocorticoid receptor content in rat adipocytes during aging. Endocrinology. 1976;99:831–839.
49. Roth GS. Reduced glucocorticoid responsiveness and receptor concentration in splenic leucocytes of senescent rats. Biochim Biophys Acta. 1975;399:144–156.
50. Dillon N, Chung S, Kelly J, O'Malley K. Age and beta-adrenoceptor-mediated function. Clin Pharmacol Ther. 1980;27:769–772.
51. Day RO, Furst DE, Dromgoole SH, Kamm B, Roe R, Paulus HE. Relationship of serum naproxen concentration to efficacy in rheumatoid arthritis. Clin Pharmacol Ther. 1982;31:733–740.
52. Orme M. Plasma concentrations and therapeutic effect of anti-inflammatory and anti-rheumatic drugs. Pharmacol Ther. 1982;16:167–180.
53. Porter RS. Factors determining efficacy of NSAIDs. Drug Intell Clin Pharm. 1984;18:42–51.
54. Perucca E, Grimaldi R, Crema A. Interpretation of drug levels in acute and chronic states. Clin Pharmacokinet. 1985;10:498–513.
55. Day RO, Graham GG, Williams KM. Pharmacokinetics of non-steroidal anti-inflammatory drugs. Baillière's Clin Rheumatol. 1988;2:363–393.
56. Furst DE, Caldwell JR, Klugman MP, Enthoven D, Rittweger K, Scheer R, Sarkissian E, Dromgoole S. Serum concentration and dose-response relationships for carprofen in rheumatoid arthritis. Clin Pharmacol Ther. 1988;44:186–194.
57. Dunagan FM, McGill PE, Kelman AW, Whiting B. Quantitation of dose and concentration effects relationships for fenclofenac in rheumatoid arthritis. Br J Clin Pharmacol. 1986;21:409–416.

58. Day RO, Furst DE, Dromgoole SH, Kama B, Roe R, Paulus HE. Relation of serum naproxen concentration to efficacy in rheumatoid arthritis. Clin Pharmacol Ther. 1982;31:733–740.

59. Dunagan FM, McGill PE, Kelman AW, Whiting B. Naproxen dose and concentration: response relationship in rheumatoid arthritis. Br J Rheumatol. 1988;27:48–53.

60. Mandelli M, Tognoni G. Monitoring plasma concentrations of salicylate. Clin Pharmacokinet. 1980;5:424–440.

61. Tugwell P, Hart L, Kraag G, Park A, Dok C, Bianchi F, Goldsmith C, Buchanan WW. Controlled trial of clinical utility of serum salicylate monitoring in rheumatoid arthritis. J Rheumatol. 1984;11:457–461.

62. Helleberg L. Clinical pharmacokinetics of indomethacin. Clin Pharmacokinet. 1981;6:245–258.

63. Halla JT, Hardin JG. Salicylate ototoxicity in patients with rheumatoid arthritis: a controlled study. Ann Rheum Dis. 1988;47:134–137.

64. Grigor RR, Spitz PW, Furst DE. Salicylate toxicity in elderly patients with rheumatoid arthritis. J Rheumatol. 1987;14:60–66.

65. Dahl S, Coleman ML, Williams JH et al. Lack of correlation between blood gold concentrations and clinical response in patients with definite or classic rheumatoid arthritis receiving auranofin or gold sodium thiomalate. Arthritis Rheum. 1985;28:1211–1218.

66. Gurwich EL, Raees SM, Skosey J, Niazi S. Unbound plasma salicylate concentration in rheumatoid arthritis patients. Br J Rheumatol. 1984;23:66–73.

67. Rudge SR, Perrett D, Swannell AJ. Free thiomalate levels in patients with rheumatoid arthritis treated with disodium aurothiomalate therapy: relationship to clinical outcome of therapy. Ann Rheum Dis. 1984;43:698–702.

68. Hande KR, Noone RM, Stone WJ. Severe allopurinol toxicity: description and guidelines for prevention in patients with renal insufficiency. Am J Med. 1984;76:47–56.

69. Kremer JM, Galivan J, Streckfuss A, Kamen B. Methotrexate metabolism analysis in blood and liver of rheumatoid arthritis patients. Association with hepatic folate deficiency and formation of polyglutamates. Arthritis Rheum. 1986;29:832–835.

70. Nolan L, O'Malley K. Prescribing for the elderly. Part 1. Sensitivity of the elderly to adverse drug reactions. J Am Geriatr Soc. 1988;36:142–149.

71. A report of the Royal College of Physicians. Medication for the Elderly. J Roy Coll Physicians (Lond.). 1984;18:7–9.

72. Steel K, Gertman PM, Crescenzi C et al. Iatrogenic illness on a general medical service at a university hospital. N Engl J Med. 1981;304:638–642.

73. Sheldrake FE, Webber JM, Marsh BD. A long-term assessment of flurbiprofen. Curr Med Res Opin. 1977;5:106–116.

74. Panayi GS, Wooley P, Batchelor JR. Genetic basis of rheumatoid disease: HLA antigens, disease manifestations and toxic reactions to drugs. Br Med J. 1978;2:1226–1238.

75. Pullar T, Hunter JA, Capell HA. Effect of acetylator phenotype on efficacy and toxicity of sulphasalazine in rheumatoid arthritis. Ann Rheum Dis. 1985;44:831–837.

76. Ayesh R, Mitchell SC, Waring RH, Withrington RH, Seifert MH, Smith L. Sodium aurothiomalate toxicity and sulphoxidation capacity in rheumatoid arthritis patients. Br J Rheumatol. 1987;26:197–201.

77. Boston Collaborative Drug Surveillance Programme Adverse Drug Interactions. J Am Med Assoc. 1972;220:1238–1239.

78. Puckett WH, Visconti JA. An epidemiologic study of the clinical significance of a drug-drug interaction in a private community hospital. Am J Hosp Pharm. 1971;28:247–253.

79. Tonkin AL, Wing LMH. Interactions of non-steroidal anti-inflammatory drugs. Baillière's Clin Rheumatol. 1988;2:455–483.

80. Abramowicz M, ed. Clinically established interactions with antirheumatic drugs. Med Lett. 1981;23:17–28.

81. Abramowicz M, ed. Clinically established interactions with antirheumatic drugs. Med Lett. 1984;26:11–14.

82. Day RO, Graham GG, Champion GD, Lee E. Antirheumatic drug interactions. Clin Rheum Dis. 1984;10:251–257.

83. Pullar T, Birtwell AJ, Wiles PG, Hay A, Feely MP. Use of a pharmacologic indicator to compare compliance with tablets prescribed to be taken once, twice and three times daily. Clin Pharmacol Ther. 1988;44:540–555.

84. Beck NC, Parker JC, Frank RG, Geden EA, Kay DR, Gamache M, Shivvers M, Smith E, Anderson S. Patients with rheumatoid arthritis at high risk for non-compliance with salicylate treatment regimens. J Rheumatol. 1988;15:1081–1084.

85. Elion GB, Benezra FM, Beardmore TD et al. Studies with allopurinol in patients with impaired renal function. Adv Exp Med Biol. 1980;122A:263–267.

86. Brooks PM, Buchanan WW. Prediction of the clinical efficacy of and intolerance to antirheumatic drug therapy. In: Bellamy N, ed. Prognosis in the rheumatic diseases. Dordrecht: Kluwer Academic Publishers; 1991:347–402.

87. Buchanan WW, Brooks PM. Prediction of organ system toxicity with antirheumatic drug therapy. In: Bellamy N, ed. Prognosis in the rheumatic diseases. Dordrecht: Kluwer Academic Publishers; 1991:403–450.

88. Ivey KJ, Rooney PJ. Non-steroidal anti-inflammatory drugs and the gastrointestinal tract. Baillière's Clin Rheumatol. 1989;3:393–409.

89. Rooney PJ, Hunt RH. The risk of upper gastrointestinal haemorrhage during steroidal and non-steroidal anti-inflammatory therapy. Bailliere's Clin Rheumatol. 1990;4:207–217.

90. Levy M, Miller DR, Kaufman DW et al. Major upper gastrointestinal tract bleeding. Relation to the use of aspirin and other non-narcotic analgesics. Arch Intern Med. 1988;109:359–363.

91. Semble EH, Wu WC. Anti-inflammatory drugs and gastric mucosal damage. Semin Arthritis Rheum. 1987;16:271–286.

92. Kilander A, Doterall G. Endoscopic evaluation of the comparative effects of acetylsalicylic acid and choline magnesium trisalicylate on human and gastric duodenal mucosa. Br J Rheumatol. 1983;22:36–40.

93. Preston SJ, Arnold MH, Beller EM et al. Comparative analgesic and anti-inflammatory properties of sodium salicylate and acetylsalicylic acid (aspirin) in rheumatoid arthritis. Br J Clin Pharmacol. 1989;27:607–611.

94. Rainsford KD, Buchanan WW. Aspirin versus the non-acetylated salicylates. Bailliere's Clin Rheumatol. 1990;4:247–268.

95. Schwartz JA. Lower gastrointestinal side effects of nonsteroidal anti-inflammatory drugs. J Rheumatol. 1981;8:952–954.

96. Charuzi L, Ovnat A, Zirkin H, Peiser J, Sukenik S. Ibuprofen and benign caecal ulcer. J Rheumatol. 1985;12:188–189.

97. Duggan DE, Hooke KF, Noll RM, Kwann KC. Enterohepatic circulation of indomethacin and its role in intestinal irritation. Biochem Pharmacol. 1975;25:1749–1754.

98. Goulston K, Cooke AR. Alcohol, aspirin and gastrointestinal bleeding. Br Med J. 1978;4:664–665.

99. Paulus HE. Government affairs: FDA arthritis advisory committee meeting. Arthritis Rheum. 1982;25:1124–1125.

100. Schlegel SI, Paulus HE. Non-steroidal and analgesic therapy in the elderly. Clin Rheum Dis. 1986;12:245–273.

101. Hart D, Ward M, Lifschitz MD. Suprofen-related nephrotoxicity. A distinct clinical syndrome. Ann Intern Med. 1987;106:235–238.

31

NSAIDs and human cartilage metabolism

J.T. Dingle

Strangeways Research Laboratory, Cambridge, CB1 4RN, UK

INTRODUCTION

It is now generally accepted that the extracellular matrix of human articular cartilage is in a state of dynamic equilibrium. The synthesis of both proteoglycan and collagen by the chondrocytes and the natural turnover of these molecules by enzymes released from these cells maintains a balance which is essential for the structural integration and function of the extracellular macromolecules. Under pathological conditions this balance may be disturbed by changes in the anabolic or catabolic activity of the indigenous chondrocytes or by the actions of surrounding connective tissues [1]. Thus, in rheumatoid arthritis (RA), where pannus erosion of cartilage is one of the prime causes of articular damage, it is likely that the extrinsic proteases, and in particular, metalloproteinases, of the synovial fibroblasts and inflammatory cells are responsible for much of the erosive process. This effect is probably compounded by the action of cytokines on the cartilage chondrocytes inhibiting proteoglycan (GAG) synthesis and hence diminishing repair processes. This effect of cytokines in inhibiting synthesis is now well documented but has still not received the attention that it probably warrants. Studies by Dingle et al. [2] have demonstrated that human cartilage is extremely sensitive to inhibition of GAG synthesis – $< 0.01 \, \text{ng ml}^{-1} \text{h}^{-1}$ IL1a will give $> 50\%$ inhibition of chondrocytic matrix synthesis in normal, osteoarthritic (OA) and RA cartilage, the most severe effects being seen in those tissues with high metabolic activity.

Human cartilage, unlike animal cartilage, is much less sensitive to catabolic activation by cytokines. The IL1 dose response for the stimulation of catabolism and the inhibition of synthesis may differ by three orders of magnitude. This differential effect is not seen in most animal tissues studied. The consequences of this great sensitivity to the inhibitory action of cytokines is probably of most importance in the prolonged development of OA. The local release of subnanogram quantities of IL1 and similar cytokines may lead to disturbance of the balance between

Side-effects of Anti-inflammatory Drugs 3. Rainsford KD, Velo GP (eds),
Inflammation and Drug Therapy Series, Volume V.

synthesis and degradation simply by inhibiting chondrocyte matrix reactions, gradually leading to the diminution of matrix integrity and lessening the resistance to mechanical stress.

It has been suggested that in OA this local release of cytokines may be an episodic process [1], perhaps due to micro-inflammation or to local mechanical trauma leading to local bursts of synthesis and release of cytokines inhibiting synthesis of GAG and collagen, the accumulative effect being a loss of matrix in those areas where cytokine activation has repeatedly occurred. It is thought likely that chondrocyte catabolic activation by cytokines is less important in this disease than is the fibroblast catabolic activation in inflammatory diseases such as RA [3].

If one accepts the hypothesis that episodic release of cytokines influences the development of OA by disturbing the natural matrix repair processes, it is important to consider how control of such cytokine action can be modulated by drug intervention and, even more important, to ensure that the therapy itself does not add to the problem.

The effect of NSAIDs on animal cartilage has been studied by Brandt and others [1,5,6] over a number of years and evidence has been accumulating that certain of these agents may interfere with the synthetic activity of cartilage chondrocytes. Little work, however, has been done on human cartilage until very recently. The finding that human cartilage is extremely sensitive to inhibition by IL1 [2] has led to the realization that the action of NSAIDs and other agents must be studied on human tissues rather than the animal tissue alone.

The present paper outlines an on-going investigation of the metabolism of human normal OA and RA cartilage and details some effects of NSAIDs on this metabolism. Some investigations of new agents that may be compatible with the general thesis that the repair process must be encouraged in arthritic cartilage are briefly reported.

RESULTS AND DISCUSSION

The metabolism of human cartilage

Table 1 demonstrates the results of an investigation of some 135 human normal and arthritic cartilages for their anabolic and catabolic activities. Cartilage GAG synthesis was measured by $^{35}SO_4$ incorporation into CPC precipitable material and GAG turnover was measured under standard *in vitro* conditions by the assaying of the release of GAG as a percentage of the total present.

It may be seen that in normal cartilages from both young and adult patients the GAG turnover rate is relatively low, whereas in OA cartilage there is a small but statistically significant increase, and in RA the cartilage GAG turnover rate is relatively high. In contrast the GAG synthesis of

Table 1. Comparison of normal and pathological human cartilage metabolism

Tissue	n	Mean age	GAG synthesis $^{35}SO_4$ cpm/mg × 10^{-3}	GAG turnover %8 d
Normal	25	13 [6–18]	6.65 (0.71)	12 (3)
Normal	49	55 [20–66]	3.80 (0.59)	14 (4)
OA	40	65 [50–55]	2.75 (0.36)	18 (4)
RA	22	69 [49–77]	1.51 (0.33)	40 (7)

n = number of patients (SEM)
av replicates/patient = 9 [range]

young normal cartilage is high but this diminishes in adult life and is substantially less in OA and RA. Whilst the GAG synthesis assays in Table 1 were on a dry weight basis, more recent studies using DNA content to give measurements of GAG synthesis on a cellular basis, show essentially the same results. The work indicates, therefore, that the ratio of GAG synthesis to GAG turnover is high in normal tissue and diminishes in arthritic tissue, and particularly in RA.

The concept of repair

The data in Table 1 illustrate the importance of GAG synthetic activity in relation to GAG turnover and the general point that repair processes may be made possible, and indeed probable, in human cartilage [1]. This has been demonstrated thoroughly *in vivo* in animals treated with IL1. Page-Thomas et al. [7] have shown that recovery can take place in severely GAG-depleted rabbit joints over the course of approximately four weeks and that this is related to increases in the indigenous chondrocyte GAG synthetic activity. Others have recognized that some cases of OA may improve both symptomatically and radiographically. Thus Perry and co-workers [8] reported on 14 patients' joint recovery observed after 10 years, whilst Danielsson [9] in a series of 91 patients followed up after the same period showed evidence of regression of arthritic changes in 7% of these cases. Dieppe [10] has also noted that joints can heal spontaneously and that this healing process could possibly be aided by drugs. Unfortunately at the present time there is no *in vivo* means of quantitating the ability of human cartilage to regenerate. Hence one has to turn to *in vitro* methods, using short-term cultures of normal and arthritic cartilage to determine what drugs may be doing to diminish or potentiate the cartilage repair activity.

263

Table 2. Effect of NSAIDs on GAG synthesis in cartilage from a normal young human population

	Drug concentration $\mu g/ml$									
Control	*Ibuprofen*		*Indomethacin*		*Diclofenac*		*Aspirin*		*Naproxen*	
	50	100	10	30	0.3	1.0	10	30	100	300
$^{35}SO_4$ incorporation into GAG [SEM]										
7.21	6.62	4.47	5.78	5.11	6.13	5.58	6.01	5.67	3.87	3.43
[1.9]	[1.8]	[1.1]	[1.5]	[1.3]	[1.5]	[1.3]	[1.4]	[1.2]	[1.2]	[1.1]
p —	ns	xx	ns	x	ns	ns	ns	ns	x	xx

Analysis of variance
Difference from control
x $p < 0.01$; xx $p < 0.001$; ns > 0.01

The effects of NSAIDs on GAG synthesis

Table 2 shows the effect of a number of NSAIDs at various dosages on GAG synthesis in cartilage from a young normal population. Similar studies on OA and RA cartilages have been carried out and will be reported elsewhere. It can be seen in Table 2 that in the population [$n = 10$] studied, diclofenac and aspirin were not statistically significant in inhibiting GAG synthesis, though there was inhibition by indomethacin at the higher concentration. Whilst ibuprofen and naproxen give significant inhibition of GAG synthesis, this action of some NSAIDs in inhibiting GAG synthesis is shown up particularly in the recovery (repair) of cartilage matrix after an *in vitro* episode of IL1.

In Table 3 the cartilage was treated briefly with hrIL1a and the GAG synthesis measured at intervals over a period of four days after the IL1 treatment had ceased. It can be seen that in the controls the recovery was complete by four days – cartilage synthetic activity was back to the normal

Table 3. Effect of NSAIDs on recovery after IL1 (OA cartilage) GAG synthesis (cpm/ mg $\times$ 10^{-3} $^{35}SO_4$ uptake)

		Time post-IL1	
	1d	*2d*	*4d*
Drug conc			
Control	1.08 (0.10)	2.01 (0.16)	2.25 (0.21)
Ibuprofen			
50 $\mu g/ml$	0.94 (0.10)	0.74 (0.09)	0.92 (0.08)
Aspirin			
30 $\mu g/ml$	1.22 (0.14)	0.56 (0.08)	0.43 (0.05)
Diclofenac			
1 $\mu g/ml$	1.20 (0.28)	1.24 (0.11)	2.63 (0.3)

(GFM); $h = 10$; (IL1 0.05 ng/ml; 2d); [untreated 2.4 (0.30) cpm/mg x 10^{-3}]

value; whereas with both ibuprofen and aspirin this recovery did not take place. On the other hand, in the presence of diclofenac, recovery had taken place by four days. These experiments tend to confirm the data on NSAID action shown in Table 2. Other recovery experiments have been made on both normal cartilage and RA cartilage, and give similar results.

It should be stressed that not all NSAIDs show this inhibitory action on human cartilage matrix synthesis. As already pointed out, diclofenac has relatively little inhibitory action on most arthritic cartilage, though there may be some inhibition in cartilage of high metabolic activity. Another agent, piroxicam, also has little effect on human normal and arthritic cartilage, and it is probable that other NSAIDs are also less potentially damaging than some shown here, though this has yet to be confirmed on human cartilage.

Another NSAID with interesting properties is the Pfizer drug, tenidap. Investigations of some 40 OA cartilages have shown that this agent at concentrations between 1 and 5 μg/ml not only does not inhibit GAG synthesis but will in fact stimulate cartilage chondrocyte synthetic activity and gives some protection against the action of IL1. Unpublished data has shown that tenidap was most effective in protecting those OA patients' cartilage with a high matrix turnover rate. Recent investigations have shown that replicate samples of cartilage from each patient may vary in metabolic activity quite considerably. These have been examined individually taking up to 70 samples from each joint. In 1400 cartilage samples assayed for GAG synthesis, those with a high metabolic turnover were most susceptible to protection by tenipad. This agent, therefore, must be considered to have significant potential for the treatment of arthritic diseases whilst allowing, and indeed encouraging, natural repair processes to take place.

It should be stressed that in the development of new NSAIDs, such properties should be a prime aim, leading to improved agents for the prolongation of the structure and mechanical integrity of the diseased joint as well as diminishing pain and inflammation.

Modulation of NSAID-induced damage

Another approach is to attempt to influence the inhibitory activity of some NSAIDs on cartilage. The action of many of these NSAIDs is important to clinical management of patients since they are very effective clinically in diminishing inflammation and increasing joint movement. Therefore it would be of considerable advantage to the patient if it were possible to continue the use of these agents at the same time ensuring that the joint integrity was not being impaired.

Investigations of the actions of IL1, as stated above, has shown that human cartilage is particularly sensitive to this cytokine. Whilst no definitive hypothesis for the natural control of IL1 synthesis or secretion has been advanced, one possibility is that the local levels of prostaglandins may influence cytokine synthesis and activation [11]. If this is the case, then the action of some of the most effective NSAIDs that have been developed may lead to a local diminution or abolition of prostaglandins and hence may effectively abolish the control of cytokine production. If this is the case, it was reasoned that the use of prostaglandin analogues might control IL1 production in arthritic cartilage. To follow through this idea, the PGE_1 analogue, misoprostol (Cytotec®, Searle), was investigated on human cartilage in the presence of a number of NSAIDs. It was found that misoprostol at 50 ng/ml gave a significant protection in terms of increasing GAG synthesis and it was most effective against the inhibition of GAG synthesis seen by naproxen, ibuprofen and indomethacin. The action of misoprostol in influencing repair after IL1 is illustrated in Table 4. In this experiment the tissue was treated with IL1 and allowed to recover in the presence and absence of ibuprofen. It can be seen that as in Table 3, ibuprofen abolished the natural recovery that takes place after IL1 inhibition of synthesis. However, in the presence of ibuprofen and misoprostol, recovery was substantial and statistically significant, illustrating that this agent has potential for modulating one aspect of NSAID action on human cartilage metabolism.

Table 4. Matrix synthesis by OA cartilage. Recovery after IL1 treatment in the presence of NSAID and misoprostol $^{35}SO_4$ cpm/mg $\times 10^{-3}$

Treatment	Control	0.1 ng/ml IL1	Post-IL1 1d	Post-IL1 2d	Post-IL1 4d
–	1.08 (0.2)	0.61 (0.05)	0.65 (0.01)	0.70 (0.06)	0.96 (0.08)
Ibuprofen	–	–	0.50 (0.05)	0.50 (0.04)	0.56 (0.06)
Ibuprofen + misoprostol 100 ng/ml	–	–	0.51 (0.04)	0.67 (0.09)[x]	1.25 (0.02)[x]

[x] $p < 0.01$

Assaying drug action on human cartilage *in vitro*

It should be emphasized that whilst it is important to assay the action of NSAIDs and other agents on human normal, OA and RA cartilage, there are difficulties in so doing. The variation between patients is an obvious factor which has to be taken into account and means that a number of patients must be assayed with every drug, but the variation across individual joints is also an important factor. As stated above, in a recent study it was found necessary to investigate some 40 patients and to look at each individual replicate from the joint. This meant investigating some 2400 replicates for their metabolic activity before and after drug treatment. The variation is obviously marked in severe inflammatory disease, but there is a consistent finding that replicates with similar GAG turnover rates tend to respond similarly to the action of a drug. This means not only that most patients will respond to drugs to some degree, but also that the local response to drugs may vary across a joint. It is possible, I suspect, to correlate the anabolic and catabolic activity of individual areas of a pathological joint with its response to NSAID activity, but this is much more complicated than attempting work on the relatively uniform animal cartilages.

CONCLUSIONS

Some NSAIDs when assayed on human cartilage *in vitro* have inhibitory effects on GAG synthesis. This is not applicable to all NSAIDs – some may be relatively innocuous whilst one or two may indeed stimulate GAG synthesis. For the clinician attempting to assess the advantages and risks of NSAID therapy, these *in vitro* experiments should at least be considered. However, I would accept that, like all *in vitro* experiments, they cannot be guaranteed to give a true picture of the events *in vivo*. Nevertheless, the possibility that long-term exposure to NSAIDs such as indomethacin and naproxen could cause inhibition of synthesis and hence diminish natural repair processes must be considered. It seems possible that the very effectiveness of these agents in depressing prostaglandin level in particular may be a reason for their potential deleterious effect on human cartilage metabolism. However, it should be stressed that these *in vitro* experiments are acute and do not reflect what the regime of treatment may be *in vivo*. It would also be true to say that short-term treatment with NSAIDs would be unlikely to cause joint damage. The results of Rashed et al. [12] showing that OA of the hip progresses faster in patients treated with indomethacin, which can augment IL1 production up to seven-fold [11], tends to support the *in vitro* work however.

In an attempt to determine whether or not these *in vitro* effects are obtained *in vivo* a study has commenced on indomethacin and aspirin in which patients have been treated prior to operation with these drugs and then the cartilage metabolism measured immediately at excision. The preliminary results suggest that in many cases the cartilage metabolism is depressed and that *in vitro* incubation of the cartilage for two to three days allows recovery to take place, analogous to that which happens after *in vitro* treatment with drugs. Much further work needs to be done on this system to determine whether or not these *in vivo* findings confirm the *in vitro* work and at this time it would be premature to do more than suggest that clinicians should view the action of certain NSAIDs with caution. An *in vivo* assessment of cartilage integrity which would effectively monitor in the short term the integrity or metabolism of human cartilage *in vivo* is urgently needed. Until such a method is available the *in vitro* human cartilage organ culture assay system offers a very useful method for assessing the development of new anti-inflammatory agents that can be shown to be free of the potential disadvantages of some of the present NSAIDs.

REFERENCES

1. Dingle JT. Cartilage damage and repair: the roles of IL-1, NSAIDs and prostaglandins in osteoarthritis. In: New Frontiers in Prostaglandin Therapeutics. Princetown, USA: Excerpta Medica: 1991.
2. Dingle JT, Horner A, Shield M. The sensitivity of synthesis of human cartilage matrix to inhibition by IL1 suggests a mechanism for the development of osteoarthritis. Cell Biochem Funct. 1991;9:99–102.
3. Martin M, Resch K. Interleukin 1: More than a mediator between leucocytes. TIPS. 1988;9:171–177.
4. Brandt KD. Effects of non-steroidal anti-inflammatory drugs on chondrocyte metabolism in vitro and in vivo. Am J Med. 1987;83(Suppl. 5A);29–34.
5. Hess EV, Herman JH. Cartilage metabolism and anti-inflammatory drugs in osteoarthritis. Am J Med. 1986;77(Suppl. 5B):36–43.
6. Kalbhen DA. The influence of NSAIDs on morphology of articular cartilage. Scand J Rheumatol. 1989;77(Suppl.);13–22.
7. Page-Thomas DP, King B, Stephens T, Dingle JT. In vivo studies of cartilage regeneration after damage induced by catabolin/IL1. Ann Rheum Dis. 1987;46:527–533.
8. Perry GH, Smith MJG, Whiteside CG. Spontaneous recovery of the joint space in degenerative hip disease. Ann Rheum Dis. 1972;31:440–448.
9. Danielsson LG. Instance and prognosis of coxarthrosis. Acta Orthop Scand. 1964;66(Suppl.): 1–114.
10. Dieppe P. Osteoarthritis. The scale and scope of the clinical problem. In: Dieppe P. ed. Osteoarthritis: Current Research and Prospects for Pharmacological Intervention. London:IPC Technical Services;1988:40–66.
11. Kunkel SL, Chensue SW. Arachidonic acid metabolites regulate interleukin 1 production. Biochem Biophys Res Commun. 1985;128:892–897.
12. Rashed S, Revell P, Hemingway A et al. Effect of non-steroid anti-inflammatory drugs on the course of osteoarthritis. Lancet. 1989;2:519–522.

32

Non-steroidal anti-inflammatory drugs and the augmented lipoxygenase pathway: conceivable impact on joint conditions

Iván L. Bonta and Graham R. Elliott

Department of Pharmacology, Faculty of Medicine, Erasmus University
Rotterdam, POB 1738, 3000 DR Rotterdam, The Netherlands

BACKGROUND AND SCOPE

Eicosanoid products of arachidonic acid (AA) metabolism are involved in several aspects of immuno-inflammatory processes. Macrophages play a pivotal role in such processes. These cells can readily release both cyclo-oxygenase and lipoxygenase metabolites and are also equipped with receptors for these products. Hence eicosanoids released from macrophages not only influence surrounding cells, but feeding back on the macrophage also modulate several functions of the macrophage itself, including *i.a.* lysosomal enzyme secretion, eicosanoid discharge and production of cytokines. Observations indicating that macrophage functions appeared to be positively related to the activity of the lipoxygenase pathway and negatively related to cyclic AMP elevating cycloxygenase metabolites, led in turn to the observation that leukotrienes can stimulate PGE_2 synthesis. This indicated that leukotrienes regulate their own production through a self-induced inhibitor, PGE_2. These earlier findings warranted an investigation of the possibility that the lipoxygenase pathway is the target through which PGE_2 suppresses and cyclo-oxygenase inhibitors stimulate macrophage functions. In this article we give a brief account of the most salient results which show that inhibition of cyclo-oxygenase by NSAIDs leads to stimulation of lysosomal enzyme release and augmented activity of the lipoxygenase pathway in macrophages. Further it will be highlighted that the two intertwined effects, i.e. removal of the regulatory role of PGE_2 and augmented production of LTB_4 underlie the facilitating effects of NSAIDs on synthesis of interleukin-1 (IL-1) and/or tumor necrosis factor α (TNFα).

Side-effects of Anti-inflammatory Drugs 3. Rainsford KD, Velo GP (eds),
Inflammation and Drug Therapy Series, Volume V.

LYSOSOMAL ENZYME SECRETION IS REGULATED BY EICOSANOIDS

Release of a lysosomal enzyme, e.g. β-glucuronidase, can serve as a marker to indicate the state of activation of the macrophage. In this context resident macrophages, which are quiescent, release less β-glucuronidase than activated macrophages, such as those elicited by some inflammatory stimulus. In contrast, resident cells release more PGE_2 than do elicited macrophages. Further studies showed that, whereas PGE_2 suppresses lysosomal enzyme discharge, the lipoxygenase metabolite LTC_4 promotes this event and that the secretory response upon stimulation by LTC_4 was further enhanced by the NSAIDs indomethacin and aspirin [1]. Thus the concept emerged that, with respect to macrophage lysosomal enzyme regulation, products of the lipoxygenase pathway and PGE_2 work in opposition, lipoxygenase metabolites being stimulatory and PGE_2 suppressive [1].

PGE_2 INHIBITS AND NSAIDs ENHANCE THE RELEASE OF LTB_4

The concept that endogenous PGE_2 is a major modulator of macrophage functions prompted the assumption that inhibition of cyclo-oxygenase will ultimately lead to stimulation of macrophages. Further, it appeared conceivable that removal of an endogenous suppressive factor, as represented by PGE_2, may promote the production of leukotrienes. Indeed, with human neutrophils indomethacin was shown to increase the formation of lipoxygenase products [2]. Subsequently we have shown with peritoneal macrophages from mice that, following calcium ionophore stimulation, indomethacin enhanced the discharge of LTB_4 [3]. Results of a representative experiment are shown in Figure 1. Similarly, using rat peritoneal macrophages, indomethacin and aspirin, while inhibiting the formation of cyclo-oxygenase metabolites, augmented the calcium flux-stimulated synthesis of LTB_4 as displayed in Figure 2. In the original paper results are also described which show that PGE_2 inhibited not only the calcium ionophore-stimulated LTB_4 formation, but also the augmentation of release caused by the NSAIDs [4]. We also presented circumstantial evidence that this effect of PGE_2, as many of its other effects, is a cyclic AMP-mediated event. More explicitly, our results suggested that elevated cyclic AMP inhibits macrophage LTB_4 synthesis by limiting the availability of AA [4]. However, in the context of the present article, the prominent finding is that, NSAIDs, probably by removing the regulatory role of PGE_2, promote the synthesis of the pro-inflammatory LTB_4. These results, together with other findings [1,2], provided experimental evidence for the

270

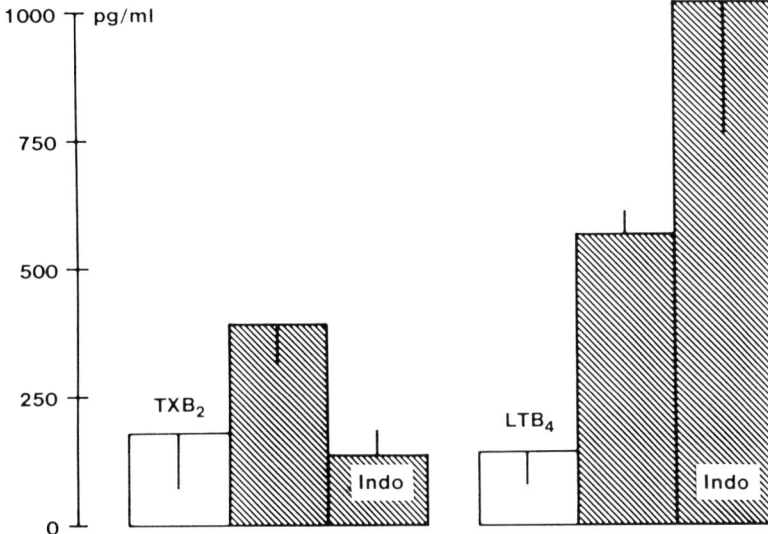

Figure 1. Effect of indomethacin (10^{-7} mol/L) on TXB_2 and LTB_4 synthesis following A23187 (10^{-6} mol/L) stimulation (hatched bars) in mouse resident peritoneal macrophages. For details see the original paper [3]

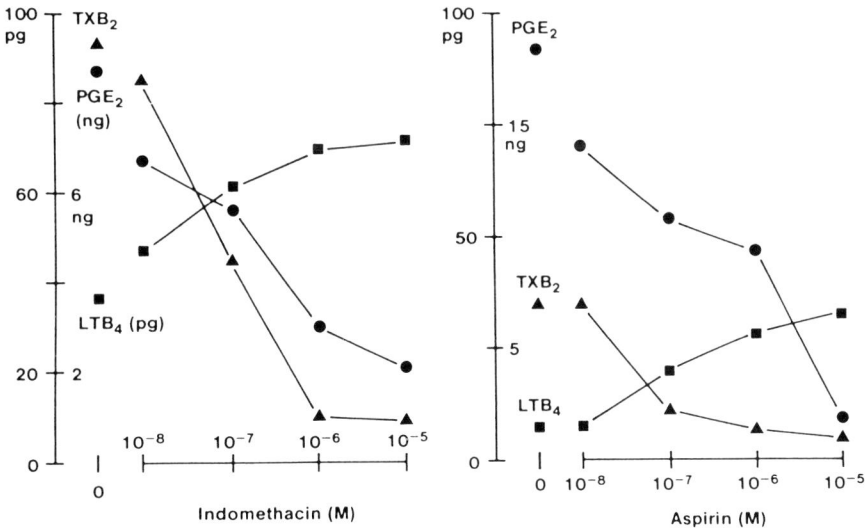

Figure 2. Effects of inhibitors of cyclo-oxygenase on A23187 (10^{-6} mol/L) stimulated release of PGE_2, TXB_2 and LTB_4 in rat elicited peritoneal macrophages. For more details see the original paper [4]. (By kind permission of Plenum Press)

theoretical proposal as forwarded in reference 5, that NSAIDs could, by inhibiting PGE_2 synthesis and stimulating leukotriene production, augment pro-inflammatory components of joint conditions.

Leukotrienes, due to their chemotactic, vascular permeability-increasing and lysosomal enzyme-discharging effects, are intrinsically pro-inflammatory. In addition, however, augmentation of the lipoxygenase pathway favours the synthesis of macrophage-derived cytokines. The ensuing part of this article turns to briefly discuss the indirect consequences of the NSAIDs-induced imbalance between PGE_2 and lipoxygenase products.

INTERACTIONS WITH SYNTHESIS OF MACROPHAGE CYTOKINES

Eicosanoids through negative-feedback interaction with the macrophage, modulate not only their own release, but also interact with the production of macrophage-derived cytokines. These complicated interactions have been recently reviewed [6]. In the context of the present article it is of importance that leukotrienes promote and PGE_2 usually downregulates the production of IL-1 and TNFα. While NSAIDs were reported to enhance the endotoxin-induced IL-1 response of macrophages [7], others showed that this enhancement was limited to cell-associated IL-1 [8]. However with TNFα there is uniformity in the reports which show that PGE_2 suppresses and indomethacin enhances its endotoxin-stimulated production [9,10]. Furthermore, in addition to the observation showing that TNFα can induce the production of IL-1 (quoted in Ref. 6), these two cytokines, synergistically with each other, were shown to be arthritogenic [11]. Figure 3 is an oversimplified view of the concept, in which PGE_2 represents a major inhibitory modulator regulating the production of LTB_4, IL-1 and TNFα, which constitute a triad of harmful mediators. Removal of PGE_2 by NSAIDs would promote this triad and may thus exacerbate tissue damage during long-term treatment of joint conditions.

CONCLUDING REMARKS

Despite several uncertainties, inherent with a network of multiple interactions, we feel at present that the following conclusions are not misplaced in the context of the enhanced production of LTB_4 following exposure of macrophages to NSAIDs: (a) endogenous PGE_2, via increased levels of intracellular cyclic AMP, limits the availability of AA and thus controls the release of lipoxygenase products; (b) NSAIDs, via inhibition of cyclo-oxygenase, remove the regulatory role of PGE_2 and thus facilitate the release of lipoxygenase products; (c) synthesis of macrophage cytokines

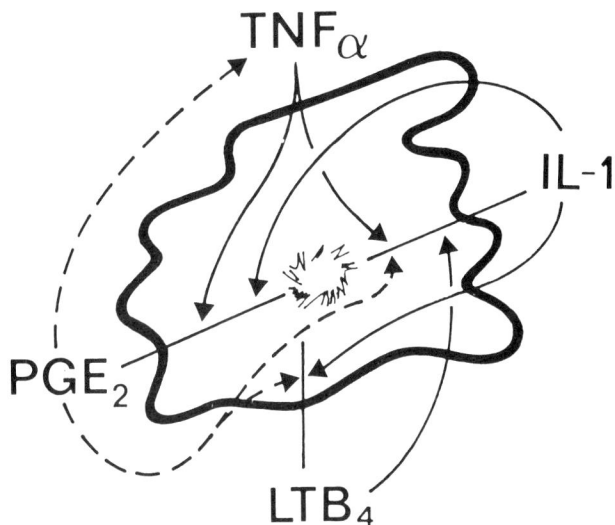

Figure 3. Heuristic model of some aspects of balanced regulation of mediator producing functions of the macrophage. Dotted lines represent inhibitory influences. Endogenous PGE_2 controls the synthesis of LTB_4, IL-1 and $TNF\alpha$. The latter two are important stimulators of PGE_2, which thus is their self-induced inhibitor. This balanced regulation represents a homeostatic process-loop system. Removal of PGE_2 by NSAIDs causes a breakdown of the homeostasis and accordingly results in uncontrolled production of the triad of harmful mediators. This oversimplified model, in common with other models, is a poor replica of the reality, in which many other factors contribute to homeostasis and the pathologic or iatrogenic breakdown thereof.

IL-1 and $TNF\alpha$ is enhanced by lipoxygenase products and downregulated by PGE_2; (d) NSAIDs augment the production of macrophage cytokines by two intertwined mechanisms: first, via inhibiting the synthesis of PGE_2 and second, via augmentation of the lipoxygenase pathway; (e) promotion of the triad (LTB_4, IL-1 and $TNF\alpha$) by NSAIDs may contribute to erosion of cartilage and resorption of bone in arthritic conditions. In view, however, that several observations leading to these conclusions have been made either *in vitro* and/or with cells harvested from laboratory animals and from sites remote from joints, the extrapolation of these conclusions to clinical conditions requires great caution.

ACKNOWLEDGEMENTS

The original experiments discussed in this article were sponsored by Sigma-Tau Pharmaceutical Co., Rome. Support was also obtained from the Emil Starkenstein Foundation.

REFERENCES

1. Schenkelaars EJ, Bonta IL. Cyclo-oxygenase inhibitors promote the leukotriene C_4 induced release of β-glucuronidase from rat peritoneal macrophages: prostaglandin E_2 suppresses. Int J Immunopharmacol. 1986;8:305–311.
2. Docherty JC, Wilson TW. Indomethacin increases the formation of lipoxygenase products in calcium ionophore stimulated human neutrophils. Biochem Biophys Res Commun. 1987;2:534–538.
3. Elliott GR, Tak C, Pellens C, Ben-Efraim S, Bonta IL. Indomethacin stimulation of macrophage cytostasis against MOPC-315 tumor cells is inhibited by both prostaglandin E_2 and nordihydroguaiaretic acid, a lipoxygenase inhibitor. Cancer Immunol Immunother. 1988;27:133–136.
4. Elliott GR, Lauwen APM, Bonta IL. Prostaglandin E_2 inhibits and indomethacin and aspirin enhance, A23187-stimulated leukotriene B_4 synthesis by rat peritoneal macrophages. Br J Pharmacol. 1989;96:265–270.
5. Rang HP, Dale MM. Drugs used to suppress inflammatory and immune reactions. In: Rang HP, Dale MM, eds. Pharmacology. Edinburgh: Churchill Livingstone; 1987:204–224.
6. Bonta IL, Ben-Efraim S. Interactions between inflammatory mediators in expression of antitumor cytostatic activity of macrophages. Immunol Lett. 1990;25:295–302.
7. Kunkel SL, Chensue SW, Phan SH. Prostaglandins as endogenous mediators of interleukin-1 production. J Immunol. 1986;136:186–192.
8. Bahl AK, Foreman JC, Dale MM. Effect of non-steroidal anti-inflammatory drugs on interleukin-1 production. In: Abstracts of 7th International Conference on Prostaglandins and Related Compounds. Florence;1990:90.
9. Scales WE, Chensue SW, Otterness I, Kunkel SL. Regulation of monokine gene expression: prostaglandin E_2 suppresses tumor necrosis factor but not interleukin-1α or β in RNA and cell-associated bioactivity. J Leuk Biol. 1989;45:416–421.
10. Spatafora M, Chiappara G, D'Amico D, Volpes D, Melis M, Pace E, Merendino A, Bonsignore MR. Indomethacin alters the kinetics of tumor necrosis factor alpha production by human blood monocytes. In: Abstracts of 7th International Conference on Prostaglandins and Related Compounds. Florence;1990:100.
11. Henderson B, Pettipher ER. Arthritogenic actions of recombinant IL-1 and tumor necrosis factor in the rabbit: evidence for synergistic interactions between cytokines *in vivo*. Clin Exp Immunol. 1989;75:306–310.

33

Therapeutic potential of 5-lipoxygenase inhibitors: the discovery and development of MK-886, a novel-mechanism leukotriene inhibitor

J.W. Gillard, R. Dixon, D. Ethier, J. Evans, A.W. Ford-Hutchinson, R. Fortin, Y. Girard, Y. Guindon, P. Hamel, T. Jones, C. Leveillé, A. Lord, D. Miller, H. Morton, C. Rouzer and C. Yoakim

Merck Frosst Centre for Therapeutic Research, Kirkland, Québec, Canada

THERAPEUTIC STATUS OF 5-LO INHIBITORS AND LT ANTAGONISTS

Two approaches toward developing anti-leukotriene therapy have led to clinical candidates at the present time. Specific potent leukotriene antagonists (MK-571 [2], MK-679 and ICI-204,219 [3]) have entered clinical trials for asthma and display efficacy in early studies of induced bronchoconstriction (allergen or exercise). These results are encouraging in supporting the thesis of leukotriene-induced pathology in asthma. Inhibitors of leukotriene biosynthesis inhibit the entire cascade of lipoxygenase products, removing simultaneously the contractile and oedemagenic peptido-leukotrienes as well as the chemotactic pro-inflammatory dihydroxy-leukotrienes. The therapeutic implications of such treatment are significant in diseases where an inflammatory response is also associated with, or causes, the pathological effect. Two agents have been examined in clinical trials to date. A-64077 (zileuton) is a 5-lipoxygenase enzyme inhibitor from Abbott [1]. It is an N-hydroxy area derivative which has demonstrated tolerability and efficacy in humans [4]. MK-886 [5], from Merck, is a novel-mechanism agent which acts at an independent site from 5-lipoxygenase, on the 5-lipoxygenase-activating protein, FLAP. This highly potent agent has been evaluated in preliminary studies in man and has been shown to be well tolerated and efficacious in

Side-effects of Anti-inflammatory Drugs 3. Rainsford KD, Velo GP (eds), Inflammation and Drug Therapy Series, Volume V.

inhibiting urinary and whole-blood leukotriene levels, concomitantly with reduction of antigen-induced bronchoconstriction. The discovery and development of this agent forms the substance of this presentation.

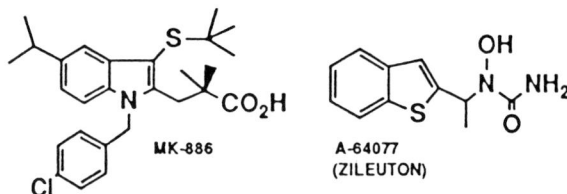

Figure 1. Clinical candidate inhibitors of leukotriene biosynthesis

LTB_4 may have a singular role in certain diseases or syndromes. For example, the role of LTB_4 in inflammatory bowel disease (IBD) is strongly inferred from the observation of elevated levels of LTB_4 in rectal dialysate and the enhanced capacity of colonic mucosa from IBD patients to synthesize LTB_4. The chemotactic properties of LTB_4 may play a key role in the induction or maintenance of neutrophilic infiltration and degranulation which characterize this disorder. The primary agent to treat this disease, sulphasalazine, has been shown to inhibit LT synthesis and the 5-LO inhibitor A-64077 (zileuton) is currently in clinical trials to determine efficacy.

The role of leukotrienes in psoriasis as a causative agent is not clear. LTB_4 is found in higher concentrations in psoriatic lesions than are found in normal or uninvolved skin. LTB_4, when injected intradermally, can produce formation of micro-abcesses containing PMN leucocytes, reminiscent of psoriatic lesions. Peptido-leukotrienes have also been detected in psoriatic skin and the vasodilative and oedematous properties of these mediators may account for the associated erythema in psoriasis. In clinical trials with very weak inhibitors of 5-LO such as Syntex lopoxalin, some clinical improvement was seen. No such clinical improvement was seen in the case of MK-886 when dosed orally, at levels sufficient to achieve 60–70% reduction in urinary leukotriene levels in psoriasis.

In rheumatoid arthritis and gout, synovial fluid exudates contain increased concentrations of LTB_4 and are neutrophil-rich. The responsiveness of these cells *in vitro* to LTB_4-induced chemotaxis and degranulation studies may imply a contribution of this mediator to the maintenance of inflammatory lesions *in vivo*. Despite the generally negative results of 5-LO inhibitors in animal models of inflammatory joint disease, zileuton, has been claimed to improve qualitative symptoms in arthritic joints in an open trial.

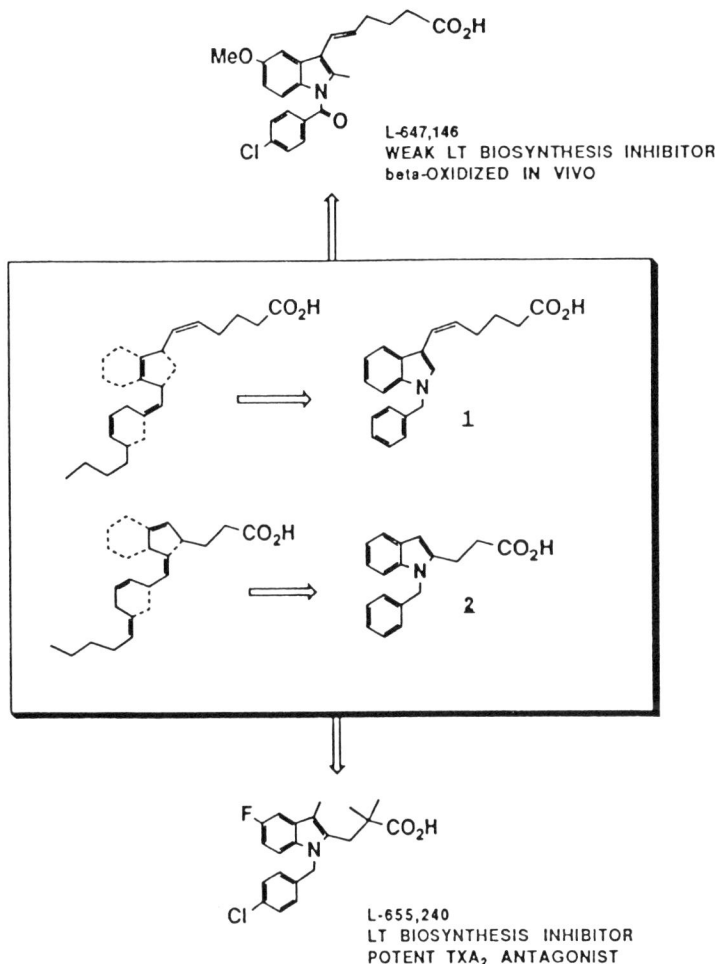

Scheme 1: Arachidonate conformers as precursors to the indole class of eicosanoid inhibitors

THE DISCOVERY AND CHEMICAL DEVELOPMENT OF MK-886

A new class of compounds, the indole-2-propanoic acids, exemplified by L-655,240 [6,7], has been recently described which has dual properties, namely thromboxane antagonism and leukotriene biosynthesis inhibition. The initial compounds in this series (1) or (2) were designed on the rationale that they might interact with the 5-LO enzyme in a manner similar to the substrate, arachidonic acid, and that they may inhibit the enzyme in a competitive manner. This mechanistic rationale for leukotriene biosynthesis was proven to be totally unfounded as will be evident from the discussion which follows; nevertheless, it served to identify new structural

277

classes with potent activity in two areas of eicosanoid biology. L-647,146, although showing some LT inhibitory activity, was not pursued due to metabolic instability. L-655,240, the product of an extensive structure activity study around the indole nucleus, showed potent thromboxane antagonism in addition to sub-micromolar inhibition of leukotriene biosynthesis.

Thromboxane antagonists

The initial aim of the chemistry programme in this series was to separate the biological activity by identifying the structural factors responsible for each property. Through an analysis of structure-activity relationships, particularly as they were influenced by molecular conformation, it was possible to synthesize molecules which were pharmacologically specific for thromboxane antagonism. Structure-analysis studies, as shown in Scheme 2, led to a second series of compounds with exclusively leukotriene inhibitory properties.

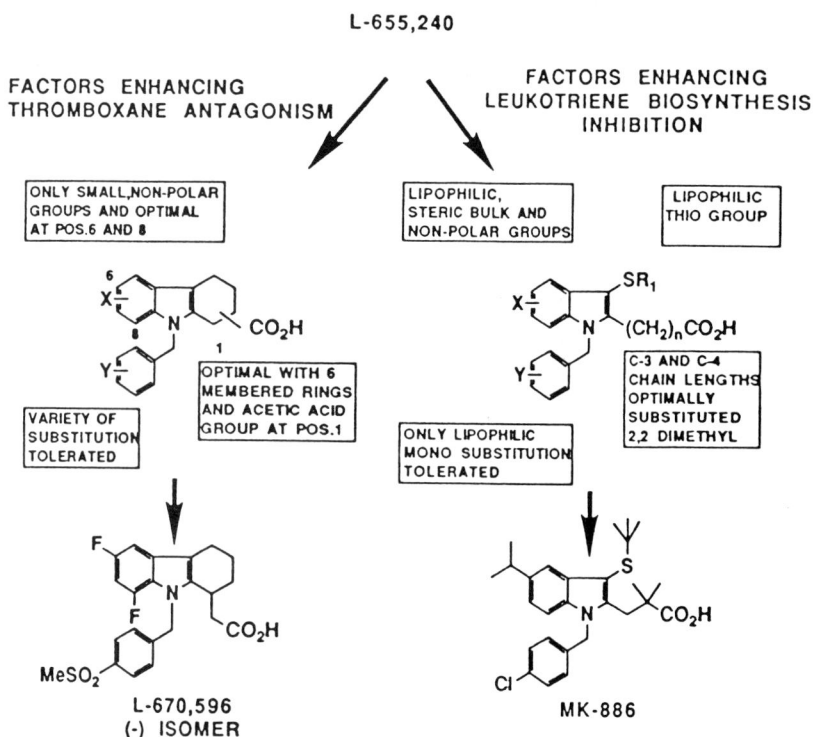

Scheme 2. Optimization of structural features to enhance TXA$_2$ antagonism and LT biosynthesis inhibition

From the tetrahydrocarbazole series, L-670,596 [8], a potent specific thromboxane antagonist with excellent pharmacokinetic parameters, has been derived. It is currently being investigated in numerous models of disease in which thromboxane is believed to be involved.

Leukotriene biosynthesis inhibitors

Using structure/activity considerations from the original lead compound, as shown in Scheme 2, a second chemical series of leukotriene biosynthesis inhibitors was defined and optimized. Highly specific, and totally devoid of TXA_2 activity, nanomolar leukotriene biosynthesis inhibitors have been found which are systemically active in *in vivo* studies. MK-886 represents the compound selected for further development as a leukotriene biosynthesis inhibitor. Its intrinsic potency in a number of cellular systems is given in Table 1. Despite the high potency in inhibiting cellular leukotriene synthesis, MK-886 is inactive in inhibiting the enzyme in purified or semi-purified preparations.

In all cases, there is inhibition of LT synthesis at the low nanomolar level, independent of the method of stimulus. The specificity of the compound for inhibition of leukotriene synthesis was demonstrated by its inability to inhibit *in vitro* or *in vivo* the concomitant synthesis of prostaglandins induced by ionophore or zymosan, PAF, or of thromboxane, or 12-HETE in human platelets, when stimulated by ionophore or thrombin.

In vivo studies on MK-886

MK-886 was examined in models of allergic bronchoconstriction in which the compound was a potent inhibitor. In the hypersensitive rat, MK-886 dosed orally reduces dyspnoea (ED_{50} = 0.015 mg/kg) with concomitant

Table 1. Inhibition of leukotriene synthesis in inflammatory cells by MK-886

Cell type	Stimulus, IC_{50} (nM)					
	Ionoph. ± PMA	Anti-IgE	Zymo.	Staph.	FMLP cyto.	PAF
Human PMN (LTB$_4$)	2.7				< 20	
Rat PMN (LTB$_4$)	3.5				5–20	
Human mast (LTC$_4$)	3–5	3–5				
Rat RBL-1 (LTC$_4$)	3–5					
Human eosinophil						50
Macrophage (LTC$_4$)						
Mouse peritoneal	4.3		10			
Human peritoneal	40			2.4		

279

inhibition of antigen-induced biliary leukotriene secretion, (ED_{50} = 0.05 mg/kg p.o.). In a primate model of antigen-induced bronchoconstriction, the compound is capable of completely blocking changes in respiratory resistance and dynamic compliance at a 0.3 mg/kg oral dose.

In a rat model of colonic inflammation using trinitrobenzene sulphonic acid (TNB), MK-886 was found to cause acute reduction of colonic leukotriene synthesis as well as significant reductions in adhesions, macroscopic ulceration and histological scores in studies following chronic dosing [9]. The maximum therapeutic effect of the compound was found to be dependent on the time of inhibition of therapy. In cases where treatment was initiated at the onset of the TNB induction and continued for the next seven days, both LT synthesis and histological improvement was seen. In protocols in which drug treatment was withheld to within seven days of final examination, histological improvement was not significant, despite >80% inhibition of colonic LTB_4 synthesis. Sulphasalazine 100 mg/kg was ineffective in any treatment protocol in reducing symptom scores or LT synthesis.

MK-886 is extremely potent topically in a skin model of leukotriene synthesis in the guinea pig ear, with a topical ED_{50} of 0.001 mg/ear. Acute systemic administration of MK-886 (ED_{50} = 2.5 mg/kg p.o.) 2 hrs prior to ionophore administration afforded identical protection. In a model of plantar inflammation of the rat paw, induced by thioglycolate, the compound was shown to be capable of total inhibition of leukotriene biosynthesis induced by subsequent stimulation with A-23187 when dosed orally at a dose of 3 mg/kg. The ED_{50} in this model was found to be 0.8 mg/kg.

MK-886 is extensively protein bound (99.9%). Oral bioavailability has been demonstrated in two species (rat and dog) to be of the order of 30%. MK-886 has undergone early clinical evaluation in man and has shown inhibition of LTB_4 production in whole blood following *ex vivo* challenge with ionophore A-23187. Furthermore, MK-886 produced significant attenuation of the early and late phase of antigen-induced bronchoconstriction in asthmatic patients [10], as shown in Figure 2.

NOVEL MECHANISM OF ACTION OF MK-886

Despite the fact that MK-886 inhibits leukotriene production in all intact cells examined to date, the compound has no effect on either 5-lipoxygenase itself or on the availability of the substrate, arachidonic acid. The absence of additional effects and the specificity for the inhibition of 5-lipoxygenase suggested a totally novel mechanism of action of this compound. One possibility was that in the intact cell, 5-lipoxygenase required an activation step before leukotriene synthesis could occur. In fact Rouzer and Kargman [11] demonstrated that following neutrophil

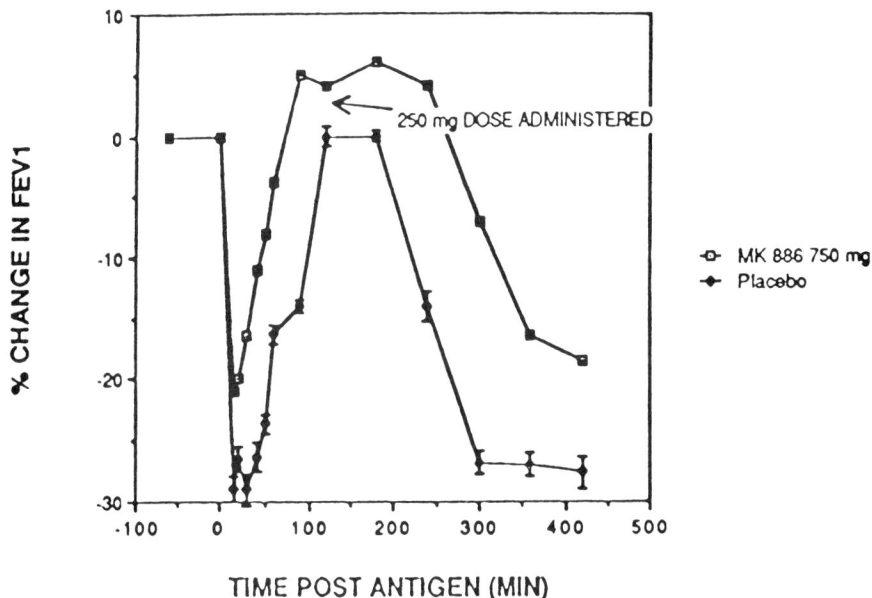

Figure 2. MK-886 (500 mg/250 mg) antigen-induced bronchoconstriction in humans

activation, 5-lipoxygenase translocated from the cytosol to the cell membrane where it could be detected as dead enzyme, presumably having undergone turnover-associated suicide inactivation. When MK-886 was added to the cell incubation mixtures, inhibition of translocation occurred. This inhibition of translocation was shown to be correlated with inhibition of leukotriene synthesis over a range of drug concentrations using both MK-886 and structurally related analogues [12]. This suggested that translocation to the membrane was a key activation step for 5-lipoxygenase.

MK-886 is active in cell incubations at nanomolar concentration, suggesting that it binds to its molecular target with a high affinity. In order to search for a putative binding protein, two series of chemical tools were synthesized at Merck Frosst. The first were radioactive photoaffinity probes based on the structure of MK-886, shown in Figure 3 as L-689,083, and the second, a series of affinity chromatography columns to which MK-886 or structurally related compounds were coupled through a variety of linkages, MK-886 gel being used for the final preparation.

Using the photoaffinity probe, we were able to show that specific binding occurred to a single 18 kD protein, present in the membranes of leucocytes, but not present in a variety of other cell types not known to contain 5-lipoxygenase. Purification of the protein was achieved from CHAPS-solubilized extracts of rat neutrophil membranes [13]. Using the affinity columns, with elution by MK-886 and subsequent purification

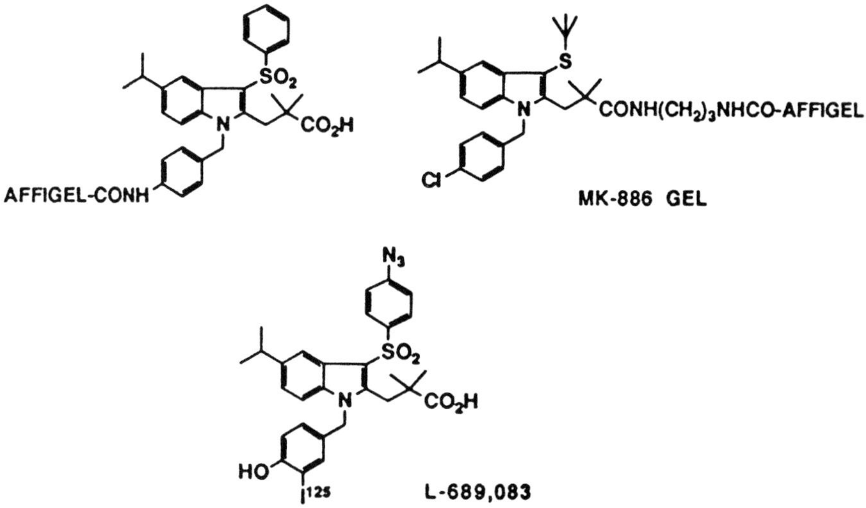

Figure 3. Affinity gels and photoaffinity labels used for FLAP identification and purification

through size exclusion columns, sufficient protein was isolated to determine partial sequence information. Both native protein as well as tryptic and cyanogen bromide cleavage products yielded useful sequence data. Oligonucleotide probes were constructed and Dixon [14] and his group utilized these to screen rat basophil leukaemia cell libraries to obtain the corresponding rat cDNA. The rat cDNA was then used to screen a human dimethylsulphoxide-differentiated HL60 cell library to obtain the human cDNA. Both cDNA clones encoded proteins of 101 amino acid residues which were 92% identical and contained all the peptide sequence derived from the previously purified rat protein. It is proposed from a hydrophobicity analysis that the structure of the protein consists of 3 transmembrane-spanning regions connected by two hydrophilic sections with the C and N-terminus on the opposite sides of the membrane (Figure 4). There appears to be no significant sequence homologies with other known proteins.

The next step was to correlate the presence of this novel 18 kD protein with cellular leukotriene synthesis. This was achieved in a series of transfection experiments in osteosarcoma cells. In cells transfected with either 5-lipoxygenase [14] or the 18 kD protein alone (unpublished data) and stimulated with ionophore A-23187 alone, no leukotriene synthesis was observed. However, in cells transfected with both proteins and exposed to the ionophore, cellular leukotriene synthesis was observed and this synthesis could be inhibited by MK-886. These results indicate that the 5-

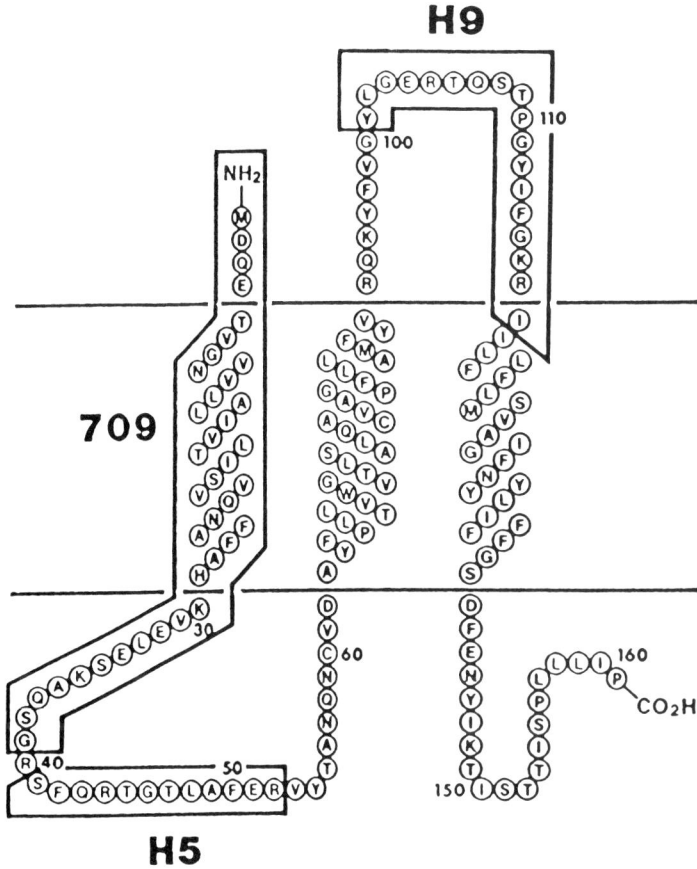

Figure 4. Proposed structure for human FLAP

LO requires the presence of the 18 kD protein to effect cellular LT synthesis. For this reason, we refer to the 18 kD protein as Five Lipoxygenase Activating Protein (FLAP).

The current hypothesis is outlined in Figure 5. Following receptor activation and elevations in intracellular calcium levels, 5-lipoxygenase is activated. This causes 5-lipoxygenase to translocate to the 'docking' protein, FLAP. This model would require a stable complex to be formed between activated 5-lipoxygenase and FLAP as well as possibly other proteins such as phospholipase A_2. This complex would regulate the interaction of 5-lipoxygenase with its substrate arachidonic acid. MK-886 would interfere with this process by binding to FLAP and preventing the formation of the complex. This mechanism may be of more widespread

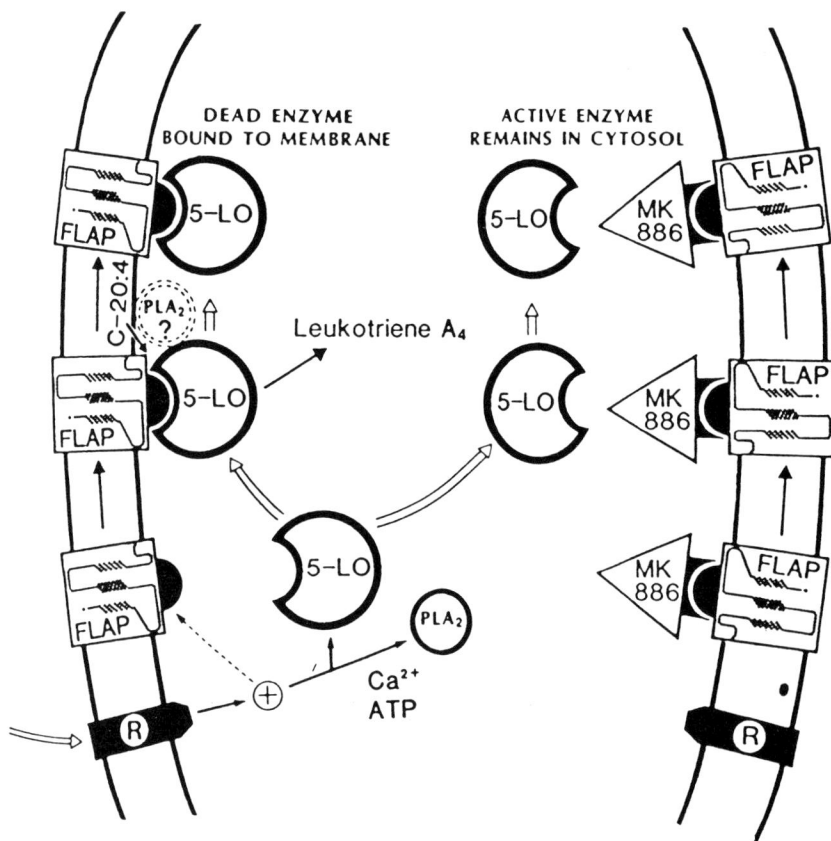

Figure 5. Proposed mechanism of action of MK-886

interest as a number of other proteins, such as protein kinase C and phospholipase C, may also be activated by translocation to the cell membrane. If this represents a general process then other 'docking' proteins may serve as novel therapeutic targets. Clearly this mechanism represents a new approach to inhibition of leukotriene biosynthesis which overcomes a number of the problems of direct 5-lipoxygenase inhibitors, many of which appear to act through redox based mechanisms which have been associated with toxicities related to methaemoglobinaemia.

CONCLUSIONS

Structure-activity studies, using classical medicinal chemistry principles, have played a vital role in the discovery of two new highly potent and specific therapeutic agents. It would now appear that the two biological activities of action observed in the early lead compound, L-655,240 were entirely coincidental. The structure-activity studies were pursued, in the absence of certainty, with the belief that specific molecular interactions could be optimized so as to greatly improve specificity. In so doing, considerable enhancements in potency were also achieved. This permitted the design of new related chemical agents as tools to further investigate the underlying biochemical mechanisms. Further advances in the biochemistry of the leukotriene pathway through the identification of the FLAP protein have been achieved through the use of the photoaffinity technique based on MK-886.

It is unlikely that this protein would have been discovered by other means, hence the value of using drugs as tools for in-depth investigation of macromolecular interactions is demonstrated. In the future, new targets for drug design for the inhibition of leukotrienes may be generated from knowledge of the nature of the tertiary structure of this protein. At present, screening assays based upon the binding of radiolabelled ligands to FLAP offer the prospect of rapid examination of novel structures which may lead to new leads as indirect inhibitors of leukotriene biosynthesis.

REFERENCES

1. For leading reviews see: Ford-Hutchinson AW. In: Rokach J, ed. Leukotrienes and lipoxygenases. New York: Elsevier;1989:405–425 and O'Donnell M, Welton A. In: Lewis AJ, Doherty NS, Ackerman NR, eds. Therapeutic approaches to inflammatory disease. New York: Elsevier; 1989:169

2. Manning PJ, Watson RM, Margolskee BJ, Williams VC, Schwartz JI. Inhibition of exercise-induced bronchoconstriction by MK-571 a potent leukotriene D_4-receptor antagonist. N Engl J Med. 1990;323:1736–1739.

3. Taylor IK, O'Shaughnessy KM, Fuller RW, Dollery CT. Effect of cysteinyl leukotriene receptor antagonist ICI-204,219 on allergen induced bronchoconstriction and airway hyperactivity in atopic subjects. Lancet. 1991;337:690.

4. Israel E, Dermarkarian R, Rosenberg M, Sperling R, Taylor G, Rubin P, Drazen J. The effects of a 5-lipoxygenase inhibitor on asthma induced by cold, dry air. N Engl J Med. 1990;323:1740–1741.

5. Gillard JW, Ford-Hutchinson AW, Chan C et al. L-663,536 (MK-886) (3-[1-(4-chlorobenzyl)-3-t-butyl-thio-5-isopropylindol-2-yl]-2,2-dimethylpropanoic acid), a novel, orally active leukotriene biosynthesis inhibitor. Can J Physiol Pharmacol. 1989;67:456–464.

6. Hall RA, Gillard JW, Guindon Y et al. Pharmacology of L-655,240 (3-[1-(4-chlorobenzyl)-5-fluoro-3-methyl-indol-2-yl]2,2-dimethylpropanoic acid); a potent, selective thromboxane/prostaglandin endoperoxide antagonist. Eur J Pharmacol. 1987;135:193.

7. Gillard JW, Guindon Y, Fortin R et al. Indole-2-alkanoic acids: a new class of biologically active molecules. Thromboxane antagonists. J Med Chem. 1991 [submitted]

8. Ford-Hutchinson AW, Girard Y, Lord A et al. The pharmacology of L-670,596, a potent and selective thromboxane/prostaglandin endoperoxide receptor antagonist. Can J Physiol Pharmacol. 1989;67:989–993.

9. Wallace JL, Kennan CM. An orally active inhibitor of leukotriene synthesis accelerates healing in a rat model of colitis. Am J Physiol. 1990;258:G527–G534.

10. Bel EH, Tanaka W, Spector R, Friedman B. MK-886, an effective oral leukotriene biosynthesis inhibitor on antigen induced early and late asthmatic reactions in man. Am Rev Resp Dis. 1990;A31:141.

11. Rouzer CA, Kargman S. Translocation of 5-lipoxygenase to the membrane in human leucocytes challenged with ionophore A23187. J Biol Chem. 1988;263:10980–10988.

12. Rouzer CA, Ford-Hutchinson AW, Morton HE, Gillard JW. MK-886, a potent and specific leukotriene biosynthesis inhibitor blocks and reverses the membrane association of 5-lipoxygenase in ionophore-challenged leucocytes. J Biol Chem. 1990;265:1436–1442.

13. Miller D, Gillard JW, Vickers PJ et al. Identification and isolation of a membrane protein necessary for leukotriene production. Nature. 1990;343:282–284.

14. Dixon RAF, Diehl RE, Opas E et al. Requirement of a 5-lipoxygenase-activating protein for leukotriene synthesis. Nature. 1990;343:282–284.

34

Mechanisms of rash formation and related skin conditions induced by non-steroidal anti-inflammatory drugs

K.D. Rainsford

Department of Biomedical Sciences and Pathology, McMaster University Faculty of Health Sciences, Hamilton, Ontario L8N 3Z5, Canada

INTRODUCTION

The occurrence of skin rashes and eruptions is a frequent and troublesome side-effect associated with the use of many non-steroidal anti-inflammatory drugs (NSAIDs) [1–4]. This problem is so severe as to be a frequent cause of cessation from therapy with certain NSAIDs [2–4]. Furthermore, a number of NSAIDs have been withdrawn in a large part because the frequency of pruriginous skin rashes, including those from photosensitivity reactions, and other manifestations of skin reactions (e.g. vasculitis, Stevens–Johnson and Lyell's syndromes), was so high as to be regarded as unacceptable. Among the drugs withdrawn have been alclofenac, clobuzarit (Clozic®), benoxaprofen, feprazone, isoxicam and zomepirac [3,4,6–8]. Each of these had a varying spectrum of skin toxicity and, in some cases (e.g. benoxaprofen) other toxic properties were regarded as unacceptable and contributed to the decision to withdraw these drugs from the market.

In this paper the conditions under which rashes and related states develop and probable mechanisms of selected NSAIDs in producing these reactions will be considered. Unfortunately, the mechanisms of NSAID-induced skin reactions has not been extensively investigated and the studies reported to date have been restricted to only a few types of NSAIDs. Recent investigations which we have performed on the mechanisms and clinical management of fenbufen-associated rash will be reported as well as some theoretical considerations of how this and some other NSAIDs (e.g. azapropazone) may cause these conditions.

Side-effects of Anti-inflammatory Drugs 3. Rainsford KD, Velo GP (eds), Inflammation and Drug Therapy Series, Volume V.

DEFINING WHAT CONSTITUTES RASHES

Rashes comprise part of the spectrum of inflammatory skin disorders associated with NSAIDs which are collectively termed *dermatitis medicamentosa* or so-called 'drug eruptions' [5,6]. These can be summarized as follows:

(a) Erythemata

(b) Urticaria

(c) Morbilliform or macupapular eruptions

(d) Mucocutaneous reactions grading in severity to bullous-type, e.g. Stevens–Johnson syndrome

(e) Toxic epidermal necrolysis (Lyell's syndrome)

(f) Photosensitivity reactions

(g) Fixed drug eruptions

(h) Lichen planus and lichenoid eruptions, and

(i) Purpura

While the occurrence of rashes *per se* from NSAIDs may have the relatively mild outcome of being merely inconvenient and unpleasant to live with, it is important to recognize that these manifestations may in some individuals with undefined susceptibility have potentially severe consequences, e.g. toxic epidermal necrolysis, and Stevens–Johnson syndrome, which are frequently fatal. The grading of pathology between rashes and other more severe skin reactions is both difficult to define and highly variable and may even include a variety of reactions in the one individual [6].

Details of the histopathological features of drug eruptions of the skin are shown in Table 1.

VARYING PROPENSITY OF NSAIDs TO INDUCE RASHES

NSAIDs appear to vary in their propensity to produce rashes but alcofenac*, aspirin, azapropazone, benoxaprofen*, fenclofenac*, fenbufen, feprazone*, isoxicam*, piroxicam and tiaprofenic acid feature particularly as being most frequently associated with these reactions [3,4,6–8].

It should also be noted that many disease-modifying antirheumatic drugs (DMARDs) such as the gold salts and D-penicillamine also produce rashes in arthritic patients. Since many such patients with rheumatoid arthritis may be receiving one or more ·of the NSAIDs with a particular

---

* now withdrawn

Table 1. Principal histopathological features in drug-induced skin reactions

I. **Urticaria**

Characteristic recurrent wheals comprising raised erythematous areas of oedema; accompanied by intense itching

Large wheals are angioedema

Histopathology – dermal oedema, sparce perivascular lymphocytic infiltrate with eosinophils

In angioedema infiltrate extends into subcutaneous tissue; various subtypes depending on associated pathology and causes

II. **Phototoxic drug eruptions**

No diagnostic histological picture

Essentially non-specific dermal inflammatory cell infiltrate

III. **Drug-induced photosensitivity eruptions**

Distinction made between this and II above

Cell-mediated reaction with epidermal spongliosis and microvesiculation, perivascular lymphoid cell infiltrate and exocytosis

IV. **Fixed drug eruptions**

Circumscribed lesions occurring persistently at same site(s) associated with drug ingestion. Commonly slightly elevated erythematous patches which may become bullous and on healing leave pigmented areas

Histopathology – cell infiltrate of most inflammatory cells

V. **Erythema multiforme**

Acute self-limiting dermatosis with periodicity of attack but sometimes resolving in 3–6 weeks. Lesions often haemorrhagic, may be idiopathic or drug-related. Two types (both with high mortality):

(1) Stevens–Johnson – with high fever, prostration and extensive eruptions. Severe involvement of mucous membranes.

(2) Lyell's syndrome (toxic epidermal necrolysis) – with subepidermal involvement initially with widespread blotchy oedema, then large flaccid bullae detachment of epidermis in large sheets giving dermal-layer scalded appearance. Mucous membrane involvement less severe than in Stevens–Johnson syndrome.

Histopathology – variably characterized as (1) dermal type (in macular – papular lesions) with perivascular infiltrate of mononuclears and eosinophils, oedema of papillary dermis. Bullae involve PAS basement membrane and extravasated red cells.

(3) Mixed dermal–epidermal type: as for (1) above with epidermis showing necrotic keratinocytes and mononuclear infiltrate therein, (3) epidermal type in Stevens–Johnson and Lyell's syndromes with mononuclear infiltrate in blood vessels around superficial blood vessels of epidermis, groups of keratinocytes with eosinophilic necrosis, neutrophil accumulation hydropic degeneration of basal cells.

VI. **Drug-induced vasculitis**

With either lymphocytic vasculitis limited to skin of extremities (macupapular rather than purpuric) or lymphocytic vasculitis in all skin areas with mainly purpuric lesions.

Histopathology shows leucocytoclastic vasculitis; leucocytes predominate with fibrinoid deposits in vessel walls, mononuclear and eosinophilic infiltrate.

Based on Lever and Schaunberg-Lever [5]

propensity to produce skin rashes together with a DMARD then the problem is exacerbated further. In some case reports it is difficult to ascribe a causal basis to the ingestion of one of these groups of drugs alone.

Most mild rashes from NSAIDs are essentially reversible inasmuch as the condition ablates upon cessation of therapy. Thus aside from inconvenience to the patient the problem is relatively manageable by simply withdrawing from the drug. The problem is, however, what to choose for therapy among the NSAIDs because many, if not all, could produce rashes.

HYPOTHESES FOR THE MECHANISMS OF NSAID-ASSOCIATED SKIN RASHES

Simple erythematous rashes and associated urticarial conditions are probably Type I immediate-type hypersensitivity reactions (of Gell and Coombs) involving the B-cell production of IgE which upon binding to mast cells and subsequent sensitization yields histamine and leukotrienes [6]. Thus antihistamines find some place in treatment of these states though in general this therapy is often limited or even ineffective. Drug-induced rashes may also have a non-allergic basis as a result of accumulation of production of photoproducts or metabolites in the skin.

Types III and IV delayed-type hypersensitivity reactions are manifest prespectively in formation of immune complexes which induce complement-activated tissue damage (vasculitis, agranulocytosis and anaphylactoid reactions), or of production of sensitized T-cells which elaborate lymphokines [6]. These states commonly underlie the development of most other drug-associated skin reactions aside from simple rashes and urticarial conditions [6].

Fundamental to the understanding of how different NSAIDs produce skin reactions is to know if these drugs accumulate in skin and what, if any, photoproducts or metabolites are produced therein. Autoradiographic and biochemical studies have shown that a range of NSAIDs do accumulate in the skin of rats [9]. Particular note should be taken that the acetyl-group of aspirin appears to be retained in the skin for long periods of time [9,10]. The covalent modification by the acetyl-group of aspirin of proteins and other macrolecules might be responsible for the long-lived retention of this moiety of aspirin in the skin and lead to a number of immunological reactions.

The underlying chemical features and actions responsible for the initiation of the range of immunological reactions responsible for skin rashes, eruptions and other severe skin reactions appears, from the limited studies performed to date, to vary from one NSAID to another. For specific drugs studied so far it appears that for the purpose of discussing their individual action, they may be grouped as follows:

290

Table 2. Putative photoproducts or metabolites of NSAIDs implicated in skin rashes and related toxicities

Drug	Toxic product(s) or photoproducts
Benoxaprofen [11,12]	(1) 2,-(4-dichlorophenyl-5-ethyl) benzoxazole (DPEB)

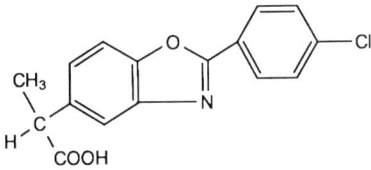

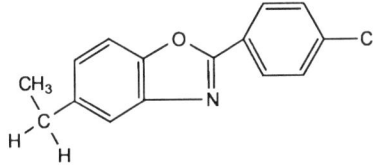

CH$_3$ C H COOH — (benoxaprofen structure)

CH$_3$ C H H — (DPEB structure)

(2) Superoxide, singlet oxygen and hydroxyethyl radicals from UV + O$_2$. Possibility of hydroxyethylperoxyl radical as intermediate during UV activation of benoxaprofen

Piroxicam [13]

Metabolite C: UV-A-induced phototoxicity

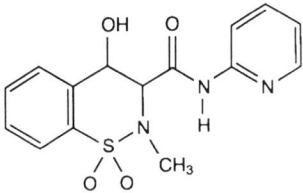

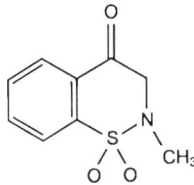

Alclofenac [8,19,20]

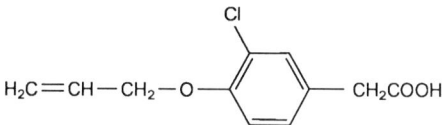

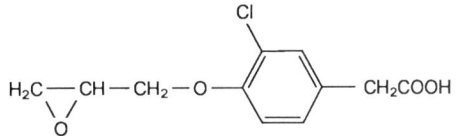

$H_2C=CH-CH_2-O-$ ... $-CH_2COOH$

$H_2C-CH-CH_2-O-$ ... $-CH_2COOH$ (with epoxide O)

Naproxen [14–16] [=(1)]

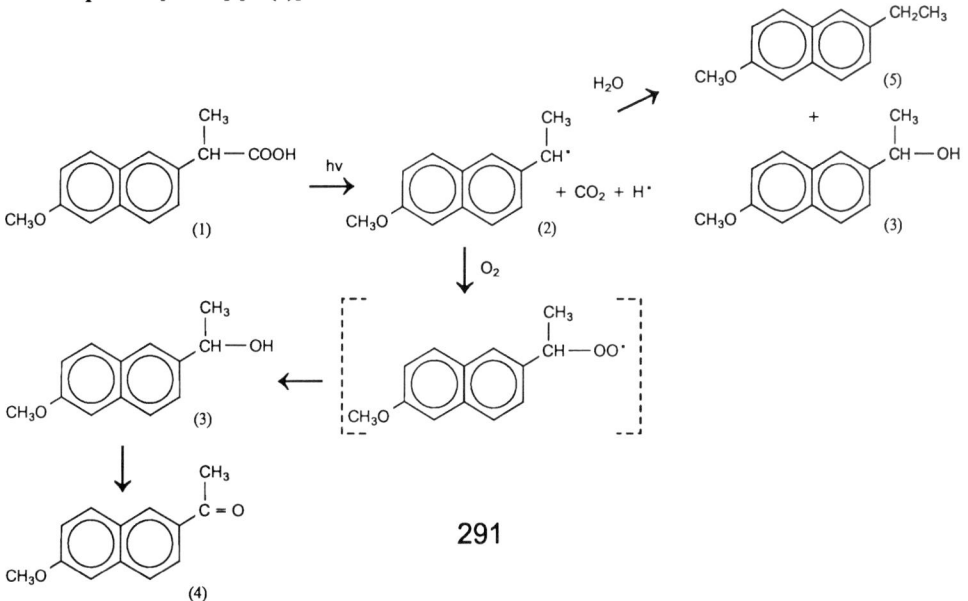

CH$_3$ CH—COOH (1)

$\xrightarrow{h\nu}$

CH$_3$ CH· (2) + CO$_2$ + H·

$\xrightarrow{H_2O}$

CH$_2$CH$_3$ (5)

+

CH$_3$ CH—OH (3)

$\downarrow$ O$_2$

CH$_3$ CH—OO· (dashed box)

CH$_3$ CH—OH (3)

$\downarrow$

CH$_3$ C=O (4)

291

Table 2. *(continued)*

Drug	Toxic product(s) or photoproducts
Pyrazolones [17] e.g. **phenylbutazone**	STRUCTURES NOT KNOWN

Azapropazone [17,18] [= APZ]

APZ $\xrightarrow[\text{H}_2\text{O}]{\text{UV}}$ Mi307

Mi306 $+CO_2$

Mi306 PHOTOPRODUCT(S) OR METABOLITES PROPOSED

(1) Those for which the development of *photo-degradation product(s)* have been implicated. The best studied examples are the photoxic products derived from benoxaprofen [1,12] and piroxicam [13]. In both these cases a photo-degradation product has been identified and cellular reactions identified (Table 2). Other examples include naproxen [14,15], various pyrazolones [16,17] and azapropazone [18,19] (Table 2) but in these cases the cellular and biochemical reactions produced by photoproducts or metabolites has not been identified.

(2) Drugs which have been found to have manufacturing impurities or excipients present which appear to have been associated with the occurrence of severe skin reactions. These include toxic epidermal necrolysis (Lyell's syndrome) with the production impurity in isoxicam; Stevens–Johnson syndrome with an excipient in clobuzarit

(Clozic®), and skin rashes and vasculitis produced from a reaction with an excipient which was developed in tablets but not capsules of alclofenac [8,19].

(3) Direct *chemical modification* has been proposed. Thus hypersensitivity reactions attributed to aspirin, some of which involve skin reactions have been attributed to formation of (a) aspirinyl or salicyl antibodies, or (b) acetylation of biomolecules by aspirin [7,10]. Likewise the skin rashes produced by alclofenac [19] might (in addition to No. 2 above) be attributed to an epoxide metabolite which is produced by alclofenac. However, to the author's knowledge no skin reactions of this alkyl-epoxide metabolite have been demonstrated although this is hepatotoxic [20].

Among the biochemical and immunological mechanisms postulated to occur during the development of skin reactions to NSAIDs are:

(1) The *eliciting of non-self antigen production* by the reaction of photoproduct(s) with endogenous proteins which could then set up the immunological reactions [17,18]. Thus, for example, photodegradation of azapropazone and its 8-hydroxy-metabolite has been demonstrated [17,18], and it has been suggested that a non-self antigen is derived from the reaction of the photoproduct (as yet undefined) with self proteins.

(2) The diversion of arachidonic acid through lipoxygenase (LO) pathways following cyclo-oxygenase inhibition by the NSAID; the excess LO products being presumed to affect the reactions of Langerhans cells in the skin (e.g. production of leukotriene B_4 (LTB_4)) [21–24].

(3) The effects of NSAIDs in enhancing production of interleukin-1 as observed in monocytes [25–27]. Studies suggest that this effect could be related to the effects of NSAIDs in reducing production of prostaglandins [25] and in enhancing production of leukotrienes especially LTB_4 [26]. PGE_2 (but not $PGF_{2\alpha}$) has been shown to reduce IL-1 production by stimulated monocytes or macrophages [25,27] whereas LTB_4 has been shown to markedly elevate IL-1 production by these cells [26]. There is also the possibility that the type and severity of arthritic disease could influence the actions of NSAIDs on the production of interleukin-1. Thus, it has been shown that the production of interleukin-1 in mononuclear cells from patients with scleroderma is markedly increased by indomethacin [28]. The response of antibody-producing cells to Il-1 may also be influenced by the type of arthritic disease (e.g. increased IgG production by IL-1 in patients with systemic lupus erythematosus [29]) and this may influence the pattern of sensitivity in different arthritic diseases towards skin reactions from NSAIDs.

That IL-1 production can occur in different cells in the skin and under the influence of diseases or various stimuli has been shown in a number of studies. Thus, for example, increased IL-1 (syn. ETAF) production has been shown in psoriatic skin lesions [30] and during allergic patch skin reaction in type IV allergy patients [31], and this has been considered important in manifestations of the inflammatory reactions in these conditions. Moreover, IL-1 (ETAF) is produced by normal keratinocytes and other cells of the skin [32,33], though in much lower quantities than in skin from diseased individuals. IL-1 can also elicit marked effects on skin cells e.g. Langerhans cells can elicit cytotoxic T-cell responses against normal epidermal cells [34]. Moreover, circulating mononuclear cells appear to have importance in skin reactions [35]. It is also possible that other inflammatory mediators e.g. platelet-activating factor (PAF) and complement C5a could be generated with infiltration of leucocytes during the development of the inflammatory process [36].

Genetic predisposition to skin conditions will inevitably play a major part in the development of rashes and more severe reactions. This may take the form of (a) alterations in the genetic control of drug metabolism (e.g. slow vs fast acetylators of sulphonamides, hydralazine, procainamide) [37,38], (b) presence of HLA antigens on immune cells (which are known to be important in DMARD-associated skin reactions) so altering their susceptibility to responsiveness [39,40], and (c) other disease states of genetic origin [37].

FENBUFEN RASH

The key features involved in the development of rashes induced by fenbufen are:

(1) Rashes of the maculopapular-type are produced by fenbufen. However, the topical application of the active cyclo-oxygenase metabolite (1,1'-biphenyl)-4-acetic acid (BPAA) does not produce an appreciable incidence of rashes [41]. It is, therefore, presumed that the development of rashes has little or no consequence for drug-induced cyclo-oxygenase inhibition by BPAA [42,43].

(2) The rashes predominate in women: in general practice the incidence is 8.2% (range 7.5–8.9%) in females and 2.4% (range 1.9–2.9%) in males (based on analysis in 8,640 subjects) [44]. There is no predisposition in any age group [44].

(3) The rashes occur most frequently within the first month of therapy and are reversible upon cessation of the drug [42,44]. Thus, there are no delayed sensitizing reactions which are prolonged at least for other development of rashes *per se* though of course there is the rash of type III or IV hypersensitivity reactions developing.

294

(4) None of the known described metabolites of fenbufen including the hydroxyl-derivative of fenbufen, nor fenbufen itself appear to be intrinsically capable of covalent modification *per se*.

POSTULATES FOR SKIN TOXICITY FROM FENBUFEN

Logically, an unknown intermediate between the metabolism of fenbufen to BPAA might be a likely candidate for a reactive metabolite if it could be shown to have intrinsic chemical reactivity. To the author's knowledge little is known about the biochemical steps involved in the metabolism of fenbufen to BPAA. The puzzling feature is what enzyme(s) system could be implicated in the removal of the γ-hydroxyl group of γ-hydroxy-(1,1'-biphenyl)-4-butanoic acid (GH-BPBA). One possibility is the linked liver microsomal reductions with mitochondrial fatty acid oxidations, which could proceed thus:

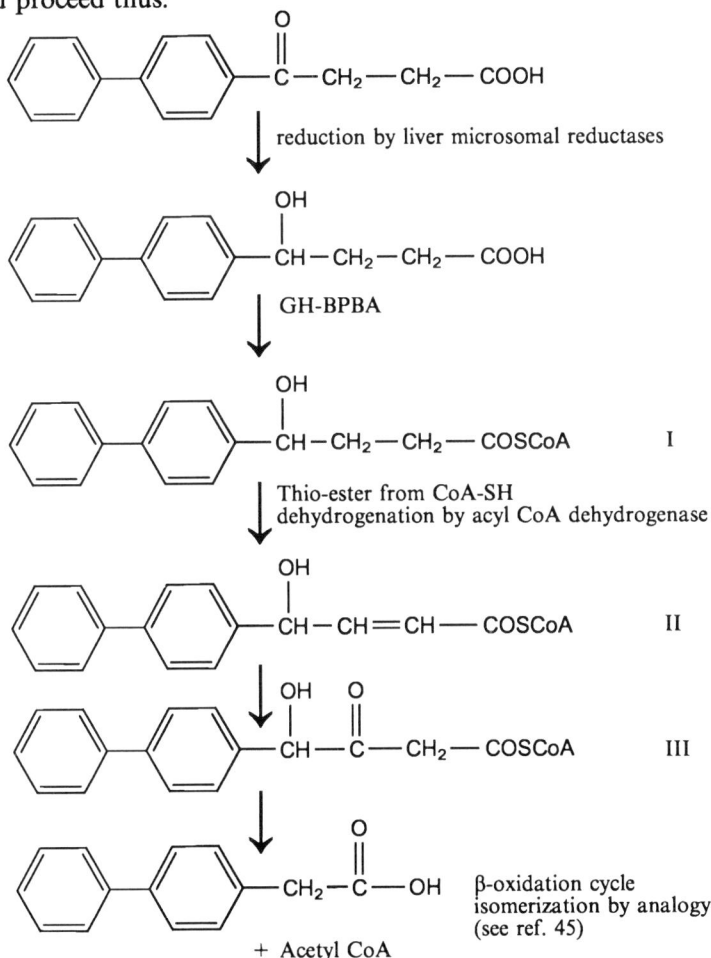

295

Intermediate no. III offers some potential for being a reactive intermediate especially with its keto-enol group.

An alternative is to consider the possibility of aromatic hydroxylation of the biphenyl group of fenbufen. In view of the lack of any substituents on the biphenyl group (other than at the point of the side chain) this leaves open the possibility that aromatic diols could form via epoxide.

The intermediates could for example comprise:

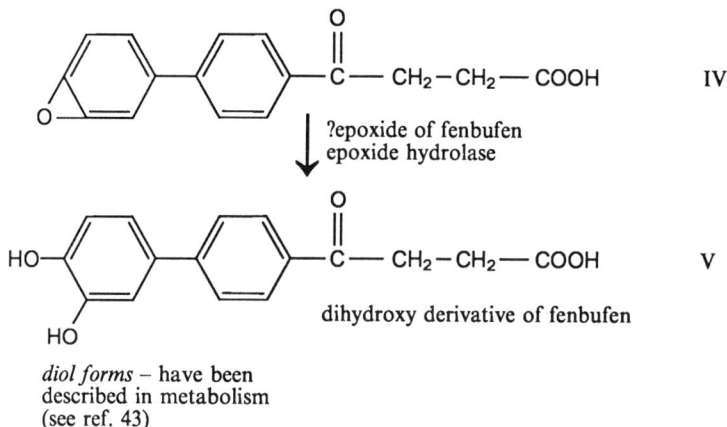

IV

?epoxide of fenbufen
epoxide hydrolase

dihydroxy derivative of fenbufen

V

diol forms – have been
described in metabolism
(see ref. 43)

It should be noted that mono-aryl derivatives of fenbufen have been described [43].

Identification of the latter dihydroxy-metabolites would imply the formation of the epoxide intermediate. This intermediate would be expected to be particularly reactive and capable of forming covalent derivatives with immuno-cellular reactivity. Simple identification of these metabolites would at least give a good lead as well. Likewise, production of UV-activated intermediates could be determined by conventional chemical procedures.

The involvement of fatty acid metabolism in the formation of the postulated intermediate III could theoretically be tested by employing selective inhibitors of fatty acid oxidation (for review see ref. 45,46).

ANTIOXIDANTS AS PUTATIVE PROTECTANTS AGAINST SKIN RASHES FROM FENBUFEN

The theoretical possibility was considered that active oxygen species are generated during the metabolism of fenbufen, or in the actions of this drug or a metabolite during the induction of rashes. Based on this premise, and the need to obtain a practical means of preventing rashes by fenbufen, a clinical trial was undertaken in collaboration with Lederle Laboratories (UK) to determine the effects of concomitant treatment with two antioxidants, vitamin E (400 iu daily) or paracetamol (2 g daily) in preventing rashes while receiving fenbufen (900 mg daily). The study design was that of a prospective, single-blind, parallel group with three approximately equal-sized treatment groups in 457 centres in General Practice. Patients who had previously received fenbufen therapy were excluded from the study. A total of 2961 evaluable patients with various arthritic conditions were recruited for the trial and were randomly allocated to three treatment groups:

Treatment A: Fenbufen (900 mg) plus vitamin E (400 iu) b.d. (the dose of this vitamin comprises that recommended daily as a normal supplement)

Treatment B: Fenbufen (900 mg) plus paracetamol (2 g) b.d.

Treatment C: Fenbufen (900 mg) plus placebo b.d.

The subjects recorded the occurrence of skin reactions, gastrointestinal side-effects and other adverse reactions. The results of this study are shown in Table 3. It can be seen that:

(a) The overall incidence of rashes in both females and males in the fenbufen and the placebo group was higher than previously reported [44] in General Practice observations.

(b) In female patients, who received paracetamol and fenbufen, the incidence of rash was 2.6% lower than in those who received fenbufen and placebo. However, the incidence in males receiving these treatments was about the same.

(c) Vitamin E did not confer any protective effects in either females or males receiving fenbufen compared with placebo-treated subjects.

The results suggest that paracetamol conferred a marginal, non-statistically significant benefit in preventing rashes from fenbufen in females. The lack of benefit from vitamin E may have been due to the dosage being inadequate to control oxyradicals since the daily dose of 400 iu was only the recommended daily dose.

SEARCH FOR PUTATIVE REACTIVE METABOLITES OF FENBUFEN

We have initiated a study design to compare the metabolism of ^{3}H-fenbufen with that of ^{3}H-BPAA (recall this is not implicated in rash development) in (a) human keratinocytes (Clonetics Corps, San Diego, California, USA) cultured *in vitro*, and (b) the skin of adjuvant arthritic rats and UV-irradiated guinea pigs *in vivo* following oral administration of the radiolabelled drugs. The results of thin layer chromatography of the organic solvent extracts of keratinocytes is shown in Figure 1. From this it can be seen that extensive metabolism of the drug occurred and notably

Table 3. Effects of antioxidant treatment on the development of cutaneous side-effects from fenbufen

	Treatment A Fenbufen 900 mg + vitamin E 400 iu	Treatment B Fenbufen 900 mg + paracetamol 2g	Treatment C Fenbufen 900 mg + placebo
Females			
Total patients	526	538	566
Cutaneous rash	65	49	66
pruritus	4	2	3
Gastrointestinal	69	78	64
Others	29	53	38
Males			
Total patients	448	423	422
Cutaneous rash	19	19	15
pruritus	1	2	1
Gastrointestinal	46	45	44
Others	30	26	15
Percentage rash incidence			
Females	12.4%	9.1%	11.7%
Males	4.2%	4.5%	3.6%

Notes on study results
Of the 2961 patients recruited, 38 did not have their gender recorded. Amongst these, there were 10 adverse events reported from a total of 5 patients, all of which were in treatment group A; 2 of these events were the occurrence of a rash. Doses are daily b.d.

All of the cutaneous and gastrointestinal side-effects reported in the study were described as 'non-serious'. Amongst events classified as 'Others', 8 events were reported under the category of 'Serious/Unexpected'. These events were typical of those reported in previous studies; 1 was of 'unknown' relationship to the study drug, 4 were 'definitely not' related to the study drug and 3 were 'remotely related'.

UV irradiation of the cells resulted in two fast-migrating metabolites. Similar metabolites were found in the skin of rats and guinea pigs which received the radiolabelled drugs. Currently we are trying to identify the structure of these two metabolites by combined gas chromatography/mass spectrometry. Given identity of these metabolites it should be possible to explore their actions on producing inflammatory mediators in skin; from this possible mechanisms of the action of fenbufen rash may emerge.

ACKNOWLEDGEMENTS

The author would like to thank Dr Jan Povey, Dr Roger Newberry and Dr Ewan Millar of Lederle Laboratories (UK) Ltd for their valuable cooperation in preparing the antioxidant clinical trial and to Lederle

298

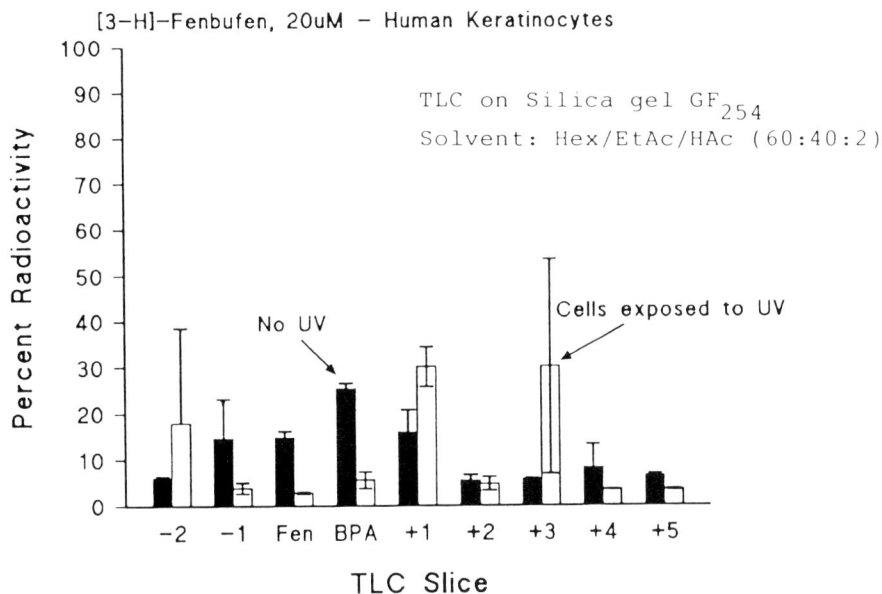

Figure 1. Thin layer chromatography of radioactive fenbufen (20 μM) cultured in human keratinocytes for 24 h showing the presence of two fast-migrating peaks in zones (+1) and (+3) in cells exposed initially for 30 mins to UV light. The identity of fenbufen (FEN) and BPAA (BPA) was confirmed by co-chromatography with authentic standards. None of the fast-migrating components was present in cells incubated with ³H-BPAA with or without UV light cultured under the same conditions

Laboratories for financial support of these studies. My thanks also to Mrs Chiyan Ying for valuable technical help in the ongoing studies of the mechanisms of skin toxicity from fenbufen.

REFERENCES

1. Weber JCP. Epidemiology of adverse reactions to non-steroidal anti-inflammatory drugs. In: Rainsford KD, Velo GP, eds. Side-effects of anti-inflammatory analgesic drugs. New York: Raven Press; 1984:1–7.
2. Wilholm BE, Myhred M, Ekman F. Trends and patterns in adverse drug reactions to non-steroid anti-inflammatory drugs reported in Sweden. In: Rainsford KD, Velo GP, eds. Side-effects of anti-inflammatory drugs. Vol. I. Lancaster: MTP Press; 1987:55–70.
3. Inman WHW, Rawson NSB. Prescription event monitoring of five non-steroidal anti-inflammatory drugs. Vol. I. In: Rainsford KD, Velo GP, eds. Side-effects of anti-inflammatory drugs. Vol. I. Lancaster: MTP Press; 1987:118–123.
4. Cox NL, Doherty SM. Non-steroidal anti-inflammatories: outpatient preferences and side-effects in different diseases. In: Rainsford KD, Velo GP, eds. Side-effects of anti-inflammatory drugs, Vol. I. Lancaster: MTP Press; 1987:137–148.
5. Lever WF, Schaumberg-Lever G. Histopathology of the skin. Philadelphia: Lippincott; 1983:259–270.
6. Bork K. Cutaneous side-effects of drugs. Philadelphia: Saunders; 1988.

7. Rainsford KD. Aspirin and the salicylates. London: Butterworths; 1987.
8. Rainsford KD. Concepts of the mode of action and side-effects of anti-inflammatory drugs. A basis for safer and more selective therapy, and for future drug developments. In: Rainsford KD, Velo GP, eds. New developments in antirheumatic therapy. Lancaster: Kluwer Academic Publishers; 1989:37–92.
9. Rainsford KD, Schweitzer A, Brune K. Autoradiographic and biochemical observations on the distribution of non-steroid anti-inflammatory drugs. Arch Int Pharmacodyn. 1981;250:180–194.
10. Rainsford KD, Schweitzer A, Brune K. Distribution of the acetyl salicyl moiety of acetylsalicylic acid. Acetylation of biomolecules in organs wherein side-effects are manifest. Biochem Pharmacol. 1983;32:1301–1308.
11. Reszka K, Chignell CF. Spectroscopic studies of cutaneous photosensitizing agents – IV. The photolysis of benoxaprofen, an anti-inflammatory drug with phototoxic properties. Photochem Photobiol. 1983;38:281–291.
12. Sik RH, Pasehall CS, Chignell CF. The phototoxic effect of benoxaprofen and its analogs on human erythrocytes and rat peritoneal mast cells. Photochem Photobiol. 1983;38:411–415.
13. Kochevar IE, Morison WC, Lamm JL, McAuliffe DJ, Western A, Hood AF. Possible mechanisms of piroxicam-induced photosensitivity. Arch Dermatol. 1986;122:1283–1287.
14. Ljunggren B. Propionic-acid-derived non-steroidal anti-inflammatory drugs are phototoxic in vitro. Photodermatology. 1985;2:39–43.
15. Moore DE, Chappuis PE. A comparative study of the photochemistry of the non-steroidal anti-inflammatory drugs, naproxen, benoxaprofen and indomethacin. Photochem Photobiol. 1988;47:173–180.
16. Diffey BL, Daymond TJ, Fairgraves H. Phototoxic reactions to piroxicam, naproxen and tiaprofenic acid. Br J Rheumatol. 1984;22:239–242.
17. Jones RA, Vavaratnam S, Parsons BJ, Philips GO. Photosensitivity due to anti-inflammatory analgesic drugs: a laser flash photolysis study of azapropazone. In: Rainsford KD, Velo GP, eds. Side-effects of anti-inflammatory drugs, Vol. II. Lancaster: MTPP Press; 1987:345–354.
18. Jones RA, Navaratnam S, Parsons BJ, Philips GO. One-electron oxidation and reduction of azapropazone and phenylbutazone derivations in aqueous solution: a pulse radiolysis study. Photochem Photobiol. 1988;48:401–408.
19. Hort JF. Adverse reactions to alclofenac. Curr Med Res Opin. 1975;3:333–337.
20. Ford-Hutchinson AW. Personal communication; 1980.
21. Aked D, Foster SJ, Howarth A, McCormick ME, Potts HC. The inflammatory responses of rabbit skin to tropical arachidonic acid and its pharmacological modulation. Br J Pharmacol. 1986;89:431–438.
22. Chang J, Carlson RP, O'Neill-Davis L, Lamb B, Sharma RN, Lewis AJ. Correlations between mouse skin inflammation induced by arachidonic acid and eicosanoid synthesis. Inflammation. 1986;10:205–214.
23. Aked J, Foster SJ. Leukotriene and prostaglandin E_2 mediate the inflammatory responses of rabbit skin to intradermal arachidonic acid. Br J Pharmacol. 1987;92:545–552.
24. Ring J, Przybilla B, Ruzicka T. Non-steroidal anti-inflammatory drugs induce UV-dependent histamine and leukotriene release from peripheral human leucocytes. Int Arch Allergy Appl Immunol. 1987;82:344–346.
25. Kunkel SL, Chensue SW, Phan SH. Prostaglandins as endogenous mediators of interleukin 1 production. J Immunol. 1986;136:186–192.
26. Rola-Pleszczynski M, Lemaire I. Leukotrienes augment interleukin 1 production by human monocytes. J Immunol. 1985;135:3958–3961.
27. Brandwein SR. Regulation of interleukin 1 production by mouse peritoneal macrophages. J Immunol. 1986;261:8624–8632.
28. Sandborg CI, Berman MA, Andrews BS, Friou GJ. Interleukin-1 production by mononuclear cells from patients with scleroderma. Clin Exp Immunol. 1985;60:294–302.
29. Jaudl RC, George JL, Dinarello CA, Schur PH. The effect of interleukin-1 on IgG synthesis in systemic lupus erythematosus. Clin Immunol Immunopathol. 1987;45:384–394.

30. Camp RDR, Fincham NJ, Cunningham FM, Greaves MW, Morris J, Chui A. Psoriatic skin lesions contain biologically active amounts of an interleukin 1-like compound. J Immunol. 1986;137:3469–3474.

31. Larsen CG, Temowitz T, Larson FG, Thestrup PK. Epidermis and lymphocyte interaction during an allergic patch test reaction. Increased activity of ETAF/IL-1, epidermal derived lymphocyte chemotactic factor and mixed skin lymphocyte reactivity in persons with type IV allergy. Invest Dermatol. 1988;90:230–233.

32. Gahring LL, Buckley A, Daynes RA. Presence of epidermal-derived thymocyte activating factor/interleukin 1 in normal human stratum corneum. J Clin Invest. 1985;76:1585–1591.

33. Hsu S.-M., Zhao X. Localization of interleukin-1 in normal or reactive lymphoid tissues and skin: abundance of IL-1 in interdigitating reticulum cells. Lymphokine Res. 1987;6:13–18.

34. Faure M, Dezutter-Dambuyant C, Schmitt D, Gaucherand M, Thivolet, J. Langerhans cell induced cytotoxic T-cell responses against normal epidermal cell targets: in vitro studies. Br J Dermatol. 1985;113(Suppl. 28):114–117.

35. Morley J, Sanjar S, Page CP, Bretz U. The role of circulating cells in skin reactions. Br J Dermatol. 1985;113(Suppl. 28):86–90.

36. Yancey KB, Hammer CH, Horvath L, Renfer L, Frank MM, Lawley TJ. Studies of human C5a as a mediator of inflammation in normal human skin. J Clin Invest. 1985;75:486–495.

37. Shear NH, Bhimji S. Pharmacogenetics and cutaneous reactions. Semin Dermatol. 1989;8:219–226.

38. Shear NH, Spielberg SP, Grant DM, Tang BK, Kalow W. Differences in metabolism of sulfonamides predisposing idiosyncratic toxicity. Ann Intern Med. 1989;105:179–184.

39. Dequeker J, Van Wanghe P, Verdickt W. A systematic survey of HLA-A, B, C and D antigens and drug toxicity in rheumatoid arthritis. J Rheumatol. 1984;11:282–286.

40. Ford P. HLA antigens and drug toxicity in rheumatoid arthritis. J Rheumatol. 1984;11:259–261.

41. Millar ED. Personal communication. Lederle (UK) Ltd; 1987.

42. Greenberg BP, Berstein J. Fenbufen. In: Rainsford KD, ed. Anti-inflammatory and antirheumatic drugs, Vol. II. Boca Raton: CRC Press; 1985:87–103.

43. Sloboda AE, Oransky AL, Kerwar SS, Greenberg BG. Fenbufen. In: Lewis AJ, Furst DE, eds. Non-steroidal anti-inflammatory drugs. Mechanisms and clinical use. New York: Marcel Dekker; 1987:371–392

44. Anonymous. Fenbufen related skin rash. Questions and answers relating to this side-effect. The Medical Information Department, Lederle Laboratories, a Division of Cyanamid of Great Britain, Ltd, Fareham Road, Gosport, Hants, UK; 1987.

45. Schulz H, Kunau W-H. Beta-oxidation of unsaturated fatty acids: a revised pathway. TIBS. 1987;12:403–405.

46. Schulz H. Inhibitors of fatty acid oxidation. Life Sci. 1987;40:1443-1449.

35

Cyclosporin: clinical efficacy and toxicity in patients with rheumatoid arthritis

W. Watson Buchanan

Rheumatology Unit, Department of Medicine, McMaster University Health Sciences Centre, 1200 Main Street West, Hamilton, Ontario L8N 3Z5, Canada

Cyclosporin is a naturally-occurring, neutral, lipophilic cyclic undecapeptide, in which some of the amino acids are methylated [1]. The drug was first isolated from the fungus *Tolypocladium inflatumgams* in 1971 [2], from which it is now commercially produced by fermentation and currently marketed by Sandoz Ltd, Basle, Switzerland under the trade name Sandimmun® [3]. A number of cyclosporins have been identified, but none so far has proven superior to cyclosporin A [4]. Originally cyclosporin was tested for antibiotic and antifungal activities, which were found to be minimal, but in 1972 Borel [5] showed marked immunosuppressive effect in a murine leukaemia model. Subsequently cyclosporin was shown to have immunosuppressive activity with its main site of action on T-lymphocytes and inhibition of interleukin-2 production [2,6–9]. The drug has gained acceptance as the immunosuppressant of choice for organ transplantation [2,3,10,11]. In addition, cyclosporin has been extensively explored in the treatment of autoimmune disorders [2,3], including rheumatoid arthritis [12–24]. Its use in rheumatoid arthritis was prompted by the demonstration of not only anti-arthritic activity [25–29] but effects on subsets of T cells [26,27] in experimentally-induced arthritis in animals. Furthermore, Del Pozo et al. [29] demonstrated an impressive dose-related regression in bone and cartilage destruction in adjuvant arthritis in rats.

This paper will review toxicity of cyclosporin when prescribed in low dosage, i.e. less than 5 mg kg^{-1} day^{-1}, in patients with rheumatoid arthritis. A few comments on clinical pharmacology and evidence of clinical efficacy with low dosage seem in order.

Side-effects of Anti-inflammatory Drugs 3. Rainsford KD, Velo GP (eds), Inflammation and Drug Therapy Series, Volume V.

CLINICAL PHARMACOLOGY

Because of its lipophilic nature cyclosporin's absorption is facilitated by bile [30,31]. The drug undergoes biotransformation in the liver by the P-450 III A enzyme system, involving especially hydroxylation, but also demethylation, and cyclization [32]. A sulphate conjugate has, however, also been identified [33]. Excretion is mainly by the bile, mostly metabolites, with only 1% of the drug being excreted by this route [34]. Less than 6% of cyclosporin is excreted by the kidney [35]. Approximately 40–60% of cyclosporin is bound to plasma proteins, especially lipoproteins, and some 35–55% to erythrocytes and 5% to leucocytes: only 1–5% circulates as free drug [36–38]. High concentrations of cyclosporin have been found in fat, pancreas, liver and kidney [35]. No current immunoassay is capable of determining the individual metabolites of cyclosporin, and the current 'gold standard' is high performance liquid chromatography [39–41]. A genetic deficiency of P-450 III activity may lead to cyclosporin toxicity despite therapeutic blood concentrations [32]. Some 29 metabolites of cyclosporin in man have been identified [42], and Lucey et al. [32] have suggested that deficiency in P-450 III A enzyme may cause a 'shunt' to alternate biotransformation pathways leading to the formation of toxic metabolites. Induction of the enzyme with rifampicin has been shown to eliminate toxicity [32]. In clinical trials in rheumatoid arthritis [29] serum cyclosporin has been measured by a polyclonal antibody radioimmunoassay [43] which is less satisfactory than high performance liquid chromatography [39–41].

CLINICAL EFFICACY

A number of open studies of cyclosporin in rheumatoid arthritis indicated therapeutic benefit [9–16] and prompted controlled clinical trials [20,29]. Initially high daily doses of cyclosporin, i.e. more than 5 mg/kg, were employed in the latter, but were found to be associated with an unacceptable incidence of nephrotoxicity [20,22,44–46]. The double-blind trials with less than $5 \, mg \, kg^{-1} \, day^{-1}$ have demonstrated clinical efficacy and much less nephrotoxicity [21,29]. In the trial by Dougados et al. [21], 52 patients participated in a four-month study, half of whom received cyclosporin and the other half placebo. The starting dose of cyclosporin was $5 \, mg \, kg^{-1} \, day^{-1}$, but half this dose in those patients receiving cimetidine. At the end of the trial the mean cyclosporin dose was $4.6 \pm SD$ $1.8 \, mg \, kg^{-1} \, day^{-1}$ (range 1.2 to $7.5 \, mg \, kg^{-1} \, day^{-1}$). All of the clinical outcome measures including pain, Ritchie articular index, number of swollen joints, proximal interphalangeal joint circumference in the hands, morning stiffness and Lee functional index showed statistically significant improvement. Overall assessment by both patients and physicians also

303

showed significant improvement. The platelet count, α_1-glycoprotein, and C-reactive protein determinations demonstrated statistically significant reduction but the erythrocyte sedimentation rate remained higher, 48.0 mm 1st hour in the cyclosporin-treated patients compared with those who received placebo, 37.5 mm 1st hour. In the randomized trial reported by Tugwell et al. [19] in 144 patients, half of whom received cyclosporin and the remainder placebo, the study period was longer, 6 months, and the trial involved a number of different Canadian centres. The starting dose of cyclosporin was 2.5 mg kg^{-1} day^{-1}, the dose being increased by 25% every week until serum trough levels of 75–150 ng/ml were obtained, as determined by a polyclonal antibody radioimmunoassay [43]. The results of this trial also showed significant improvements in the cyclosporin-treated patients compared to the controls of 23% in active joint counts, 24% in pain relief, 16% in functional status, and 27% in global improvements. These improvements are all the more impressive when one takes into consideration that more than half the patients had previously taken two or more second-line drugs, approximately two thirds were in Functional Class III, and 40% had subcutaneous nodules. The patients also had had their arthritis for a considerable time, mean approximately 10 years. The mean dose of cyclosporin in this trial was 3.79 mg kg^{-1} day^{-1}. As in the trial reported by Dougados et al. [21], no effect was noted on the erythrocyte sedimentation rate. Neither of these short-term trials attempted to determine radiological change in articular joint erosions.

Dougados et al. [23] continued to follow 49 of their 52 patients in an open study for a period of one year. Ten patients discontinued treatment due to lack of effect and a further 9 for a combination of lack of effect and side-effects. However, in the 17 patients who continued therapy, clinical improvement was maintained.

Both of the double-blind trials failed to take into account the effects of adverse reactions on the efficacy of treatment. To meet modern-day ethical standards patients must be informed of side-effects they might experience. How many of the patients in these two trials were able to identify when they were receiving cyclosporin? How double-blind is double-blind, one may rightly ask [47]? In addition, both mild and severe adverse reactions potentiate analgesia [48].

CLINICAL ACCEPTANCE

A relatively large percentage of patients in the two double-blind trials using low daily doses of cyclosporin developed adverse drug reactions [21,24]. Particularly troublesome were hypertrichosis, dyspepsia, tremor and paraesthesiae, and gingival hyperplasia. Mammary hypertrophy was observed in one patient in the trial by Dougados et al. [21]. In the one-year open study in 49 patients by these authors [23] the same pattern of adverse effects was observed although one patient also developed herpes zoster. Treatment with cyclosporin has been associated with the development of viral and opportunistic bacterial infections [49], and a patient with rheumatoid arthritis has been described who developed Legionnaire's disease while receiving treatment with cyclosporin [50].

As mentioned above, higher doses of cyclosporin in patients with rheumatoid arthritis i.e. more than 5 mg kg^{-1} day^{-1}, were associated with unacceptable nephrotoxicity [18,20,22,44–46]. The mechanisms of nephrotoxicity are complex and involve inhibition of renal PGE$_2$ production [51–58]. Nephrotoxicity may be exacerbated by cyclo-oxygenase inhibition by non-steroidal anti-inflammatory analgesics [19,59]. Berg et al. [44] found that serum creatinine concentrations were increased by approximately 27%, and creatinine clearances reduced by 8% by non-steroidal anti-inflammatory analgesics in patients with rheumatoid arthritis receiving cyclosporin therapy. No effect, however, was observed by these authors on serum cyclosporin levels, suggesting that the effect was pharmacodynamic. Whether this effect of non-steroidal anti-inflammatory analgesics on renal function is mediated by cyclo-oxygenase remains controversial [59], and whether it could be prevented by administration of fish oil [61] or misoprostol [62] remains to be tested. Regular consumption of non-steroidal anti-inflammatory analgesics is a risk factor for chronic renal failure [63] and renal complications may occur in rheumatoid arthritis, such as secondary amyloidosis, which may make patients more susceptible to cyclosporin nephrotoxicity [49,64,65].

With long-term low-dose cyclosporin therapy i.e. less than 5 mg kg^{-1} day^{-1} a rise in serum creatinine levels and a reduction in creatinine clearance have been observed in a high proportion of patients with rheumatoid arthritis [21,23,24,60,66]. Predisposing factors include patients over 60 years of age and those whose serum creatinine exceeds 88 μmol/L [23]. Increase in both diastolic and systolic blood pressures also occurs with low-dose cyclosporin therapy [21,24]. Although improvement in both renal function, as determined by serum creatinine levels and creatinine clearance, and blood pressure, occur following discontinuation of cyclosporin therapy [21,24], the claim that it is reversible [67] should be considered with caution. The serum creatinine levels, although significantly reduced, have not always returned to baseline [21,24]. Serum creatinine determinations do not accurately reflect renal function, especially in patients with severe rheumatoid arthritis who have lost lean body mass [67–69]. Renal biopsies have rarely been reported in patients who have had cyclosporin therapy [24,70]. The potential for interaction of calcium channel blockers and cyclosporin [71,72] have not as yet been reported in patients with rheumatoid arthritis.

Nephrotoxicity with low-dose cyclosporin therapy in patients with rheumatoid arthritis appears to be manageable, but not negligible, and until further data is available limits wide application. Perhaps some of the novel macrolides which have selective anti-T-cell effects similar to cyclosporin may prove less toxic [73].

The development of neoplasms with continuous cyclosporin therapy remains a potential risk, especially since patients with rheumatoid arthritis are more prone to develop malignancies, especially lymphomas. One patient with severe rheumatoid arthritis treated with low-dose cyclosporin has been observed who developed a pseudo-lymphoma of the duodenum. This disappeared completely on discontinuation of cyclosporin therapy. Patients with Sjögren's syndrome are much more likely to develop lymphomas, and the use of cyclosporin in such patients [74] cannot be recommended.

Acceptability of a medication is largely determined by clinical efficacy and lack of toxicity and is best measured by life-table analysis of treatment termination [75]. In the short-term trials of low-dose cyclosporin, discontinuation of therapy at four months, 15.4% [21] and at six months, 13.5% [24] compares favourable with those reported with gold, 37%, D-penicillamine 38%, and sulphasalazine, 38%, by Situnayake et al. [75]. However, in the one-year open study of Dougados et al. [23] the drop-out with cyclosporin was 65.3%, which is higher than that of 50% reported for gold. D-penicillamine and sulphasalazine [76].

In transplant recipients an association has been observed between cyclosporin toxicity and blood cholesterol levels [77]. Since cyclosporin circulates in the blood largely bound to lipoproteins, low levels of serum lipids might be associated with a larger amount of unbound, biologically active drug [32]. Surprisingly, in none of the studies of low-dose cyclosporin therapy in rheumatoid arthritis has this been considered, especially as it is well known that patients with rheumatoid arthritis have low serum cholesterol levels [78]. In addition, it might have been useful to know the concentrations of cyclosporin achieved in synovial fluid with long-term therapy. Cyclosporin readily penetrates into the joint [79] where it and its metabolites will be largely bound to synovial lipids. These latter can attain extremely high levels so that the synovial fluid may have the macroscopic appearance of milk [80]. Could cyclosporin be sequestered in such joints, and its intermittent release account for toxicity with long-term therapy?

REFERENCES

1. Gilman SC, Lewis AJ. Immunomodulatory drugs in the treatment of rheumatoid arthritis. In: Rainsford KD, ed. Anti-inflammatory and anti-rheumatic drugs, Vol. 3, Anti-rheumatic

drugs, experimental agents and clinical aspects of drug use. Boca Raton, FL: CRC Press; 1985:127–154.

2. Keown PA. Emerging indications for the use of cyclosporin in organ transplantation and autoimmunity. Drugs. 1990;40:315–325.

3. Shand N, Richardson B. Sandimmum® (cyclosporin A): mode of action and clinical results in rheumatoid arthritis. Scand J Rheumatol (Suppl 76). 1988:265–278.

4. Harding MW, Handschumacher RE. Cyclosporin and its receptor, cyclophilin. In: Lewis A, Ackerman N, Otterness I, eds. New perspectives in anti-inflammatory therapies. Advances in inflammation research, Vol. 12. New York: Raven Press; 1988:283–294.

5. Borel JF. The history of cyclosporin A and its significance. In: White D, ed. Cyclosporin A. Amsterdam: Elsevier; 1982:5–17.

6. Handschumacher RE, Harding MW, Rice J et al. Cyclophilin: a specific cytosolic binding protein for cyclosporin A. Science. 1984;226:544–546.

7. Granelli-Piperno A, Andrus L, Steinman RM. Lymphokine and nonlymphokine in RNA levels in stimulated human T-cells: kinetics, mitogen requirements and effects of cyclosporin A. J Exp Med. 1986;163:922–937.

8. Kahan BD. Cyclosporin. N Engl J Med. 1989;321:1725–1737.

9. Kasaian MT, Biron CA. Cyclosporin A inhibition of interleukin 2 gene expression, but not natural killer cell proliferation, after interferon induction in vivo. J Exp Med. 1990;171:745–762.

10. White DJG, Calne RY. The use of cyclosporin A immunosuppression in organ grafting. Immunol Rev. 1982;65:115–131.

11. Borel JF. Immunosuppression: building on cyclosporin (Sandimmun®). Transplant Proc. 1988;20(Suppl. 1):149–153.

12. Herman B, Muller W. Die therapie der chronischen polyarthritis mit cyclosporin A, einen neuen immunsuppressivum. Akt Rheumatol. 1979;4:173–186.

13. Graf U, Marbet U, Muller W et al. Cyclosporin A: effects and side-effects in the treatment of rheumatoid arthritis and psoriatic arthritis. Immun Inpekt. 1981;9:20–28.

14. Amor B, Dougados M. Cyclosporin in rheumatoid arthritis: open trials with different dosages. In: Schindler R, ed. Cyclosporin in autoimmune diseases. Berlin: Springer; 1985:283–287.

15. Bombardier C, Tugwell P, Gent M et al. A pilot of CyA in patients with rheumatoid arthritis. In: Schindler R, ed. Cyclosporin in autoimmune diseases. Berlin: Springer; 1985:288.

16. Herog Ch, Gross D. Low dose cyclosporin A and prednisone: a step in the direction of selective immunosuppression in rheumatoid arthritis refractory of treatment (6-month follow-up). In: Schindler R, ed. Cyclosporin in autoimmune diseases. Berlin: Springer; 1985:289–296.

17. Madhok R, Capell HA. Cyclosporin in rheumatoid arthritis. In: Schindler R, ed. Cyclosporin in autoimmune diseases. Berlin: Springer; 1985:197–298.

18. Dougados M, Amor B. Cyclosporin A in rheumatoid arthritis: preliminary clinical results of an open trial. Arthritis Rheum. 1987;30:83–86.

19. Tugwell P, Bombardier C, Gent M et al. Low dose cyclosporin in rheumatoid arthritis: a pilot study. J Rheumatol. 1987;14:1108–1114.

20. Weinblatt ME, Coblyn JS, Fraser PA. Cyclosporin: a treatment of refractory rheumatoid arthritis. Arthritis Rheum. 1987;30:11–17.

21. Dougados M, Awada H, Amor B. Cyclosporin in rheumatoid arthritis: a double blind, placebo controlled study in 52 patients. Ann Rheum Dis. 1988;47:127–133.

22. Yocum DE, Klippel JH, Wilder RL et al. Cyclosporin A in severe, treatment-refractory rheumatoid arthritis. A randomized study. Ann Intern Med. 1988;109:863–869.

23. Dougados M, Duchesne L, Awada H, Amor B. Assessment of efficacy and acceptability of low dose cyclosporin in patients with rheumatoid arthritis. Ann Rheum Dis. 1989;48:550–556.

24. Tugwell P, Bombardier C, Gent M et al. Low dose cyclosporin versus placebo in patients with rheumatoid arthritis. Lancet. 1990;335:1051–1055.

25. Borel JF, Feuer C, Gubler HU, Stahelin H. Biological effects of cyclosporin A: a new antilymphocyte agent. Agents Actions. 1976;6:468–475.

26. Yocum DE, Allen JB, Wahl SM, Calandra GB, Wilder RL. Inhibition by cyclosporin A of streptococcal cell wall-induced arthritis and hepatic granulomas in rats. Arthritis Rheum. 1986;29:262–274.

27. Bersani-Amado CA, Duart AJ daS, Tanji MM, Cianga M, Jancar S. Comparative study of adjuvant induced arthritis in susceptible and resistant strains of rats. III. Analysis of lymphocyte subpopulations. J Rheumatol. 1990;17:153–158.

28. Cannon W, McCall S, Cole BC, Griffiths MM et al. Effects of indomethacin, cyclosporin, cyclophosphamide, and placebo on collagen-induced arthritis of mice. Agents Actions. 1990;29:315–323.

29. Del Pozo E, Graeber M, Elford P, Payne T. Regression of bone and cartilage loss in adjuvant arthritis rats after treatment with cyclosporin A. Arthritis Rheum. 1990;33:247–252.

30. Tachinski RJ, Venkataramanan R, Burckart GJ. Because of its lipophilic nature CyA's absorption is facilitated by bile. Clinical pharmacokinetics of cyclosporin. Clin Pharmacokinet. 1986;11:107–132.

31. Borel JF. The cyclosporins. Transplant Proc. 1989;21:810–815.

32. Lucey MR, Kolars JC, Merion RM, Campbell DA, Aldrich M, Watkins PB. Cyclosporin toxicity at therapeutic blood levels and cytochrome P-450 IIIA. Lancet. 1990;335:1–15.

33. Herricsson S. A sulfate conjugate of cyclosporin. Pharmacol Toxicol. 1990;66:53–55.

34. Venkataramanan R, Starzi YE, Yang S et al. Biliary excretion of cyclosporin in liver transplant patients. Transplant Proc. 1985;17:286–289.

35. Maurer G, Lemaire M. Biotransformation and distribution in blood of cyclosporin and its metabolites. Transplant Proc. 1986;18(Suppl. 5):25–34.

36. Lemaire M, Tillement JP. Role of lipoproteins and erythrocytes in the *in vitro* binding and distribution of cyclosporin A in the blood. J Pharm Pharmacol. 1982;34:715–718.

37. Handschumacher RE, Harding MW, Rice J et al. Cyclophilin: a specific cytosolic binding protein for cyclosporin A. Science. 1984;226:544–547.

38. Akagi H, Reynolds A, Hjelm M. Cyclosporin A and its metabolites, distribution in blood and tissues. J Int Med Res. 1991;19:1–18.

39. Critical issues in cyclosporin monitoring: report of the task force on cyclosporin monitoring. Clin Chem. 1987;33:1269–1288.

40. Christians U, Schlitt HJ, Bleck JS et al. Measurement of cyclosporin and 18 metabolites in blood, bile and urine by high-performance liquid chromatography. Transplant Proc. 1988;20(Suppl. 2):609–613.

41. Consensus Document: Hawk's Cay meeting on therapeutic drug monitoring of cyclosporin. Clin Chem. 1990;36:1510–1516.

42. Kahan BD, Grevel J. Optimization of cyclosporin therapy in renal transplantation by a pharmacokinetic strategy. Transplantation. 1988;46:631–644.

43. Donatsch P, Abisch E, Homberger M et al. A radioimmunoassay to measure cyclosporin in plasma and serum samples. J Immunoassay. 1982;2:19–32.

44. Berg KJ, Forre O, Bjerkhoel F et al. Side-effects of cyclosporin. A treatment in patients with rheumatoid arthritis. Kidney Int. 1986;29:1180–1187.

45. Rijthoven AWAM, Dijkmans BAC, The HSG, Hermans J, Montnor-Beckers ZLMB, Jacobs PCJ, Cats A. Cyclosporin treatment for rheumatoid arthritis: a placebo controlled, double blind, multicentre study. Ann Rheum Dis. 1986;45:726–731.

46. Forre O, Bjerkhoel F, Salvesem CF et al. An open, controlled, randomized comparison of cyclosporin and azathioprine in the treatment of rheumatoid arthritis: a preliminary report. Arthritis Rheum. 1987;30:88–92.

47. Huskisson EC, Scott J. How double-blind is double-blind? And does it matter? Br J Clin Pharmacol. 1976;3:331–332.

48. Max MB, Schafer SC, Culnane M et al. Association of pain relief with drug side-effects in post herpetic neuralgia. Clin Pharmacol Ther. 1988;43:363–371.

49 Palestine AR, Nussenblatt RB, Chan CC. Side-effects of systemic cyclosporin in patients not undergoing transplantation. Am J Med. 1984;77:652–656.

50. Pillemer SR, Webb D, Yocum DE. Legionnaire's disease in a patient with rheumatoid arthritis treated with cyclosporin. J Rheumatol. 1989;16:117–120.

51. Mihatsch MJ, Oliviere W, Marbet U, Thiel G et al. Giant mitochondria in renal tubular cells and cyclosporin A. Lancet. 1981;1:1162–1163.

52. Jung K, Pergande M. Influence of cyclosporin A on the respiration of rat kidney mitochondria. FEBS Lett. 1985;183:167–169.

53. Stahl RAK, Kudelka S. Chronic cyclosporin A treatment reduces prostaglandin E-2 formation in isolated glomeruli and papilla of rat kidney. Clin Nephrol. 1986;25(Suppl. 1):S78–S82.

54. Jung K, Reinholdt C, Scholz P. Inhibitory efficiency of the kidney mitochondria from rats treated with cyclosporin A. Neprhon. 1987;45:43–45.

55. Crompton M, Ellinger H, Costi A. Inhibition by cyclosporin A of a Ca^{2+}-dependent pore in heart mitochondria activated by inorganic phosphate and oxidative stress. Biochem J. 1988;255:357–360.

56. Broekemeier KM, Dempsey ME, Preiffer DK. Cyclosporin A is a potent inhibitor of the inner membrane permeability transition in liver mitochondria. J Biol Chem. 1989;264:7826–7830.

57. Erman A, Chen-Gal B, Rosenfeld J. Cyclosporin treatment alters prostanoid and thromboxane production by rat isolated kidney mitochondria. J Pharm Pharmacol. 1990;42:181–185.

58. Kopp JB, Klotman PE. Cellular and molecular mechanisms of cyclosporin nephrotoxicity. J Am Soc Nephrol. 1990;1:162–179.

59. Kahan BD. Cyclosporin nephrotoxicity: pathogenesis, prophylaxis, therapy and prognosis. Am J Kid Dis. 1986;8:323–331.

60. Berg KJ, Forre O, Djoseland O, Mikkelsen M, Narverud J, Rugstad HE. Renal side-effects of high and low cyclosporin A doses in patients with rheumatoid arthritis. Clin Nephrol. 1989;31:232–238.

61. Elzinga L, Kelley VE, Houghton DC et al. Modification of experimental nephrotoxicity with fish oil as the vehicle for cyclosporin transplantation. Transplantation. 1987;43:271–274.

62. Paller M. The prostaglandin E-1 analog misoprostol reverses acute cyclosporin nephrotoxicity. Transplant Proc. 1988;20(Suppl. 3):634–637.

63. Buchanan WW, Brooks PM. Prediction of organ system toxicity with anti-rheumatic disease therapy. In: Bellamy N, ed. Prognosis in the rheumatic diseases. Dordrecht, Kluwer; 1991: 403–490.

64. von Graffenried B, Harrison WB. Renal function in patients with autoimmune diseases treated with cyclosporin. Transplant Proc. 1985;17(Suppl. 1):215

65. Ludwin, D, Bennett KJ, Grace EM, Buchanan WW, Bensen W, Bombardier C, Rugwell PX. Nephrotoxicity in patients with rheumatoid arthritis treated with cyclosporine. Transplantation Proc. 1988;20 (Suppl 4):367—370

66. Hannedouche TP, Delago AG, Gnionsahe AD et al. Nephrotoxicity of cyclosporine in autoimmune diseases. Adv Nephrol. 1990;19:169—186

67. Boers M, Diskmans BAC, Andre WAM, van Rijthoven HS. The HSG Cats A. Reversible nephrotoxicity of cyclosporine in rheumatoid arthritis. J Rheumatol. 190;17 : 38—42

68. Gabriel R. Time to scrap creatinine clearance? Br med J. 1986; 293:1370—1373

69. Levey A, perrone RD, Madias NE. Serum creatinine and renal function. Ann. Rev Med. 1988;39:465—490

70. Pitty MH. Safety of long term cyclosporine therapy in rheumatoid arthritis. ILAR 1989 Proceedings. Sao Paulo. Compania Melhoramentos de Sao Paulo;1989:491—492

71. Nagineni CN, Misra BC, Lee BDN et al. Cyclosporine A — a calcium channels interaction: a possible mechanism for nephrotoxicity. Transplant Proc.1987;19:1358—1362

72. Wagner K, Henkel M, Heinemeyer G et al. Interaction of calcium blockers and cyclosporine. Transplant Proc.1988;20 (Suppl 2) :561—568

73. Macleod AM, Thomson AW. FK 506: an immunosuppressant for the 1990'2? Lancet. 1991;337:25—27

74. Drosos AA, Skopouli FN, Costopoulos JS, Papadimitriou CS, Moutsopoulos HM. Cyclosporin A (CyA) in primary Sjogren's syndrome: a double-blind study. Ann. Rheum Dis. 1986;45:732—735

75. Capell HA, Rennie JAN, Rooney PJ et al. Patient compliance: a novel method of testing non-steroidal anti-inflammatory analgesics in rheumatoid arthritis. J Rheumatol. 1979;6:586—593

76. Situnayake RD, Grindulis KA, McConkey B. Long term treatment of rheumatoid arthritis with sulphasalazine, gold, or penicillamine: a comparison using life-table methods. Ann Rheum Dis. 1987;46:177—183

77. de Groen PC, Aksanut AJ, Rakel J et al. Central nervous system toxicity after liver transplantation: the role of cyclosporine and cholesterol. N Engl J Med.1987;317:861—866

78. London MG, Muirden KD, Hewitt JV. Serum cholesterol in rheumatic diseases. Br Med J. 1963;1:1380—1383

79. Rijthoven AWAM, Dijkmans BAC, The HSG, Boers M, Cats A. Penetration of cyclosporin into synovial fluid in rheumatoid arthritis. Eur J Clin Pharmacol. 1989;37:321—322

80. Newcome DS, Cohen AS. Chylous synovial effusion in rheumatoid arthritis. Clinical and pathogenetic significance. Am J Med. 1965;38:156—164

81. Jaffe IA. The technique of penicillamine administration in rheumatoid arthritis. Arthritis Rheum. 1975;18:513—514

36

Risk factors and risk–benefit problems in the use of DMARDs

R. Numo*, M. Covelli** and G. Lapadula**
*Centre for Rheumatic Diseases, Policlinico, Bari, Italy
**Chair of Rheumatology, University of Bari, Bari, Italy

The observation of the great discrepancies in the general strategy for the use of disease-modifying antirheumatic drugs (DMARDs) by rheumatologists amply reflects their evaluation of the relative potential risk factors.

Even though it is assumed that they are capable of modifying the course of the disease [1,2], agreement among rheumatologists as to when and how the treatment should be commenced has yet to be reached. Many problems still remain to be understood about the use of DMARDs.

The following questions still remain to be answered

1. Are there factors which can be predicted for their efficacy?
2. Are there factors predictive for the appearance of toxic or side-effects?
3. What is the impact of concurrent drug load?
4. Is the role of immunogenetics and immune profile the most relevant one?
5. Is there any relationship between the appearance of toxic effect and the type of rheumatic disorder?

In view of the increasing use of combined therapy with DMARDs in different rheumatic diseases it is clear that some new problems will arise and new data will have to be gathered.

On the other hand every new acquired knowledge will influence the overall evaluation of the risk–benefit aspects in the use of DMARDs. This latter aspect demands a wider retrospective reappraisal of all data coming from the different studies [3,4].

RISK FACTORS RELATED TO THE HOST

The main features associated with risk factors are:

i.   The immunogenetic profile of the patient;

Side-effects of Anti-inflammatory Drugs 3. Rainsford KD, Velo GP (eds), Inflammation and Drug Therapy Series, Volume V.

ii. The acetylator phenotype;

iii. Other factors.

The immunogenetic profile

The data gathered in the literature unanimously indicate the association between HLA-DR3 [5] and toxic effects from gold salts and D-penicillamine [6,7]. The relative risk (RR) itself seems to vary considerably from study to study but, since the RR is quite low, the practical implimentation on everyday therapeutical choices seems to be of minor relevance [8].

It appears that the DR3 antigen [9] alone does not account for the appearance of toxic effects but requires enhancing factors from the host which are poorly understood to date.

Other related antigens of both class II and class I [10] have not been thoroughly investigated even though an agranulocytosis from levamisole in B27-positive individuals was described long time ago [11]. DR3 is associated with development of proteinuria. Thus DR3-positive RA patients exhibit an eleven-fold higher risk of having proteinuria from injectable gold salts when compared to DR3-negative patients. On the other hand, patients with classical erosive RA exhibit a higher risk of haematological adverse reaction associated with DR3 [9].

The presence of B8, B12 and B40 has been found to be associated with drug toxicity [10].

The role of sex differences has not yet been evaluated, but the presence of gold stomatitis is higher in the female than in the male [6].

The acetylator phenotype

It has been shown that the rate of acetylation activity (due to a liver enzyme N-acetyltransferase) is strictly related to the occurrence of toxic effects with drugs such as sulphasalazine. The distribution of acetylator phenotype does vary in different ethnic groups but there is general agreement on the increased frequency of slow acetylator in drug-induced SLE, SLE, RA and Sjögren's syndrome [12]. In RA, even though an increased frequency of slow acetylator phenotype has been shown in classical erosive forms [13] in comparison with healthy donors, nonetheless no association was found between that increased frequency of slow acetylator phenotype and the appearance of adverse reactions, which is higher in male patients [14,15].

Other factors

It has become more intriguing to investigate these factors as our knowledge of them becomes more extensive.

Aside from acetylation a further way of inactivation of both gold salts and penicillamine is the oxidation of their sulphydryl groups. It is certainly well established in RA patients that the sulphoxidation rate is lower than in normal controls [5].

Unlike the acetylation status, which is a genetically determined phenotype, sulphoxidation seems to be influenced by the disease activity and perhaps by some drugs. Among other factors, age is an important one as is the need for concurrent use of different drugs for different purposes, when the possibility of development of adverse reactions for drug interactions is definitely higher.

Further enhancing factors (which are difficult to quantitate) are the roles of:
– concomitant diseases
– low compliance
– altered pharmacokinetics due to acquired metabolic disorders.

Elderly patients have shown a reduced tolerance to injectable gold salts, but other studies have failed to confirm this [16]. In addition, side-effects from oral gold were not more frequent in patients older than 65 when compared to younger patients [6]. Furthermore, there is a higher incidence of skin rashes in smokers (40% of 99 smokers developed dermatitis versus 17% of 109 non-smokers). Smoking enhances the uptake of gold into red blood cells, regardless of its plasma concentrations, and this increases the development of skin sensitivity, the most common reason for withdrawal from gold therapy.

The relationship between smoking and the development of skin rash was not confirmed in other studies.

Other risk factors evaluated such as weight, concurrent drug therapy and biochemical parameters were not predictive of potential development of adverse reactions.

The influences of the duration of the disease, and the sex status (female) are important but their level of significance was lower than smoking.

RISK FACTORS RELATED TO THE MOLECULE

Because of the high frequency of side-effects, some DMARDs have a predictably higher intrinsic risk. This is the case with methotrexate (MTX), D-penicillamine (PA) and other immunosuppressive molecules such as cyclophosphamide (CY), chlorambucil (Ch) and azathioprine (AZA).

Generally it can be said that the higher the dose the greater the risk; but with some drugs the possibility of accumulation is critical. This is why the prospect of inducing long-term side-effects is highly probable. This is the case with injectable gold salts. High doses of gold salts have been shown to induce albuminuria more frequently than low dose [17], whilst gold therapy can provoke both hepatocyte damage and cholestatic reaction. These reactions have been found to be milder than those to methotrexate (MTX). The outstanding question arises as to whether it will be possible to have a complete remission of the lesion after suspension of the drug.

Oral gold salts are responsible for less severe side-effects than injectable salts [18]; the lack of these with auranofin is mainly related to contact action with the mucosa of the intestine. The effects of injectable salts are basically related to both the partial function failure of entero-hepatic recirculation and to prolonged intrahepatic cholestasis and skin and mucosal sensitization. Hence the development of skin rash, pruritus and gastrointestinal complaints, while dose-related, may not seem to be relevant to abnormal liver function test. Thus, a liver function even though not apparently impaired or alternatively a liver gallbladder dysfunction can evoke or facilitate the appearance of skin manifestations.

Chloroquine (CQ) and hydrochloroquine (HCQ) [19, 20] still carry the legacy of a historical attribution of enhanced retinal damage. More recent appraisal in large retrospective studies has failed to show a correlation between dose and this side-effect, but in the absence of data for a normal population. It appears that proper tailoring of the dosage in relation to body weight is able to prevent the development of the severe retinopathy.

All data from literature are consistent with the conclusion that a maximum daily dose of 250 mg of CQ or 400 mg of HCQ, that guarantees a clinical outcome, when properly followed-up by biannual opthalmologic examination still represents an acceptable risk/benefit ratio for the patient in view of the good and easy handling of these molecules. Special attention should be given to elderly patients for their high risk of macular degeneration specifically related to the molecule itself [21].

Though used for a long time for inflammatory bowel diseases, sulphasalazine (SASP) has only recently been introduced in the treatment of rheumatic diseases. The basis for its use rests on a theoretical premise of the potential of the gut to determine or induce flare-ups of joint lesions [22].

These views are still unproven and conflicting clinical reports have been gathered on the beneficial effect of the drug. Nonetheless the use, alone or in combined therapy, is raising extensive clinical interest.

The risk of adverse drug reactions (ADR) from sulphasalazine is quite low in severity: cases of leucopenia or pancytopenia related to high dose of SASP are anecdotal; the most usual complaints are gastric (an intestinal intolerance with high dose) and unpredictable skin rash. Both of these

314

reactions have higher risk of appearance when pharmacological supplementation is added. The observation of increased plasma levels of transaminases and gamma-GT is less rare than described, a well-known effect to clinical rheumatologists who regard it as a common reason for withdrawal. The action of SASP on folate metabolism should be more pronounced than expected judging from two main pictures of side-effects, namely macrocytic anaemia and reversible oligospermia in young males.

After some 20 years of use of penicillamine in rheumatic diseases conflicting points still exist: the starting dose with PA seems to be crucial for the development of ADR, fewer side-effects being recorded with the dose of 125 mg/day vs. the 250 mg/day dose [24].

Further analysis suggests that when patients receiving the same maximum dose were compared, those with the high initial dose tended to have higher rate of side-effects [25]. On the other hand other authors failed to demonstrate significant differences between high- and low-dose groups for ADR to PA, regardless of the starting dose.

Initially, the 'start low' strategy can be useful to identify, as soon as possible, the risk factors without any real damage to the haematopoietic or renal systems of the patient.

An underestimated risk factor in patients undergoing therapy with PA is represented by the preliminary knowledge of previous ADR (albuminuria and haematological complications) to gold salts that make the development of both intolerance and inefficacy more predictable.

Special attention should be given to the cytotoxic drugs whose use is becoming more common in the treatment of different rheumatic diseases (psoriatic arthritis, rheumatoid arthritis, SLE, Wegener's disease, etc.)

Among these MTX is gaining popularity with the possibility that it allows good therapeutic management in different inflammatory conditions [26–28]. MTX can be administered once a week by 7.5 mg injection or oral dose. Of course this is the standard dose that was originally accepted both by dermatologists and rheumatologists [26] but later a very flexible posology ranging from 5 mg to 30 mg/weekly tailored both to clinical outcome and toxic effect monitoring appeared as the proper strategy.

When using MTX the ADR are subjective (nausea, gastrointestinal complaints, pruritus) but laboratory parameter alterations which include two lines of control, namely haematological status and liver function, are equally if not more important.

MTX was first used in 1940 in the treatment of leukaemia but in the late 40s was identified as inducing a wide range of liver damage ranging from hepatocellular lesions with associated enzyme release, to liver fibrosis and even cirrhosis.

The development of liver toxicity appears to be therapy duration and dose related but certainly obesity, alcohol and renal failure enhance or increase the risk of liver toxicity.

The risk of liver fibrosis seems to be related to the cumulative dose. In patients having a cumulative dose of 3 g of MTX the overall incidence of fibrosis in biopsy specimens was 25%. However, even though fibrosis is regarded as a step toward cirrhosis, the latter has not been reported in patients with RA under MTX [30].

Again, the observation that under similar dose schedules only some patients develop fibrosis (ranging from 18 to 25%) may also involve both genetic and immunogenetic predisposing factors. Unfortunately the need for detecting liver lesions by biopsy creates an obvious limitation both for pre-screening and monitoring therapy. Also, the observations that all liver function tests are not sensitive enough in detecting early stages of fibrosis raises some perplexities on the indiscriminate use of MTX in high dose, especially in certain geographical areas with endemic B virus hepatitis. Anyway, the need to use patient-tailored dosage is now emerging along with the warning to observe a strict surveillance of the patient under MTX, which must never be used when a contraindication is already known (previous virus hepatitis, alcoholism, pills, renal failure, etc.).

The crucial point is when can liver toxicity be expected? General agreement is that liver toxicity, when developing, appears within 6 months; the use of postmarketing surveillance being regarded as of little use. In conclusion, the value of routine biopsy examination in patients on low doses of MTX is controversial mainly because different studies carried out in RA patients did not confirm liver damage. Nonetheless the need for careful monitoring is more acute when potential liver-damaging acute concurrent therapy is to be used.

Other cytotoxic drugs [29] responsible for liver damage include cyclophosphamide, azathioprine and chlorambucil. They all share some common features that are individual sensitivity-related for liver damage at low dose and dose-related for haematological alterations.

What makes MTX special is the unpredictable pneumonitis in patients who have never experienced lung problems.

One more consideration to be borne in mind when evaluating liver damage is that the basic disease might be liver-damaging *per se* by plasma modifications, low concentrations of albumin, concurrent therapy, fever, etc.

Combined therapy

A more recent trend introduced is polychemotherapy or combined therapy [30] in some rheumatic disorders. The theoretical basis for this comes from a similar strategy used in haematological disorders. Different sequential or concurrent combinations have been tried (injectable gold + hydroxychloroquine, azathioprine, and SASP, PA and SASP): the concurrent use of two or more cytotoxic drugs increase, unpredictably, the risk of lung fibrosis. Paradoxically data have been reported indicating that combination between AZA and SASP, gold and HCQ, CY and MTX does not increase significantly the rate of episodes of ADR or toxicity [31].

Of course concurrent use of NSAIDs creates problems of enhanced or potentiated and unexpected toxicity [32]. Pharmacokinetic interaction between naprosyn and MTX has been studied and it was found that neither their relative bioavailability nor their protein binding is altered unless renal function is normal or slightly impaired.

Nonetheless further studies are required for investigating other expectedly risky combinations such as MTX and indomethacin, AZA and oxyphenylbutazone, etc.

RISK FACTORS RELATED TO THE DISEASE OR PLASMA ALTERATIONS

Controversial information comes from the level of immunoglobulins [3]. IgE are present in higher concentrations in RA patients than in healthy volunteers, and a good correlation has been found between levels of IgE and the development of ADR to gold. As for IgA it has been demonstrated that decreased level of IgA correlates with ADR to gold salts but, on the other hand, many drugs induce a lowering of circulating IgA.

Thus low IgA concentration seems to represent a potential risk factor.

Data from studies on cryoglobulins, rheumatoid factor and ANA have been controversial, conflicting and finally inconclusive. Patients with important eosinophilia have been reported to be at a high risk of developing ADR to gold, PA, SASP, AZA or MTX [16].

THE RISK–BENEFIT PROBLEM

The therapeutic strategy of many rheumatic diseases has experienced dynamic and progressive change from monotherapy to the stepwise one, to the pyramid strategy and, more recently to the 'Sawtooth' strategy [33] and combined therapy [30].

All these therapeutical approaches have represented a sort of historical step, sometimes trendy if not fashionable. Of course, this creates a great deal of misleading results due to the insufficient collection of cases under the same dose-regime. Social Health Systems are continuously facing the increasingly higher costs of therapeutic strategies in rheumatic diseases, but an additive cost comes from the introduction of new procedures that are more interesting from the speculative point of view than from the practical one. This is the case with some immunomanipulative therapies using monoclonal antibodies [34] that represent a great challenge to the problem of cost benefit as they are very expensive both for therapy itself and for monitoring, while the outcome is time-limited and still to be fully proved.

Of course such considerations are strictly related to the present moment, but in a more or less far future a progressive reduction of the costs for production of monoclonal antibodies together with the reduction of undesirable effects and proper target-tailored aims will make them a therapeutic tool with greater interest than merely being speculative.

As for the general aspects of immunomanipulative therapy it must be said that, despite strong theoretical premises, clinical outcome is not encouraging to date. In some cases they may be regarded as stimulating at best, but surely they are more expensive when compared with more conventional and experienced drugs. This for example is the case with thymic hormones versus azathioprine.

Improving the cost-effectiveness ratio in the treatment of rheumatic disease means not only using cheap drugs but even economizing on simple, easy to perform and inexpensive monitoring of laboratory parameters to test both efficacy and toxicity of a given drug or combined therapy. Using less toxic and easy to handle drugs may be very convenient to monitor, but the balance of convenience will become less favourable if poor or disappointing clinical results are achieved.

Generally speaking DMARDs themselves are inexpensive (ranging from 4.7 to 14% of the overall cost) but the final cost is dramatically augmented by the necessary medical controls and all procedures related to the potential toxic effects [35]. Nonetheless they guarantee in most patients a good benefit versus an acceptable risk, the relative ratio being positive [36].

Lowering the dose-schedule to tailor clinical effect may reveal an interesting tool to further reduce the rate of toxic effects. This means both the need for periodical medical controls and the opportunity for withdrawal.

When dealing with cost-benefit analysis, two major questions arise:

a) What can be defined as an 'acceptable risk'?

b) Are DMARDs really able to influence the natural course of a given rheumatic disease?

As for 'acceptable risk' [37], the level of acceptability is different among doctors and patients, as the former are more willing than the latter to accept a high risk with major diseases, whilst doctors consider them either not acceptable or less so as a risk for non-articular rheumatism.

For instance, if the risk of renal damage from cyclosporin A (usually irreversible) can be acceptable both for doctor and patient in cases of renal transplantation, the same risk is certainly less acceptable, at least for the patient, in different clinical conditions, as, for instance, rheumatoid arthritis, or Behçet's syndrome. The aspect of benefit under special circumstances becomes notable when proven alternatives are available. Also, the need for expensive and sophisticated controls augment both medical and economic involvement.

Many risks may be acceptable if they warrant a long-standing positive outcome [38]. Some anecdotal reports raise another problem: the malignancy following or during therapy with cytotoxic drugs. Unfortunately, a full evaluation of this aspect requires a wide series of cases with properly matched normal population controls.

The question of the true influence of DMARDs on the natural history of some rheumatic diseases is still a debatable matter. The problems are the great difficulty of collecting large numbers of cases with similar clinical features, the real impossibility of a guarantee of a proper placebo-treated group, and last, but not least, the determination of adequate and reliable parameters of evaluation (radiological progression [1,2], plasma markers, etc.).

REFERENCES

1. Scott DL, Greenwood A, Davies J, Maddison PJ, Maddison MC, Hall ND. Radiological progression in rheumatoid arthritis: do D-penicillamine and hydroxychloroquine have different effects? Br J Rheumatol. 1990;29:126–127.
2. Larsen A, Dale K, Eck M. Radiographic evaluation of rheumatoid arthritis and related conditions by standard reference films. Acta Radiol (Stockh). 1977;18:481–91.
3. Wijnands MJ, van Riel PL, Dribnau FW, van de Putte LB. Risk factors of second-line antirheumatic drugs in rheumatoid arthritis. Sem Arthritis Rheum. 110;19:337–352.
4. The Research Sub-Committee of the Empire Rheumatism Council. Gold therapy in rheumatoid arthritis: final report of a multicenter controlled trial. Ann Rheum Dis. 1961;20:315.
5. Emery P, Panayi GS, Huston G. D-penicillamine induced toxicity in rheumatoid arthritis: the role of sulphoxidation status and HLA-DR3. J Rheumatol. 1984;11:626–632.
6. Kay EA, Jayson IV. Risk factors that may influence development of side-effects of gold sodium thiomalate. Scand J Rheumatol. 1987;16:241–245.
7. Gran JT, Husby G, Thorsby E. HLA-DR antigens and gold toxicity. Ann Rheum Dis. 1983;42:62–66.
8. Wooley PH, Griffin J, Panayi GS. HLA-DR antigens and toxic reaction to sodium aurothiomalate and D-penicillamine in patients with rheumatoid arthritis. N Engl J Med. 1980;303:300–302.
9. Rantapaa Dhlqvist S, Strom H, Bjelle A, Moller E. HLA antigens and adverse drug reactions to sodium aurothiomalate and D-penicillamine in patients with rheumatoid arthritis. Clin Rheumatol. 1985;4:55–61.
10. Dequeker J, Van Wanghe P, Verdickt W. A systemic survey of HLA-A, B, C, and D antigens and drug toxicity in rheumatoid arthritis. J Rheumatol. 1984;11:282–286.
11. Veys EM, Mielants H, Verbruggen G. Levamisole-induced adverse reactions in HLA-B27-positive rheumatoid arthritis. Lancet. 1978;1:148.
12. Leden I, Hansson A, Melander A, Sturfelt G, Svensson B, Wahlin-Boll E. Varying distribution of acetylation phenotypes in RA patients with and without Sjögren's syndrome. Scand J Rheumatol. 1981;10:253–255.
13. Ehrlich GE, Freeman-Narrod M, Wineburgh GS. Predominance of slow acetylators among patients with rheumatoid arthritis. Eur J Rheumatol Inflamm. 1979;2:196–198.

14. Rantapaa Dahloqvist S, Mjorndal T. Acetylator phenotypes in rheumatoid arthritis patients with or without adverse drug reactions to sodium-aurothiomalate or D-penicillamine. Scand J Rheumatol. 1987;16:235–239.
15. Molin L, Larsson R, Karlsson E. Evaluation of the sulfapyridine acetylator phenotyping test in healthy subjects and in patients with cardiac and renal diseases. Acta Med Scand. 1977;201:217–222.
16. Borg G, Allander E, Goobar JE. Disease modifying antirheumatic drug therapy. Scand J Rheumatol. 1990;19:115–121.
17. Cats A. A multicentre controlled trial of the effects of different dosage of gold therapy, followed by a maintenance dosage. Agents Actions. 1976;6:355–363.
18. Palit J, Hill J, Capell HA, Carey J, Daunt SO'N, Cawley MID, Bird HA, Nuki G. A multicentre double-blind comparison of auranofin, intramuscular gold thiomalate and placebo in patients with psoriatic arthritis. Br J Rheumatol. 1990;29:280–283.
19. Elman A, Gulberg R, Nilsson E. Chloroquine retinopathy in patients with rheumatoid arthritis. Scand J Rheumatol. 1976;5:161–166.
20. Voipio H. Incidence of chloroquine retinopathy. Acta Ophthalmol. 1966;44:349–354.
21. Graniewski-Wijnands HS, Van Lith GHM, Vijfvinkel-Bruinenga S. Ophthalmological examination of patients taking chloroquine. Doc Ophthalmol. 1979;48:231–234.
22. Amos RS, Pullar T, Bax DE. Sulphasalazine for rheumatoid arthritis. Toxicity in 774 patients monitored for 1 to 11 years. Br Med J. 1986;293:420–423.
23. Farr M, Brodick A, Bacon PA. Plasma and synovial concentrations of sulphasalazine and two of its metabolites in rheumatoid arthritis. Rheumatol Int. 1985;5:247–251.
24. Hall CL, Tighe R. The effect of continuing penicillamine and gold treatment on the course of penicillamine and gold neuropathy. Br J Rheumatol. 1989;28:53–57.
25. Magnus JH, Gran JT, Mikkelsen K, Nygaard H, Brath HK. Toxicity to D-penicillamine in rheumatoid arthritis. Scand J Rheumatol. 1987;16:441-444.
26. Warin AP, Landells JW, Levene GM. A prospective study of the effects of weekly oral methotrexate on liver biopsy. Br J Dermatol. 1975;93:321–327.
27. Kremer JM, Lee RG, Tolman KG. Liver histology in rheumatoid arthritis patients receiving long term methotrexate therapy. Arthritis Rheum. 1989;32(2):121–127.
28. Weinblatt ME, Lee Maier A. Longterm experience with low dose weekly methotrexate in rheumatoid arthritis. J Rheumatol. 1990;17(suppl. 22):33–38.
29. De Pinho RA, Goldgerg CS, Lefkowitch JH. Azathioprine and the liver. Gastroenterology. 1984;86:162–165.
30. Bitter T. Combined disease-modifying chemotherapy for intractable rheumatoid arthritis. Clin Rheum Dis. 1984;10(2):417–428.
31. Lewis P, Hazleman B, Bulgen D. Clinical and immunological study of high dose azathioprine combined with gold therapy. In: Rheumatoid arthritis, cellular pathology and pharmacology. Amsterdam: North Holland; 1977:280.
32. Furst DE. Clinically important interactions of non-steroidal antiinflammatory drugs with other medications. J Rheumatol. 1988;suppl 17;15:58–62.
33. Fries JF. Reevaluating the therapeutic approach to rheumatoid arthritis: the 'Sawtooth' strategy. J Rheumatol. 1990;17(suppl.22):12–15.
34. Kingsley G. Monoclonal antibody treatment of rheumatoid arthritis. Br J Rheumatol. 1991;30(suppl.2):33–35.
35. Harris GB. Costs of monitoring chrysotherapy. Arizona Med. 1977;24,4 April.
36. Block SR. The cost of parenteral gold vs oral gold in the long term treatment of rheumatoid arthritis. J Rheumatol. 1986;13:3.
37. Pullar T, Wright V, Feely M. What do patients and rheumatologists regard as an 'acceptable' risk in the treatment of rheumatic disease? Br J Rheumatol. 1990;29:215–218.
38. Thompson MS. Willingness to pay and accept risks to cure chronic disease. Am J Public Health. 1986;76:392–396.

37

Gold toxicity: chemical, structural, biological and clinical experimental issues

Walter F. Kean, C.J.L. Lock, W. Watson Buchanan, Helen Howard-Lock and M.G. Hogan

Rheumatic Disease Unit and Laboratories for Inorganic Medicine, McMaster University, Hamilton, Ontario, Canada

INTRODUCTION

Gold compounds have been used in the treatment of rheumatoid arthritis since 1929 [1]. but to date the mechanisms of efficacy and toxicity have not been established. Forestier's original study of 15 patients treated with gold thiopropanol sodium sulphonate identified adverse effects in 11 patients, 3 of whom were stated to have serious side-effects [1]. Today, the incidence of gold therapy associated toxicity is in the order of 30–50% with approximately 10% of patients experiencing a significantly severe problem which requires withdrawal from therapy [2]. However, clinical interpretation of severity varies, and author bias is a major factor in identification of frequency of adverse reactions. An experienced clinician may continue gold treatment even after the development of a mild skin rash or small degree of proteinuria whereas the inexperienced clinician may immediately discontinue therapy. In a clinical trial such outcomes will be recorded differently. Of equal importance to the problem of interpretation, is the fact that the pharmacodynamics of gold compounds are poorly understood. Several factors contribute to this problem: the nature of gold chemistry, the structural formulation of the compounds and the biological activity of gold and the ligands. The following review of the literature outlines some of the basic science experimental issues we have encountered in the study of gold toxicity and outlines our clinical research experience with adverse reactions to gold complexes.

GOLD CHEMISTRY

A knowledge of gold chemistry is essential in order to accurately study the mechanisms of gold compounds.

Side-effects of Anti-inflammatory Drugs 3. Rainsford KD, Velo GP (eds), Inflammation and Drug Therapy Series, Volume V.

Gold is in group 1b of the periodic table, and has the common oxidation states of I, II, III and V, although complexes with metal/metal bonds exist in which it is difficult to assign a formal oxidation state to the atom. The halides form the true salts of Au(I) but they are unstable in the presence of water and disproportionate to Au(0) and Au(III) [3]. Au(I) compounds form stable complexes with 'soft' ligands [4] such as the thiolates [5–7] and phosphines [5,8,9]. All anti-arthritic gold complexes are Au(I) thiol or phosphine compounds [10]. Elder and colleagues have shown that if gold sodium thiomalate is administered to laboratory animals, the gold recovered from the tissues and urine exists in the Au(I) oxidation state [11]. If Au(III)Cl$_3$ is administered to laboratory animals, only Au(I) is recovered in tissues and urine as detected by X-ray absorption near edge spectroscopy (XANES) and extended X-ray absorption fine structure (EXAFS). Elder and colleagues have shown that in rats chronically treated with gold sodium thiomalate, the gold within particles obtained from the rat kidney cells was Au(I) and was bound to two sulphur atoms with a gold–sulphur bond length of 2.3 A [11]. The Au(I) oxidation state therefore appears to be the primary oxidation state in the biological milieu and *in vivo*. Reduction from Au(III) to Au(I) is most likely caused by the powerful sulphydryl-containing reducing enzymes present *in vivo*.

The molecular weight of gold sodium thiomalate based on the empirical formula is usually assumed to be 390.12. This is incompatible with the known chemical properties of Au(I) [3,12–14] and a more likely structure is a polymer. Both Shaw, and Sadler and colleagues, support the concept that the gold sodium thiomalate structure is a polymer [12,15–17]. Based on model building, a possible structural formula is a hexamer. The chirality of the thiomalic acid, means that if gold sodium thiomalate is a cyclic hexamer, then it exists as thirteen different structural and chiral isomers. The thiomalate ligand is bound to two gold atoms through the sulphur atom, which acts as a bridge. Since thiomalic acid is chiral, each ligand could be either d(+) or l(–) if a racemic mixture of thiomalic acid is used to make the gold sodium thiomalate. Complexes would be formed in which all the ligands in a molecule are d(+), or 1l(–) and 5d(+), or 2l(–) and 4d(+) and so on, all the way to 6l(–). The amount of each type is given by probability theory and they are in the ratios 1:6:15:20:15:6:1. There are further complications within the groups. If we take the case of 2l(–) and 4d(+) ligands and number the positions around the ring structure, one can have molecules with the l(–) ligands at positions 1,2 or 1,3 or 1,4 as distinct species. Similarly for the 3l(–) and 3d(+) compounds the l(–) ligands can be at 1,2,3:1,2,4; or 1,3,5. In our laboratory we have prepared gold sodium thiomalate from d(+)-thiomalic acid only (or alternatively from l(–)-thiomalic acid only). When the resulting gold complexes are mixed, however, one does not obtain a mixture of gold sodium thiomalate containing molecules with 6d($+$) or 6l($-$) ligands only. The ligands exchange very rapidly ($t_{1/2} < 10^{-2}$ s) so the 1:6:15:20:15:6:1 mixture is obtained.

Normally when one mixes two chiral compounds to get a racemic mixture, the chemical and biological properties of the racemate are the average of the properties of the individual enantiomers. This does not however happen in the case of gold sodium thiomalate. The biological properties of 'all-d' and 'all-l' thiomalate, as measured by the suppression of platelet aggregation, are quite different, but the properties of a 50:50 mixture of 'all-l' and 'all-d' are substantially different from the expected average. The reason is quite simple. Because of exchange the amount of 'all-l' and 'all-d' in the resultant mixture is very small (one part each in 64 parts) and the properties of the mixture are determined by the more common 2l($-$),4d($+$), 3l($-$),3d($+$) and 4l($-$),2d($+$) compounds.

Lack of knowledge of the structural formulae of gold sodium thiomalate and related complexes has contributed to the lack of understanding of the biological activity of the Au(I) anti-arthritic complex. Attention to the structural forms and their properties of the gold sodium thiomalate compound and related gold thiol compounds is essential for researchers studying the nature of the interaction of gold complexes with biological species. Few researchers record in their reports that compounds such as gold sodium thiomalate and gold thioglucose are polymers, or that gold sodium thiosulphate and auranofin are monomers.

PROBLEMS OF INTERPRETATION

A common misconception amongst clinicians is that D-penicillamine can chelate gold, and can be used as a protective agent if a toxic reaction occurs during or following the administration of the anti-arthritic gold complexes [18–21]. There is no theoretical or biochemical evidence that D-penicillamine chelates Au(I) *in vivo* [22]. Au(I) compounds have a linear geometry in which the Au(I) atom is attached to only two ligand atoms (X) such that the X-Au(I)-X angle is 180° [23]. Even when a ligand has two potential sulphur bonding sites, the ligand binds to two different gold atoms rather than form a chelate [24]. There is no apparent reason why D-penicillamine should show exceptional behaviour and thus one would expect D-penicillamine to bind to Au(I) only through the sulphydryl site. Thus, as supported by the studies of Davis and Barraclough [22], and as previously reported by us, there is no theoretical reason why D-penicillamine should *chelate* Au(I) [25].

Many *in vivo* and *in vitro* studies on the use of gold sodium thiomalate have compared the effectiveness of the compound to gold chloride [26–28]. In such experiments sodium thiomalate was often used as a control. In two of these studies, the results were reported to show that sodium thiomalate had no effect on inhibition of mixed lymphocyte response whereas gold sodium thiomalate and gold chloride did inhibit the mixed lymphocyte response. It was then concluded that the gold was the effective agent. In a further study it was concluded that gold was the effective agent in the inhibition of acid phosphatase since both gold chloride and gold sodium thiomalate inhibited the enzyme [26]. There are problems with these comparisons.

1. Cell viability and enzyme activity is usually pH-dependent and aqueous solutions of gold chloride are acidic. Even in buffered solutions, gold chloride can be cytotoxic.

2. Gold chloride is a Au(III) compound and gold sodium thiomalate is a Au(I) compound.

3. Gold sodium thiomalate is not monomeric but is a mixture of different chiral and structural polymers, the stability of which have not been established and the activities of the individual isomers has not been reported.

4. Most authors do not describe whether they are dealing with mono-, di- or trisodium thiomalate, all of which differ in pH stability.

PHARMACOKINETIC DISPOSITION OF GOLD COMPLEXES

Extrapolation of the pharmacokinetics of gold compounds as an interpretation of the pharmacodynamics has not been useful. Their chemical structures are unknown and the pharmacokinetic profile has largely centred on the measurement of gold only.

Injectable gold complexes

Following a 50 mg injection of gold sodium thiomalate or gold thioglucose, gold is rapidly absorbed into the circulation and peak serum levels of 700–1000 μg/100 ml are achieved in 2–6 hours. Over six days the serum level will fall to 300 μg/100 ml. The gold is excreted 75% via the kidneys and the remainder in the faeces. More than 95% of the gold is bound to albumin and the remainder of the gold is bound to macroglobulins, with a small amount bound to low molecular weight thiol species [29,30]. It has not yet been determined which part of the gold complex *in vivo* is the active species, although it is likely that it is the low molecular weight species.

Oral gold complexes

The oral gold compound auranofin contains Au(I) and binds predominantly to albumin through cysteine and histidine [13]. Following administration of [195]Au-auranofin, approximately 25% of the administered dose is detected in plasma bound to albumin. Peak concentrations of 6–9 μg/100 ml are reached within 1–2 hours [31,32]. The plasma half-life of auranofin is in the order of 15–25 days with a total body elimination rate of 55–80 days [33]. Only approximately 1% of the [195]Au is detectable by 180 days whereas up to 30% of the [195]Au from gold sodium thiomalate may be detected at this time [34].

When auranofin crosses the plasma membrane, the acetyl groups on the thioglucose are lost and some dissociation of the compound takes place [35]. Triple labelling studies with radioactive [195]Au, ^{32}P and ^{35}S show evidence of Au–S and Au–P disruption which occurs across the plasma membrane [36]. Various experimental models have shown different results as to the radioactive ligand grouping [35]. Design of *in vitro* and *ex vivo* experiments, has to incorporate the expected ligands which occur following the dissociation of the auranofin. The application of the intact auranofin molecule to an *in vitro* or *ex vivo* experiment may not provide results which reflect the *in vivo* activity of the dissociated components of the auranofin.

The study of gold kinetics has been of little value in the interpretation of the mechanisms of action of gold complexes *in vivo*.

EXPERIMENTAL PROBLEMS IN THE STUDY OF GOLD TOXICITY

In addition to the chemical and structural variables of the gold drugs, we have identified a marked variation in the physical and biological activities of gold sodium thiomalate.

Gold sodium thiomalate

The commercial solution of gold sodium thiomalate used to treat patients, is a yellow solution containing 0.05% chlorocresol (Rhône-Poulenc, Canada), phenylmercuric nitrate 0.002% (May and Baker, UK), or benzyl alcohol 0.5% (Merck Sharp & Dohme, USA) as preservatives. All contain 0.3 moles of glycerol per mole of thiomalate. However gold sodium thiomalate for experimental use, prepared by dissolving gold sodium thiomalate powder in sterile water, is a colourless solution. The yellow commercial solution is prepared by heating the colourless solution at 100°C for thirty minutes. During this procedure a yellow solution results [37]. In order to investigate the physical and biological properties of the colourless and yellow solutions of gold sodium thiomalate we studied the following:

1. ^{1}H spectroscopy
2. Ultraviolet (UV) irradiation of the colourless solution
3. Action of the solutions on platelet aggregation
4. Electronmicroscopy of platelets treated with the solutions
5. Thrombin inhibition
6. Action of the solution on the mixed lymphocyte response

1. NMR spectroscopy

^{1}H NMR spectra of freshly prepared colourless solutions of gold sodium thiomalate made from solid (3.2×10^{-2} mol/L) showed no significant difference in the spectral pattern when compared to the commercial yellow solution of gold sodium thiomalate (3.2×10^{-2} mol/L) which had been heat-sterilized for human use.

2. UV Irradiation

When the colourless solution, 3.2×10^{-2} mol/L, was irradiated with ultraviolet light at 350 nm over a prolonged time period in the 400–500 nm region, we identified curves consistent with a peak glowing in the 450–475 nm range. After 500 minutes of irradiation the colourless solution had become dark brown. We concluded that the yellow colour of the commercially available gold sodium thiomalate was caused by an absorption at 450 nm.

3. Platelet aggregation

Since sterilization procedures should not alter the chemical or biological equivalence of a drug, we decided to study the effects of the colourless and yellow solutions of gold sodium thiomalate on biological systems which might bear some relevance to the study of the rheumatic diseases in which commercial gold sodium thiomalate (yellow solution) was known to be active. Concentrations of the yellow solution ($1.3 \times 10^{-3} - 6.4 \times 10^{-3}$ mol/L) were added to washed human platelets in aggregation experiments [37]. Platelet aggregation was not observed for gold concentrations of the yellow solution of gold sodium thiomalate $< 1.3 \times 10^{-3}$ mol/L. When a range of concentrations of the colourless solution of gold sodium thiomalate $1.8 \times 10^{-5} - 6.4 \times 10^{-3}$ mol/L was added to washed human platelets no reactivity of the platelets was observed. However yellow solutions of gold sodium thiomalate caused aggregation, internal granule release and deaggregation over 2–4 minutes. Equimolar concentrations of gold thioglucose, gold sodium thiosulphate, and disodium thiomalate did not cause platelet aggregation or release. We therefore concluded that some activity in the yellow solution resulted in the platelet aggregation taking place at these concentrations.

4. Electron microscopy

Electron micrographs of platelets treated with the yellow solution of gold sodium thiomalate $1.3 \times 10^{-3} - 6.4 \times 10^{-3}$ mol/L had numerous pseudopodia and were consistent with platelets which had undergone aggregation. Fibrillar gold containing particles 100–700 nm in length were identified:

1. in the process of being phagocytosed
2. within intracellular vesicles
3. within the surrounding media

Energy dispersive spectroscopic analysis revealed the presence of gold and sulphur within these particles. Platelets treated with the colourless solution of gold sodium thiomalate $1.8 \times 10^{-5} - 6.4 \times 10^{-3}$ mol/L were oval in shape and did not appear to have aggregated. These platelets contained numerous scattered particles of less than 40 nm in diameter which were distinct from glycogen granules. Occasional particles were membrane-bound and energy dispersive analysis confirmed that these particles contained Au and S. No Au was detected in platelets treated with gold thioglucose, gold sodium thiosulphate, auranofin, or disodium thiomalate.

5. Thrombin inhibition

Gold sodium thiomalate has been shown to inhibit the serine esterase enzymes, trypsin, elastase and cathepsin G. Both the colourless and yellow solutions of gold sodium thiomalate in a concentration range of $3.8 \times 10^{-5} - 3.0 \times 10^{-4}$ mol/L inhibited the action of bovine thrombin (0.05 units/ml) on 1 ml of washed human platelets if added to the platelet suspension before or simultaneously with the addition of the thrombin [38]. A range of inhibition of platelet aggregation with colourless and yellow solutions of gold sodium thiomalate $3.8 \times 10^{-5} - 3.0 \times 10^{-4}$ mol/L was also demonstrated within the bovine thrombin concentration range of 0.025 to 0.25 units/ml. Control experiments indicated that chlorocresol had no effect on thrombin activity. Both the yellow and colourless solution were equally active in their inhibition of thrombin [37,38].

6. Mixed lymphocyte response

We studied the effects of the yellow and colourless solutions on the mixed lymphocyte response [39]. This system was used since gold sodium thiomalate is a known inhibitor of the mixed lymphocyte response by modulation of macrophage expression. The addition of the yellow and colourless solutions of gold sodium thiomalate ($3.8 \times 10^{-5} - 3.0 \times 10^{-4}$ mol/L) to the mixed lymphocyte response resulted in a significant decrease in lymphocyte response and was enhanced with the increase in gold concentration. There was no significant difference in the inhibition of the mixed lymphocyte response by either the colourless or the yellow solutions at the concentrations used. Control experiments indicated that chlorocresol had no effect on lymphocyte activity.

EXPERIMENTAL PROBLEMS – COMMENT

The inhibition of mixed lymphocyte response and the inhibition of the serine esterase enzyme thrombin, was identical for both the colourless and yellow solutions [37–39]. Thus the yellow component was not necessary for the biological expression in these studies [40]. If this type of activity of the drug *in vitro* is relevant to its *in vivo* effects, then it is possible that the colour change during sterilization does not affect the antirheumatic activity of the preparation. The only differences between the colourless and yellow solutions of the gold sodium thiomalate that we have been able to identify are in the ultraviolet absorption spectra and in platelet aggregation using supra-pharmacological concentrations [40].

ADVERSE REACTIONS

Adverse reactions are the major limiting factor to the use of disease modifying antirheumatic drugs. Approximately 30–50% of patients who receive either the injectable gold compound or the auranofin oral preparation, will develop some form of toxicity [2,41] and irrespective of any beneficial effect, the drug will have to be stopped, sometimes indefinitely.

Skin rash

Rash is the most common side-effect of the injectable gold compounds and occurs in approximately 30% of cases [2]. Up to 20% of patients may have gold discontinued because of rash. The rash is usually dry and itchy, and is approximately 1–10 cm in diameter. The slightly erythematous patches are scaly and resemble a seborrhoeic rash with a distribution in the hands, forearms, trunk, shins, and occasionally the face. The drug should be discontinued if rash occurs and should not be administered until the rash has resolved. The drug may be restarted in low dose of 10 or 25 mg intramuscularly. Severe skin rash problems such as nummular eczema, total exfoliation and intense pruritis have been known to develop. The development of exfoliation is a medical emergency and treatment with fluids and electrolytes must be given. Problems are less common when a strict monitoring system is applied.

Rash is also a common side-effect of auranofin therapy, and occurs in up to 20% of patients, half of whom also have pruritis [41]. Skin rash is most common in the first twelve months of treatment but can occur at any time. When rash develops, the drug should be stopped until the condition resolves. Approximately 2–3% of patients have to discontinue therapy because of severe skin rash [42].

It is also possible that clinicians engaged in a research protocol might be more likely to discontinue a patient from gold therapy because of rash compared to a clinician who observes a mild to moderate rash in a clinical non-research setting provided the patient is achieving benefit.

Pigmentation due to gold in the skin has been referred to as chrysiasis. On sun-exposed areas, e.g. the face, the skin takes on a bluish hue. Leonard and colleagues identified increased melanin in the skin of one patient who had received a cumulative dose of 36 g of gold sodium thiosulphate [43]. A possible mechanism of melanin production is suggested by Lewis [44] and cited by Leonard and colleagues [43]. In the early stages of melanin formation, the production of dihydroxyphenylalanine (DOPA) from tyrosine and of dopaquinone from DOPA both require the copper-containing enzyme tyrosinase. Cystine and glutathione inhibit tyrosinase but gold can bind to these low molecular weight thiols and thus inactivate these inhibitors of tyrosinase thus permitting the formation of melanin. Such a mechanism could be accepted for the appearance of chrysiasis in sun-exposed areas.

Gold depositions in skin appears to be predominantly in the phagolysosomes of the macrophage-like cells but the correlation of quantity of depositions with toxicity is questionable [45].

Oral ulcers

Oral ulceration, which may or may not be painful, occurs in 20% of patients [2,42]. The ulcers resemble aphthous ulcers in the mucous membrane and in the vestibule of the mouth. Occasionally the lesions are present on the tongue or the hard palate. The development of a mouth ulcer is a definite contraindication to gold therapy until the mouth ulcer has resolved. Oral ulceration can precede the development of pemphigoid-like bullous skin lesions.

Oral inflammation occurs in 1–12% of patients on auranofin and may be concomitant with skin rash. The ulcers are not common in the first month but like other side-effects, may occur at any time [42]. The mechanism of oral ulceration or stomatitis is unknown.

Proteinuria

Proteinuria has been reported in 0–40% of gold-treated patients [2,42,46–48]. The wide variation in the definition or lack of definition of proteinuria in the literature has resulted in a considerable difference in the reported incidence [2,42,46–48]. Proteinuria in urine in amounts of 1 + by dip stick over two to three weeks warrants a 24-hour urine protein estimation. If proteinuria is less than 500 mg for 24 hours the drug should be continued. Between 500 and 3000 mg for 24 hours, gold therapy should be withheld until it is established that renal function is normal. Patients whose proteinuria is greater than 3000 mg for 24 hours should have the gold therapy stopped until the proteinuria resolves. There are no well documented cases of long-term serious or permanent renal damage due to gold-induced proteinuria. The most common renal histological lesion is membranous glomerulonephritis with the deposition of IgG, IgM and C_3 on the glomerulus [49], although heavy metal tubular damage does occur during injectable gold therapy [50].

One postulated mechanism of the proteinuria is that the gold or a gold complex damages the renal tubule, analagous to heavy metal damage, and results in release of a 'neo-antigen' which complexes with immunoglobulin and deposits on the glomerulus to result in a glomerulonephritis. The tubular damage is characterized by the presence of β_2-microglobulin in the urine. Electron microscopy demonstrates the presence of fibrillar particulate gold-containing material within the proximal tubular cells and also the presence of degenerating mitochondria [50]. Numerous studies have suggested an association between HLA DR3 and the presence of proteinuria.

Proteinuria secondary to oral gold is extremely uncommon [42] and occurs in up to 5% of patients treated with auranofin. The drug should be withheld and assessments of renal function made in a manner similar to that for injectable gold toxicity to the kidney.

Haematuria is not a recognized side-effect of gold therapy. When microscopic haematuria develops, gold therapy should be stopped immediately and a cause for the haematuria sought.

Once proteinuria has reduced in quantity or the haematuria has resolved, gold therapy may be reinstituted at a reduced dosage.

330

Thrombocytopenia

Physicians monitoring gold therapy should observe a platelet count less than $200\,000/\text{mm}^3$ as an indication to temporarily discontinue gold therapy. Most laboratories record a value of $150\,000/\text{mm}^3$ as the lower level of normal for the platelet count. A falling platelet count even within the normal range can be a signal of early thrombocytopenia. A sudden change in a platelet count which has been steady at $400\,000/\text{mm}^3$ weekly to a value of e.g. $210\,000/\text{mm}^3$ behoves a physician to withhold gold therapy until a repeat platelet count confirms a stable value above $200\,000/\text{mm}^3$ on at least two occasions one week apart. When a fall in platelet count results in a value which is persistently less than $200\,000/\text{mm}^3$ extreme caution is advised and whenever facilities are available, blood should be tested for the presence of platelet surface-associated IgG auto-antibodies [51]. Platelet antibodies are not associated with the much rarer gold-induced thrombocytopenia secondary to bone marrow suppression. Although it has been stated that thrombocytopenia secondary to injectable gold therapy may occur precipitously, close observation of changes in platelet count even within the normal range may result in earlier identification of some patients who may develop a sudden thrombocytopenia. The development of thrombocytopenia secondary to injectable gold therapy is an absolute contraindication to the further use of the gold compound. We and others have reported that the presence of HLA DR3 may be indicative of an increased risk of thrombocytopenia associated with platelet surface antibodies [52,53].

Rarely thrombocytopenia and bone marrow suppression may occur as a result of auranofin treatment. This type of thrombocytopenia (unlike the more common type seen with gold sodium thiomalate) does not have platelet surface associated auto-antibodies and is most likely due to direct marrow suppression. The treatment of choice is immediate withdrawal of auranofin therapy. The development of thrombocytopenia and/or low white blood cell count is an absolute contraindication to therapy with auranofin.

Bone marrow suppression

Bone marrow suppression due to gold treatment is rare but is sufficiently serious to warrant strict monitoring of blood parameters on a weekly basis [2]. The marrow suppression secondary to either injectable or oral gold therapy has been postulated as due to a direct action of the drug on the marrow cells [54]. A fall in either platelet count as recorded above, or a fall in haemoglobin below 10 g/100 ml, and/or a fall in total white count below $4000/\text{mm}^3$ requires immediate discontinuation of therapy until cause and effect have been established. A reversal of the white cell differential ratio and/or a rise in monocyte count above 10% are also indications for immediate discontinuation of the gold drug until at least two normal values, one week apart, have been recorded. If any of the above indicators of haemopoiesis remain abnormal, a bone marrow examination and investigation for auto-antibodies to white cells, red cells and platelets is essential before gold therapy can be reintroduced. Bone marrow suppression secondary to gold compounds is an absolute contraindication to further continuation of therapy.

Notwithstanding the rare side-effect of bone marrow suppression, it should be noted that successful gold therapy in rheumatoid disease results in a return to normal haemoglobin levels, as one of the first indicators of clinical improvement. Dr Andrew Harvey, in our laboratory, has shown that erythroid growth colony counts derived from peripheral blood mononuclear cells were inversely proportional to the level of IgM and IgM rheumatoid factor in the peripheral blood of patients with rheumatoid disease [55]. It is therefore possible that some forms of rheumatoid anaemia have a humoral basis and therefore it can be postulated that modulation of these humoral mechanisms by gold compounds may result in improvement of rheumatoid anaemia [55].

While gold therapy associated bone marrow suppression could be a direct effect of the gold compound, an alternative postulate is that there is an alteration in the marrow feed-back system from monocytes in the peripheral blood due to an action of gold compounds on these cells or their 'cell messengers'.

In spite of the potential for gold compounds to induce marrow suppression, injectable gold compounds are now recognized as the treatment of choice for Felty's syndrome [56]. The drug should be given in exactly the same manner as described for rheumatoid disease. The recommended starting dose is 10 mg or 25 mg weekly until an observed rise in the absolute white count takes place. Treatment of Felty's syndrome should be carried out in a controlled situation where assessment of bone marrow tissue is available.

Diarrhoea

The onset of loose soft stools and a change of stool frequency and pattern, is the most common side-effect of auranofin therapy and may occur in over 40% of treated patients [57,58]. The frequency of this side-effect is highest in the first month of treatment, though many resolve spontaneously. It should be noted that the lower incidence of altered stool pattern in later months may be directly related to a pre-selected drop-out of those patients susceptible to the diarrhoea. The development of frank watery diarrhoea occurs in 2–5% of patients on auranofin and is dose-related, but some patients are totally intolerant of even 3 mg/day. Other non-specific digestive system complaints account for approximately 20% of all side-effects due to auranofin and 2% of all withdrawals [59].

Although gastrointestinal side-effects are more common with oral gold compounds, injectable compounds can result in gut problems. Mascarenhas and colleagues in their kinetic study of injectable gold compounds recorded that faecal excretion accounted for 25–64% of the total excretion of gold [60]. This was much higher than expected for an injectable compound. In one of their patients who received gold sodium thiomalate, the faecal gold excretion was much higher than the urinary gold excretion. It has not yet been established whether those patients receiving injectable gold who developed a diarrhoea are higher excretors of gold by the faecal route than the urinary route. In open studies, the frequency of side-effects with the oral gold compound was 40% but only 4% with injectable compounds [41]. In double-blind studies, the frequency of side-effects noted with injectable gold compounds was 20% although higher rates were still noted with oral gold compounds [46%]. A 20% incidence of diarrhoea caused by injectable gold is much higher than recorded by some authors [2,42].

Several mechanisms of gold compound induced diarrhoea have been proposed. Most water and solute absorption occurs in the small intestine with the large intestine, particularly the distal colon, playing the role of a final modifier. This mechanism is analogous to that observed in the renal tubule where obligatory reabsorption of salts, solutes and water occurs in the proximal segments, with the distal tubule and collecting duct being responsible for facultative reabsorption. By analogy with the renal tubule collecting ducts, the reabsorptive capacity of the distal colon is limited. Decreased reabsorption of solutes and water in the proximal segments can overwhelm the reabsorptive capacity of the distal segment, resulting in diuresis in the case of the kidney and diarrhoea in the case of the gut.

Diarrhoea can arise from:

(i) decreased normal solute and water absorption;

(ii) increased electrolyte secretion;

(iii) the presence of poorly absorbed, osmotically active solutes in the gut lumen;

(iv) abnormal intestinal motility, or

(v) inflammation or infection leading to exudation of mucus, blood or pus.

Diarrhoea secondary to drugs can be considered as arising due to alterations in transport (decreased absorption, increased secretion) or changes in motility patterns. This can be expressed as:

(a) decreased absorption,

(b) increased secretion, or

(c) abnormal motility.

Van Riel and colleagues studied the occurrence of diarrhoea during the course of a long-term clinical trial [57]. Eleven patients developed diarrhoea and in eight, faecal Na^+ concentration was elevated, K^+ was reduced and dry weight was reduced. It was postulated that auranofin could have a direct effect on absorption of salt and water by the colon.

Behrens and colleagues studied 6 patients treated with auranofin who were found to have increased intestinal transit time [61]. The concentration of Na^+ in faecal water was increased with reduction in bicarbonate but no significant changes in levels of Cl^- or K^+ were recorded. They also noted that the excretion of ^{51}Cr-EDTA and lactulose was increased with little increase in the excretion of mannitol. This suggested an increase in intestinal permeability and implied destruction of the absorptive surface; an experimental study in the rat did produce evidence of mucosal damage. In contrast, a study of a single patient given gold thioglucose suggested that a secretory type of diarrhoea could be induced [62].

Inhibition of absorption and secretory mechanisms have been reported. Hardcastle and colleagues used everted sacs from the rat colon [63,64] and showed that auranofin in the mucosal solution reduced fluid and Na^+ absorption whereas it was ineffective from the serosal side. The drug also inhibited the activity of Na^+/K^+ ATP-ase. Similar observations were made in dogs where auranofin caused significant elevations in efferent volume, osmolarity and Na^+ concentration with significant decreases in K^+ [65]. These results led to the hypothesis that auranofin and other gold compounds such as gold sodium thiomalate and chlorauric acid reduced absorptive processes by inhibiting the Na^+ pump activity of enterocytes. In contrast to the above observation, Ammon and colleagues have argued that auranofin induced net fluid and electrolyte secretion across the *in vivo* perfused rat jejunum [66]. Since gold sodium thiomalate did not produce similar effects, they suggested that it was not the gold moiety but the carrier molecule that was responsible for the effects. Later these authors showed that prolonged perfusion with auranofin produced mucosal injury whereas gold sodium thiomalate did not. It should be noted that the structural differences of gold compounds especially between the oral compound auranofin and the injectable compounds suggest that the gold moiety may not be the active species and may not be chemically available for biochemical interaction with other ligands except in conjunction with another molecule such as sulphur or with a complete ligand [see gold chemistry].

It is possible that gold compounds could alter colonic transport by modulating enteric neural activity. This was investigated by de Beaux and colleagues by using two different *in vitro* canine colon preparations [67]: (a) mucosa which had the muscularis mucosa and attendant submucous plexuses present; and (b) an epithelium that was functionally nerve-free

[68]. Both preparations responded to auranofin from both luminal and contraluminal (serosal) sides. However, the concentrations required to elicit responses from the luminal side were 100-fold greater. With the mucosal preparation, responses to auranofin were significantly reduced by tetrodotoxin, a neurotoxin. From these results, one can argue that the effects of auranofin on colonic secretion has a significant neural component, although direct effects were also noted. Auranofin traverses the epithelial lining to modulate colonic activity from the serosal side. The ionic gold compound, gold sodium thiosulphate, altered colonic transport only on serosal application but had no effects on luminal application. Thus two chemically distinct gold compounds, auranofin and gold sodium thiosulphate, produced similar effects on serosal application. It should be noted that this suggests that a Au–S complex or Au–ligand or the ligand alone is the active species. It is not appropriate to assume that 'free' gold is the active species since it could not exist in these biological conditions but would have to be bound to some other species [see gold chemistry].

Snyder and colleagues proposed that auranofin and other gold complexes stimulate the activity of phospholipase C [69]. This leads to the alteration of a number of cellular processes via the production of secondary messengers – diacylglycerol (DAG) and inositol 1,4,5 triphosphate [IP_3]. DAG can be hydrolysed to produce arachidonic acid which could in turn produce a variety of eicosanoids through the cyclo-oxygenase and lipoxygenase pathways. These metabolites (prostanoids, leukotrienes) have pronounced effects on intestinal transport [70]. The other messenger, IP_3, by releasing intracellular Ca^{2+} could stimulate Cl^- secretion by enterocytes [71]. Other possible cytotoxic mechanisms discussed by Snyder and colleagues, include lipid peroxidation leading to the production of superoxide (O_2^-) and hydroxyl radicals (OH) as well as hydrogen peroxide, and disruption of membrane fluidity etc. [69]. Which of these mechanisms is responsible for the effects of gold compounds on the epithelial cells and the enteric nerves is uncertain at present, though the activation of phospholipase C is a possibility.

The above results suggest that gold compounds can produce diarrhoea by either inhibiting absorption or stimulating secretion. Whether motility is significantly altered is uncertain. The clinical studies of Behrens and colleagues demonstrated that mean transit time decreased from 71.0 hours (off auranofin) to 40.5 hours (on auranofin) and the authors suggested that this could be due to more rapid transit through the colon [61]. In one experimental study, however, Fondacaro and colleagues found that auranofin had no effect on basal tension of isolated colonic smooth muscle strips nor did it alter KCl-induced contractions [65]. These findings need further exploration since the responses of the muscle to neurotransmitters or hormones could have been altered. Thus the evidence for an effect on gut motility is inconclusive at present.

335

Langer reviewed 29 cases of gold-induced colitis and illustrated that in addition to the diarrhoea associated with the oral gold compounds, colitis has been reported with gold thioglucose, gold sodium thiosulphate and gold sodium thiomalate [72]. The precise mechanism of the colitis is unclear. Langer and colleagues, analysing a single case, noted that rectal biopsy showed erosions of the mucosa, with a dense inflammatory infiltration of the lamina propria with 'crypt abscesses'. Electron microscopic staining for gold, demonstrated punctate black precipitates in macrophages under the bases of the glands and the periglandular stroma [72]. These are similar to gold particles identified in other phagocytic cells [37]. Langer and colleagues state that since 95% of auranofin is excreted in the faeces, constant exposure of the colonic mucosa to excreted gold could alter the antigenicity of the cells leading to the formation of antibodies against the mucosal cells [72]. Withdrawal of the drug and steroid therapy was effective in 22 of the 29 cases reviewed by Lanson [72]. It is curious to note that there is almost a 4:1 preponderance of females in the cases reported.

Since gold colitis is a potentially lethal complication, diarrhoea occurring during gold therapy should not be dismissed as trivial. In suspicious cases, proper investigations are necessary and it appears that rectal biopsy and rectosigmoidoscopy are better diagnostic tools than barium enema.

The nitritoid reaction

The immediate allergic reaction known as the nitritoid reaction is unique to gold sodium thiomalate. Patients develop flushing, sweating, headache, joint pain, hypertension or hypotension, and on occasion, chest pain which may lead to myocardial infarction as in one reported case [73]. The variable chemical structure of gold sodium thiomalate may be implicated in precipitating this toxic reaction. The nitritoid reaction is not seen with any other gold compound and is usually mild and self-limiting. Patients can be switched to the oral gold compound or gold thioglucose if they find the nitritoid reaction intolerable or becomes recurrent with each dosage. There is an unreferenced statement in the Merck Manual that the nitritoid reaction 'occurs more often if the gold is not stored in the dark' [74]. Thus whether the nitritoid reaction is secondary to the yellow component in gold sodium thiomalate which we have studied, is not proven but there is no question that there is a progressive yellow colour change on exposure to UV light and/or heat (e.g. office windows or radiator) [37]. The implications of the colour change have been discussed by us previously and are outlined above [see experimental problems in the study of gold toxicity].

336

Pulmonary injury

Anecdotal reports of pulmonary injury associated with gold therapy are scattered in the literature. The most common association reported is a form of a diffuse interstitial lung disease, usually infiltrates visible on X-ray [75–77]. Fortunately, pulmonary toxicity is rare and usually responds to the withdrawal of the injectable gold compound. The mechanism is not known and the true relationship of the gold therapy to the pulmonary injury is frequently in question.

Hepatic problems

Hepatic toxicity due to injectable gold sodium thiomalate is rare but is usually characterized as a cholestasis with frank jaundice or elevated bilirubin, with elevated alkaline phosphatase, AST and ALT [78]. The gold should be stopped immediately. The condition may appear at any time in the treatment schedule. No specific mechanism of action has been identified. The jaundice is usually self-limiting, but in 1937, Hartfall and colleagues, in a review of 900 patients treated with injectable gold compounds, recorded 85 cases of toxic jaundice, two of whom died from sub-acute necrosis of the liver [79]. This incidence is not observed in any modern study and it is not possible to determine from Hartfall's report what associated factors may have been present. In view of the rare association of hepatic toxicity with the injectable gold compounds all other causes of jaundice should be excluded before a cause and effect relationship with the gold compound can be claimed.

Eye problems

In patients who have received long-term injectable gold therapy, deposition of gold in the lens of the eye [80] and the cornea has been reported [81,82], but this does not seem to result in any specific damage to visual acuity. Depositions of particulate gold have been identified in the cornea of 2 patients treated with auranofin [83].

Conjunctivitis occurs in 4% of patients treated with auranofin and occurs with equal frequency at any time period throughout treatment. Its significance is not known [83].

Age-related toxicity

There is no evidence of apparent increased risk of toxicity due to gold therapy in elderly patients [46], but specific caution should be taken with regard to haematological toxicities, since bone marrow aplasia secondary to gold compounds or any drug is more commonly recorded in the elderly than in the young. In one study in 1983 it was shown that the elderly responded to gold sodium thiomalate just as well as young adults and that the drop-out rate for no response and toxicity was the same in both groups [46]. However, it was noted that serious haematological toxicity only occurred in patients over 42 years of age and nephrotic syndrome only occurred in patients over 52 years of age in that study. The elderly should not be denied injectable gold therapy in the treatment of rheumatoid disease.

Gold in pregnancy and lactation

Injectable gold compounds have been implicated in the cause of fetal abnormalities in humans [84,85] but this has not been substantiated due to the small numbers studied [86,87]. Since gold levels have been found in the blood of newborns [86,88,89] it would seem wise to avoid gold therapy if possible during pregnancy. Usually rheumatoid arthritis will decrease in severity or even remit during pregnancy. A small number of patients who received auranofin during pregnancy have been observed with no effect to mother or child [90]. Since auranofin has immunosuppressive-like properties and contains triethylphosphine, it would seem wise to avoid the medication during pregnancy [91].

Trace amounts of gold derived from gold thioglucose therapy have been detected in breast milk [92,93] but since gold is not readily absorbed from the gastrointestinal tract it is unlikely to be a significant problem. To date there is no data in the concentration of auranofin in breast milk. As noted above, because of its immuno-suppressive properties, auranofin should be avoided in breast-feeding mothers.

HLA system – significance

Numerous reports have suggested the possible association of toxicity to injectable gold compounds (and D-penicillamine) with the human leucocyte antigen (HLA) type [53]. HLA-D4 and HLA-DR4 are present in 25–30% of normals but are found in rheumatoid patients in a ratio of 2:1 over controls, although this is less apparent in Jewish and East Indian groups. Patients with HLA-DR3 (also claimed to be associated with increased levels of rheumatoid factor) have been shown to be at increased risk of developing toxic reactions to injectable gold sodium thiomalate and also to D-penicillamine. In 1978 Panayi and colleagues reported studies on 95 patients with rheumatoid arthritis and noted that although there was no increase in HLA-DR3 over controls, 14 out of 18 with DR3 had a toxic reaction to gold or D-penicillamine and that 7 of 8 patients with HLA-DR2 had a toxic reaction [94]. HLA-DR2 has been reported to be associated with mouth ulcers [95] but the association between HLA-DR2 and toxicity in general has been disputed. Several reports suggest that HLA-DR2 and also HLA-DR7 may be protective against the development of toxicity and like HLA-DR4, the HLA-DR2 group may be a disease modifier [96]. In a follow-up report Panayi and colleagues reported that 79% of patients with HLA-DR3/B8 developed proteinuria while on gold (14 out of 15) or on D-penicillamine (9 out of 13) [97]. Subsequent reports reviewed by Ford have claimed an association with HLA-DR3 and thrombocytopenia, HLA-DR3/B8 and proteinuria and HLA-DR3 alone for skin rash. The last association is unusual in view of the known linkage disequilibrium between HLA-DR3 and B8 [53]. DeQueker and colleagues found no association between gold thiopropanol sodium sulphonate use and HLA groups, but they did find an association between HLA-B8 (but not DR3) and proteinuria [98]. Again, an unusual outcome in view of the linkage disequilibrium between DR3 and B8. Ford has pointed out that most studies, if not retrospective, only looked at the first 6 months of therapy, when clearly side-effects due to gold or penicillamine can occur at any time [2,53]. In particular, it is our experience and that of others that proteinuria occurs predominantly between 6 and 15 months [2,42,46–48]. It is of interest that HLA-DR3 and B8 are rare in Japanese and that in a large Japanese trial of D-penicillamine, proteinuria occurred in only 2.2% of patients [99].

Most investigators agree that HLA-DR3 and HLA-B8 are associated with drug toxicity, particularly proteinuria in association with injectable gold therapy and D-penicillamine. However, patients with these antigens should not be denied therapy with these agents since the relative risk does not outweigh the clinical benefit.

In conclusion

Despite the apparent overall lower number of side-effects related to auranofin compared to injectable gold compounds, auranofin should not be considered a benign drug. A strict monitoring system as for injectable gold compounds should be undertaken for each patient. Insufficient data are available at present to determine whether there will be any long-term side-effects related to auranofin therapy and particular attention should be paid to effects on immune functions related to long-term therapy.

Toxicity to gold compounds is the major limitation to the management of the inflammatory arthritides such as rheumatoid arthritis. The mechanism of action of gold complexes *in vivo* in humans is not known. Gold chemistry is complex and the structural formulae of many gold compounds are unknown. Consequently the principle in vivo 'metabolites' or pharmacodynamic species derived from many of the gold compounds are unknown. It is therefore not surprising that the mechanisms of toxicity as outlined above are poorly understood and may be the result of several different possible interactions.

REFERENCES

1. Forestier J. L'Aurothiopie dans les rhumatisme chronique. Bull Mem Soc Méd Hopitaux Paris. 1929;53:323–327.
2. Kean WF, Anastassiades TP. Long-term chrysotherapy. Incidence of toxicity and efficacy during sequential time periods. Arthritis Rheum. 1979;22:495–501.
3. Puddephatt RJ. The chemistry of gold. New York: Elsevier;1978:1.
4. Pearsons RG. Hard and soft acids and bases. J Am Chem Soc. 1963;85:3533-3539.
5. Brown HA. Sodium aurothiosulphate: a simple method for its preparation. J Am Chem Soc. 1927;49:958–959.
6. Coates GE, Kowala C, Swan JM. Co-ordination compounds of group IB metals: triethylphosphine complexes of gold(I) mercaptides. Aust J Chem. 1966;19:539–545.
7. Reuben H, Kalkin A, Faltens MO, Templeton DH. Crystal structure of gold(I) thiosulphate dihydrate, $Na_3Au(S_2O_3)2H_2O$. Inorg Chem. 1974;13:1836–1839.
8. Kowala C, Swan JM. Co-ordination compounds of group IB metals. Some tertiary phosphine and phosphite complexes of gold(I). Aust J Chem. 1966;19:547–554.
9. Puddephatt RJ, Thompson PJ. Some reactions of methylplatinum and methylgold compounds with phenylselenol diphenylphosphine, diphenylarsine, D-bromosuccinimide and 2-nitrophenylsulphenyl chloride. J Organomet Chem. 1976;117:395–403.
10. Sadler PJ. The comparative evaluation of the physical and chemical properties of gold compounds. J Rheumatol. 1982;9(Suppl. 8):71–78.
11. Elder RC, Tepperman KG, Eidsness MK et al. EXAFS and edge studies of gold-based anti-arthritis drugs and metabolites. In: Lippard SJ, ed. Chemistry and biochemistry of platinum, gold and other therapeutic agents. ACS Symposium Series. 1983;209:385–400..
12. Sadler PJ. The biological chemistry of gold: a metallo-drug and heavy atom label with variable valency. Struct Bond. 1976;29:171–215.
13. Shaw III FC. The mammalian biochemistry of gold: an inorganic perspective of chrysotherapy. Inorg Perspect Biol Med. 1979;2:287–355.
14. Brown DH, Smith WE. The chemistry of the gold drugs used in the treatment of rheumatoid arthritis. Chem Soc Rev. 1980;9:217–240.
15. Shaw III CF, Schmitz G, Thompson HO, Witkiewicz P. Bis(L-cystenato) gold(I): chemical characterization and identification in renal cortical cytoplasm. J Inorg Biochem. 1979;10:317–330.
16. Isab AA, Sadler PJ. Hydrogen-I and carbon-13 nuclear magnetic resonance studies of gold(I) thiomalate (Myocrisin) in aqueous solution: dependence of the solution structure on pH and ionic strength. J Chem Soc [Dalton]. 1981;1657–1663.
17. Isab AA, Sadler PJ. ^{13}C nuclear magnetic resonance detection of thiol exchange in gold(I): significance in chemotherapy. J Chem Soc Chem Commun. 1976;1051–1052.
18. Moskowitz R. Clinical rheumatology. Philadelphia: Lea and Febiger;1975:266.
19. Zvaifler NJ. Gold and antimalarial therap.In: McCarty DJ, ed. Arthritis and allies conditions. Philadelphia: Lea and Febiger; 1979:362.
20. Flower RJ, Moncada S, Van JR. Analgesic-anti-pyretics and anti-inflammatory agents: drugs explored in the treatment of gout. In: Goodman LS, Gilman A, eds. The pharmacological basis of therapeutics. New York: MacMillan; 1980:716
21. Engleman EP, Shearn MA. Arthritis and allied disorders. In: Krupp MA, Chatton MJ, eds. Current medical diagnosis and treatment. California: Lange Medical Publications; 1982:490.
22. Davis P, Barraclough D. Interaction of D-penicillamine with gold salts. Arthritis Rheum. 1977;20:1413–1418.
23. Schaeffer N, Shaw CF, Thomson HO, Satre RW. In vitro penicillamine competition for protein-bound gold(I). Arthritis Rheum. 1980;23:165–171.

24. Drew MGB, Riedle MJ. Crystal and molecular structure of μ-[1,2,-bis-(phenylthio)ethanel]-bis[chlorogold(ɪ)]. J Chem Soc Dalton Trans. 1973;?:52–55.

25. Kean WF, Lock CJL. Penicillamine does not chelate gold(ɪ). J Rheumatol. 1983;10:527–530.

26. Paltemaa S. The inhibition of lysosomal enzymes by gold salts in human synovial fluid cells. Acta Rheumatol Scand. 1968;14:161–168.

27. Lipsky P, Ziff M. Inhibition of antigen- and mitogen-induced human lymphocyte proliferation by gold compounds. J Clin Invest. 1977;59:455–466.

28. Harth M, Stiller CR, Sinclair NR St C. Effects of a gold salt on lymphocyte responses. Clin Exp Immunol. 1977;27:357–364.

29. Herrlinger JD. Difference in the pharmacokinetics, protein binding and cellular distribution of gold when different gold compounds are used. In: Schattenkirchner M, Muller W, eds. Modern aspects of gold therapy. Basel: Karger; 1983.

30. Rudge SR, Perret D, Drury PL, Swannwell AJ. Determination of thiomalate in physiological fluids using high performance liquid chromatography and electrochemical detection. J Pharm Biochem Anal. 1983;1:205–210.

31. Gianninni EH, Brewer EJ, Person DA. Blood gold concentrations in children with juvenile rheumatoid arthritis undergoing long-term oral gold. Ann Rheum Dis. 1984;43:228–231.

32. Walz DT, DiMartino MJ, Griswold DE, Intoccia AP, Flanagan TL. Biologic actions and pharmacokinetic studies of auranofin. Am J Med. 1983;75:90–108.

33. Blocka AK. Auranofin versus injectable gold. Comparison of pharmacokinetic properties. Am J Med. 1983;75:114–122.

34. Gottlieb NL, Smith PM, Smith EM. Pharmacodynamics of [195]Au-labelled aurothiomalate in blood. Arthritis Rheum. 1974;17:171–183.

35. Tepperman K, Finer R, Donovan S et al. Intestinal uptake and metabolism of auranofin, a new oral gold-based antiarthritis drug. Science. 1984;225:430–432.

36. Intoccia AP, Flanagan TL, Walz DT et al. Pharmacokinetics of auranofin in animals. J Rheumatol. 1982;9:90–98.

37. Kean WF, Lock CJL, Kassam YB et al. A biological effect on platelets by the minor component of gold sodium thiomalate – a by-product of heat sterilization and exposure to light. Clin Exp Rheumatol. 1984;2:321–328.

38. Kean WF, Kassam YB, Lock CJL et al. Antithrombin activity of gold sodium thiomalate. Clin Pharmacol Ther. 1984;35:627–632.

39. Kean WF, Lock CJL, Singal D et al. Biological action of colourless and yellow solutions of gold sodium thiomalate on thrombin activity and the mixed lymphocyte reaction. J Pharm Sci. 1988;77:1033–1036.

40. Harvey D, Kean WF, Lock CJL, Singal D. Sodium aurothiomalate is a mixture. Lancet. 1983;1:470–471.

41. Blodgett RC, Heuer MA, Pietrusko RG. Auranofin: a unique oral chrysotherapeutic agent. Sem Arthritis Rheum. 1984;13:255–273.

42. Ward JR, Williams NJ, Egger MJ et al. Comparison of auranofin, gold sodium thiomalate and placebo in the treatment of rheumatoid arthritis. Arthritis Rheum. 1983;26:1303–1315.

43. Leonard PA, Moatamed F, Ward JR et al. Chrysiasis: the role of sun exposure in dermal hyperpigmentation secondary to gold therapy. J Rheumatol. 1986;13:58–64.

44. Lewis MG. Basic sciences in relation to dermatology. In: Practical Dermatology. Philadelphia: Saunders; 1969:1–77.

45. Beckett VL, Doyle JA, Hadley GA, Spear KL. Chrysiasis resulting from gold therapy in rheumatoid arthritis. Mayo Clin Proc. 1982;57:773–777.

46. Kean WF, Bellamy N, Brooks PM. Gold therapy in the elderly rheumatoid patient. Arthritis Rheum. 1983;26:705–711.

47. Cooperating Clinics Committee. A controlled trial of gold salt therapy in rheumatoid arthritis. Arthritis Rheum. 1973;16:353–358.

48. Furst D, Levine S, Srinivasan R et al. A double-blind trial of high versus conventional dosages of gold salts for rheumatoid arthritis. Arthritis Rheum. 1977;20:1473–1480.

49. Tornrot T, Skrifvars B. Gold nephropathy prototype of membranous glomerulonephritis. Am J Pathol. 1974;75:573–584.

50. Merle LJ, Reidenberg MM, Camacho MT, Jones BR, Drayer DE. Renal injury in patients with rheumatoid arthritis treated with gold. Clin Pharmacol Ther. 1980;28:216–222.

51. Kelton JG, Carter CJ, Rodger C et al. The relationship between platelet-associated IgG, platelet life-form and reticuloendothelial cell function. Blood. 1984;63:1434–1438.

52. Adachi JD, Bensen WG, Kassam Y et al. Gold induced thrombocytopenia: 12 cases and a review of the literature. Sem Arthritis Rheum. 1987;16.

53. Ford PM. Editorial. HLA antigens and drug toxicity in rheumatoid arthritis. J Rheumatol. 1984;11:259–261.

54. Howell A, Gumpel JM, Watts RWE. Depression of bone marrow colony formation in gold induced neutropenia. Br Med J. 1975;1:432–434.

55. Harvey AR, Clarke B, Chui D, Kean WF, Buchanan WW. Anaemia associated with rheumatoid disease: inverse correlation between erythropoiesis and both IgM and rheumatoid factor levels. Arthritis Rheum. 1983;26:8–34.

56. Gowans JDC, Salami M. Response of rheumatoid arthritis and leukopenia to gold salts. N Engl J Med. 1973;288:1007–1008.

57. Van Riel PL, Gribnau FW, Van De Putte LB, Yap SH. Loose stools during auranofin treatment: clinical study and some pathogenic possibilities. J Rheumatol. 1983;10:222–226.

58. Bandilla KK, Delattre M, Rahn B, Missler B. Long-term treatment of rheumatoid arthritis with auranofin: clinical results with auranofin from German and international studies which included a comparison of once and twice daily treatment. In: Capell HA, Cole DS, Manghani KK, Morris RW, eds. Auranofin. Amsterdam: Excerpta Medica; 1983:97–114.

59. Morris RW, Cole DS, Horton J, Hever MA, Pietrusko RG. Worldwide clinical experience with auranofin. Clin Rheumatol. 1984;3:105–112.

60. Mascarenhas BR, Granda JL, Freyburg RH. Gold metabolism in patients with rheumatoid arthritis treated with gold compounds – reinvestigated. Arthritis Rheum. 1972;15:391–404.

61. Behrens R, Devereaux M, Hazelman B et al. Investigation of auranofin-induced diarrhoea. Gut. 1986;27:59–65.

62. Nagler J, Paget SA. Non-exudative diarrhoea after gold salt therapy: case report and review of the literature. Am J Gastroenterol. 1983;78:12–14.

63. Hardcastle J, Hardcastle PT, Kelleher DK et al. Effect of auranofin on absorptive processes in the rat small bowel. J Rheumatol. 1986;13:541–546.

64. Hardcastle J, Hardcastle PT, Kelleher DK, Fondacaro JD. The effect of auranofin on the colonic transport of Na^+ and fluid in the rat. J Pharm Pharmacol. 1986;38:466–468.

65. Fondacaro JD, Henderson LS, Hardcastle PT et al. Effects of auranofin (SK&F 39162) on water and electrolyte flux in canine small bowel: a possible diarrhoeagenic mechanism. J Rheumatol. 1986;13:541–546.

66. Ammon HV, Fowle SA, Cunningham JA, Komorowski RA, Loeffler RF. Effects of auranofin and myochrysine on intestinal transport and morphology in the rat. Gut. 1987;28:829–834.

67. De Beaux A, Keenan CM, Tytgat K, Rangachari PK. Effect of gold salts on the canine colonic mucosa-direct and indirect effects. Physiologist. 1988;31(4):A142.

68. Rangachari PK, McWade D. Epithelial and mucosal preparations of canine proximal colon in Ussing chambers: comparison of responses. Life Sci. 1986;38:1641–1652.

69. Snyder RH, Mirabellit CK, Crooke ST. The cellular pharmacology of auranofin. Sem Arthritis Rheum. 1987;17:71–80.

70. Whittle BJR, Vane JR. Prostanoids as regulators of gastrointestinal function. In: Johnson LR, ed. Physiology of the gastrointestinal tract. 2nd ed. New York: Raven Press; 1987:143–180.

71. Powell DW. Intestinal water and electrolyte transport. In: Johnson LR, ed. Physiology of the gastrointestinal tract. 2nd ed. New York: Raven Press; 1987:1267–1305.

72. Langer HE, Hartmann G, Heinemann G, Richter K. Gold colitis induced by auranofin treatment of rheumatoid arthritis: case report and review of the literature. Ann Rheum Dis. 1987;46:787–792.

73. Harris BK. Myocardial infarction after a gold-induced nitritoid reaction [letter]. Arthritis Rheum. 1977;20:1561.

74. The Merck Manual. 14th ed. Rahway NJ: Merck; 1982;104:1181.

75. Winterbauer RH, Wilske KR, Wheelis RF. Diffuse pulmonary injury associated with gold treatment. N Engl J Med. 1976;17:919–921.

76. McCormick J, Cole S, Lahirir B et al. Pneumonitis caused by gold salt therapy. Evidence for the role of cell-mediated immunity in its pathogenesis. Am Rev Resp Dis. 1980;122:145–152.

77. Scott DL, Bradby GVH, Aitman TJ et al. Relationship of gold and penicillamine therapy to diffuse interstitial lung disease. Ann Rheum Dis. 1981;40:136–141.

78. Favreau M, Tannenbaum H, Louch J. Hepatic toxicity associated with gold therapy. Ann Intern Med. 1977;87:717–719.

79. Hartfall SJ, Garland HG, Goldie W. Gold treatment of arthritis: a review of 900 cases. Lancet. 1937;2:1459–1463.

80. Gottlieb NL, Major JC. Ocular chrysiasis – a clinical study correlated with gold concentrations in the crystalline lens during chrysotherapy. Arthritis Rheum. 1978;21:704–708.

81. Hashimoto A, Maeda Y, Ito H et al. Corneal chrysiasis – a clinical study in rheumatoid arthritis patients receiving gold therapy. Arthritis Rheum. 1972;15:309.

82. Prouse PJ, Kanski JJ, Gumpel JM. Corneal chrysiasis and clinical improvement with chrysotherapy in rheumatoid arthritis. Ann Rheum Dis. 1981;40:564.

83. Heur MA, Morris RW. Smith Kline & French worldwide clinical experience with auranofin: a review. In: Capell HA, Cole DS, Manghani KK et al. eds. Auranofin: proceedings of a Smith Kline & French international symposium. Amsterdam: Excerpta Medica; 1983:474–503.

84. Miyamoto TS et al. Gold therapy in bronchial asthma – special emphasis on blood levels of gold and its teratogenicity. J Jp Soc Intern Med. 1974;63:1190–1197.

85. Rogers JG et al. Possible teratogenic effect of gold. Aust Paediatr J. 1980;16:194–195.

86. Cohen DL, Orzel J, Taylor A. Infants of mothers receiving gold therapy. Arthritis Rheum. 1981;24:104–105.

87. Tarp U, Graudal H. A follow-up study of children exposed to gold in utero. Arthritis Rheum. 1985;28:235–236.

88. Rocker I, Hendeson MJH. Transfer of gold from mother to foetus. Lancet. 1976;2:1246.

89. Richards AJ. Transfer of gold from mother to foetus. Lancet. 1977;1:99.

90. Ostensen M, Husby G. Antirheumatic drug treatment during pregnancy and lactation. Scand J Rheumatol. 1985;14:1–7.

91. Brooks PM, Kean WF, Buchanan WW. The clinical pharmacology of anti-inflammatory agents. London: Taylor and Francis; 1986:91–97.

92. Blau SP. Metabolism of gold during lactation. Arthritis Rheum. 1973;16:777–778.

93. Ostensen M, Skavdal K, Myklebust G et al. Excretion of gold in human breast milk. Eur J Clin Pharmacol. 1986;31:261.

94. Panayi GS, Wooley P, Batchelor JR. Genetic basis of rheumatoid disease: HLA antigens, disease manifestations, and toxic reactions to drugs. Br Med J. 1978;2:1326–1328.

95. Panayi GS, Griffin AJ, Wooley PM. Genetic predisposition to gold and penicillamine toxicity. Arthritis Rheum. 1979;22:645.

96. Repice MM, Radvany RM, Schmid FR. HLA, A, BC and DR locus antigens and gold toxicity in rheumatoid arthritis. Clin Res. 1979;647A.

97. Wooley PM, Griffin J, Panayi GS et al. HLA-DR antigens and toxic reaction to sodium aurothiomalate and D-penicillamine in patients with rheumatoid arthritis. N Engl J Med. 1980;303:300–303.

98. DeQueker J, Van Wanghe P, Verdict WA. Systematic survey of HLA ABC and D antigens and drug toxicity in rheumatoid arthritis. J Rheumatol. 1984;11:282–290.

99. Shiokana Y, Horiuchi Y, Homma M et al. Clinical evaluation of D-penicillamine by multicentre double-blind comparative study in chronic rheumatoid arthritis. Arthritis Rheum. 1977;20:1464–1472.

38

A review of interaction studies between non-steroidal anti-inflammatory drugs and H$_2$-receptor antagonists or prostaglandin analogues

J.S. Dixon and M.C. Page

Division of Gastroenterology, Glaxo Group Research Limited, Greenford Road, Greenford, Middlesex, UB6 0HE, UK

INTRODUCTION

The potential for non-steroidal anti-inflammatory drug (NSAID) induced peptic ulceration in susceptible individuals [1], and the risk of complications in patients with existing ulcers [2], has led to the practice of co-prescribing these agents with H$_2$-receptor antagonists or prostaglandin analogues. The major consumers of NSAIDs are patients with arthritis who are frequently elderly and are often already receiving multiple drug therapy. Such therapy provides considerable potential for drug interactions. Furthermore, the elderly frequently have decreased renal and hepatic function together with impaired absorption from the gut [3]. Therefore any observed interaction between NSAIDs and H$_2$-receptor antagonists or prostaglandin analogues in the absence of other therapy, in young healthy subjects may be enhanced in patients, particularly in the elderly.

METHODS

Literature searches using MEDLINE and *Excerpta Medica* databases identified published pharmacokinetic interaction studies between NSAIDs and H$_2$-receptor antagonists and between NSAIDs and prostaglandin analogues. The relevant papers were inspected to determine study design, subject or patient demography, the treatments and doses used, duration and frequency of blood sampling and the pharmacokinetic and statistical results. The pharmacokinetic parameters reported included area under the plasma concentration/time-curve (AUC), apparent oral clearance (Cl$_o$),

Side-effects of Anti-inflammatory Drugs 3. Rainsford KD, Velo GP (eds), Inflammation and Drug Therapy Series, Volume V.

maximum plasma concentration (C_{max}), time to C_{max} (T_{max}), plasma elimination half life ($t_{1/2}$), elimination rate constant (k_{el}), absorption rate constant (k_{abs}) and apparent volume of distribution (VD).

RESULTS

H_2-receptor antagonists

Twenty-two studies involving H_2-receptor antagonists were identified: 17 involved cimetidine (nine used cimetidine alone, seven compared cimetidine with ranitidine and one compared cimetidine with nizatidine) and 12 involved ranitidine (five used ranitidine alone, and seven compared ranitidine with cimetidine). Sixteen of the 22 studies used a two, three or four-way crossover design. Only two studies involved patients with rheumatoid arthritis (RA), the remainder employing from six to 18 young, healthy volunteers. The NSAIDs studied comprised ibuprofen (five studies) [4–8], indomethacin (four studies) [9–13], aspirin (three studies) [14–16], flurbiprofen (two studies) [18,19], piroxicam (three studies) [20–22] and one study for each of sulindac [9], ketoprofen [23], isoxicam [24], naproxen [25], and oxaprozin [26]. The plasma (occasionally urine) samples were assayed for the NSAID using high performance liquid chromatography in each study except for the three aspirin studies, in which spectrophotometric or spectrofluorometric methods were used, and one indomethacin study in which gas liquid chromatography was employed. The design and results of all studies are summarized in Table 1.

Only seven studies directly compared the effects of cimetidine and ranitidine on the pharmacokinetics of the NSAID under investigation: ibuprofen [4,5], flurbiprofen [18,19], indomethacin [9], sulindac [9] and oxaprozin [26]. The ibuprofen and flurbiprofen studies all showed an increase in AUC with concomitant cimetidine but not with ranitidine. Both H_2-receptor antagonists showed evidence of some interaction with sulindac and oxaprozin, but neither affected indomethacin pharmacokinetics.

Prostaglandin analogues

Five studies involving misoprostol were identified, and these were carried out in healthy subjects. These included multiple dose studies with indomethacin [10,11] or piroxicam [27] and single dose studies with aspirin [28], ibuprofen and diclofenac. None of these studies has been published as a full paper, but they have been recently included in an overview of misoprostol pharmacokinetics [29]. With the exception of the indomethacin study (also in Table 1), none of these studies reported the number of blood samples taken or the period over which they were collected. Demographic details of the subjects were also generally lacking.

345

Table 1. Summary of the design and results of H_2-receptor antagonist/NSAID interaction studies

Reference	Design	Treatment NSAID	Cimetidine Dose	Ranitidine Dose	Change in NSAID kinetics[1] + Cimetidine	+ Ranitidine
Ochs et al. 1985 [4]	3-way rand. XO	Ibuprofen 600 mg	400 mg tds	150 mg bd	C_{max}↑[2]	None[2]
Conrad et al. 1984 [7]	2-way rand. XO	Ibuprofen 400 mg	300 mg qds	NA	None	NA
Stephenson et al. 1988 [5]	3-way rand. XO	Ibuprofen 600 mg qds	800 mg mane	300 mg mane	AUC↑; Cl_o↓; T_{max}↓	T_{max}↓; C_{max}↑
Forsyth et al. 1988 [6]	3-way rand. XO,DB,P	Ibuprofen 400 mg	800 mg nocte	NA	None	NA
Berardi et al. 1988[5] [8]	3-way rand. XO	SR Ibuprofen 800 mg	NA	300 mg	NA	None
Delhotal-Landes et al. 1988 [9]	3-way rand. XO, P	Sulindac 200 mg	400 mg mane	150 mg mane	AUC↑; C_{max}↑; Cl_o↓; VD↓	$t_{1/2}$↓; VD↓; C_{max}↑; T_{max}↑
Delhotal-Landes et al. 1988 [9]	3-way rand. XO, P	Indomethacin 50 mg	400 mg mane	150 mg mane	AUC↑; Cl_o↓; $t_{1/2}$↓; C_{max}↑; T_{max}↑	$t_{1/2}$↓; C_{max}↑
Howes et al. 1983[3] [13]	2-way seq.	Indomethacin 100–200 mg/day	1 g/day	NA	Steady state conc↓*; Total urinary recovery↓*	NA
Dammann et al. 1989[6] [10]	3-way XO, SB, P	Indomethacin 75 mg bd	NA	150 mg bd	NA	C_{max}↑
Muller et al. 1989 [12]	4-way rand. XO, DB	Indomethacin 50 mg tds	NA	300 mg nocte	NA	None
Corrocher et al. 1987 [14]	2-way XO, DB, P	Aspirin[4] 1g	NA	150 mg bd	NA	k_{abs}↓; k_{el}↑
Paton et al. 1983 [16]	2-way XO	Aspirin[4] 1300 mg	300 mg tds	NA	Urinary recovery↑ Bioavailability↑	NA
Trnavska et al. 1985 [15]	2-way seq.	Aspirin[4] 1g	1 g /day	NA	AUC↑; $t_{1/2}$↑; Cl_o↓	NA
Kreeft et al. 1986[3,6] [19]	2-way rand.	Flurbiprofen 50 or 100 mg tds	300 mg tds	150 mg bd	AUC↑; C_{max}↑	None
Sullivan et al. 1986 [18]	3-way rand. XO	Flurbiprofen 200 mg	300 mg qds	150 mg bd	AUC↑; T_{max}↓	None
Mailhot et al. 1986 [20]	2-way seq.	Piroxicam 20 mg	300 mg qds	NA	AUC↑; C_{max}↑; Cl_o↓; VD↓	NA
Said and Foda 1989 [21]	2 Parallel groups	Piroxicam 20 mg	200 mg tds	NA	AUC↑; $t_{1/2}$↑	NA
Dixon et al. 1991 [22]	2-way rand. XO, DB, P	Piroxicam 20 mg	NA	150 mg bd	NA	None
Verbeeck et al. 1988 [23]	2-way rand. XO	Ketoprofen 100 mg bd	600 mg bd	NA	None	NA
Scavone et al. 1986 [26]	4-way XO	Oxaprozin 1.2 g	300 mg qds	150 mg bd	AUC↑; Cl_o↓; C_{max}↑; VD↓	AUC↑; Cl_o↓; C_{max}↑; T_{max}↓; VD↓
Holford et al. 1981[6] [25]	2-way XO, DB, P	Naproxen 500 mg bd	1.2 g/day	NA	None	NA
Farnham et al. 1982 [24]	2-way XO	Isoxicam 200 mg	300 mg qds	NA	AUC↑	NA

XO = crossover
DB = double blind
SB = single blind
rand = randomized
seq = sequential
P = placebo controlled

NA = not applicable
SR = slow release
* = statistically significant increase ↑ or decrease ↓, $p < 0.05$

1 = increase ↑ or decrease ↓ of >10%
2 = a statistically significant difference was shown between the three groups for AUC and Cl_o primarily due to cimetidine
3 = study conducted in RA patients
4 = results based on salicylate concentrations
5 = this study compared SR ibuprofen, standard ibuprofen, and SR ibuprofen and ranitidine
6 = reported only in abstract form

The pharmacokinetics of misoprostol, as determined by the assay of the active metabolite 'misoprostol acid', were investigated in the three single dose studies, but a statistically significant effect was only seen on the AUC of aspirin. In the indomethacin study [10], a 20–60% reduction in steady state plasma concentration of indomethacin was reported but the correct interpretation of these results remains in doubt [11].

A solitary study with arbaprostil [30] comprised an open 3-way crossover design in 24 healthy male subjects (age 40–60 years) who received medication four times a day including arbaprostil 50 μg, aspirin 975 mg, and both treatments together. Statistically significant ($p < 0.05$) reductions in AUC and Tmax for aspirin were seen, but no significant alteration in salicylate or arbaprostil kinetics was observed.

DISCUSSION

This review suggests that H$_2$-receptor antagonists may have some effects on the pharmacokinetics of some NSAIDs. In particular, cimetidine increases the AUC, and hence decreases the Cl$_o$, of several NSAIDs when these agents are taken concurrently. Cimetidine is known to have important pharmacokinetic interactions with warfarin, phenytoin, theophylline, propranolol and benzodiazepines, resulting from its capacity to inhibit hepatic microsomal oxidative drug metabolism by binding to cytochrome P-450 to form a stable complex. Ranitidine has less affinity for cytochrome P-450 and hence does not inhibit drug metabolism to any significant extent at therapeutic concentrations. It might therefore be expected that decreased metabolism and hence decreased clearance would be seen for NSAIDs that are extensively metabolized by this system, when given with concomitant cimetidine. Most NSAIDs undergo some degree of oxidation, hydroxylation or demethylation in the liver followed by glucuronidation prior to elimination, so this may contribute to the increase in AUC in many of the cimetidine studies. However, if this was the complete explanation the t$_{1/2}$ should also increase and this was only observed in some studies. This may be because accurate determination of t$_{1/2}$ is difficult, particularly if the frequency of blood sampling or study duration is inadequate. Alternatively the observed changes in AUC and Cl$_o$ may partially reflect an increase in bioavailability, though this is likely to be a small change since most NSAIDs are readily absorbed from the gut.

The design of some of these studies, and the statistical power of most, are inadequate to draw reliable conclusions about the effects of the H$_2$-receptor antagonist on the pharmacokinetics of the NSAID. For example, Muller's study of indomethacin [12] used ranitidine at a dose of 300 mg nocte and conclusions were based on infrequent and largely irrelevant daytime blood sampling times. The apparent difference in results for ibuprofen 400 mg and 600 mg may be related to the use of males and females in the 600 mg studies but only males in the two 400 mg studies. However, it is more likely that the power of the 400 mg studies was too low with only six subjects in each study. Indeed, the two studies of piroxicam plus ranitidine [25] are the only interaction studies to date which had sufficient power to detect a 20% difference between treatments.

Long-term NSAID use results in asymptomatic, reversible impairment of renal function [31,32] which should also be taken into consideration. Disease may also influence NSAID kinetics; for example, an increase in unbound (and hence pharmacologically active) naproxen in active RA compared with inactive disease has been observed [33]. Only two interaction studies have been reported in patients with RA, one investigating indomethacin with cimetidine [13] and the other flurbiprofen with cimetidine and ranitidine [19].

In conclusion this review has highlighted the need for steady-state pharmacokinetic interaction studies between various anti-ulcer agents and NSAIDs in patients with various arthritides. The available information from young healthy subjects suggests that cimetidine may cause an increase in the AUC of several NSAIDs, although clinical sequelae resulting from an interaction between H_2-receptor antagonists and NSAIDs have not been reported. In contrast ranitidine does not appear to cause an increase in AUC in any of the marketed NSAIDs investigated and hence may represent a safer therapeutic option. The situation regarding prostaglandin analogues clearly remains uncertain, and therefore such co-prescribing should proceed with caution until more data are available.

NB: A full paper based on this review has been published in *Rheumatology International*. 1991;11:13–18.

REFERENCES

1. Duggan JM, Dobson JA, Johnson H, Fahey P. Peptic ulcer and non-steroidal anti-inflammatory agents. Gut. 1986;27:929–933.
2. CSM update. Non-steroidal anti-inflammatory drugs and serious gastrointestinal adverse reactions. 2. Br Med J. 1986;292:1190–1191.
3. Dawling S, Crome P. Clinical pharmacokinetic considerations in the elderly. An update. Clin Pharmacokinet. 1989;17:236–263.
4. Ochs HR, Greenblatt DJ, Matlis R, Weinbrenner J. Interaction of ibuprofen with the H_2-receptor antagonists ranitidine and cimetidine. Clin Pharmacol Ther. 1985;38:648–651.
5. Stephenson DW, Small RE, Wood JH et al. Effect of ranitidine and cimetidine on ibuprofen pharmacokinetics. Clin Pharm. 1988;7:317–321.
6. Forsyth DR, Jayasinghe KSA, Roberts CJC. Do nizatidine and cimetidine interact with ibuprofen? Eur J Clin Pharmacol. 1988;35:85–88.
7. Conrad KA, Mayersohn M, Bliss M. Cimetidine does not alter ibuprofen kinetics after a single dose. Br J Clin Pharmacol. 1984;18:624–626.
8. Berardi RR, Dressman JB, Elta GH, Szpunar GJ. Elevation of gastric pH with ranitidine does not affect the release characteristics of sustained release ibuprofen tablets. Biopharm Drug Dis. 1988;9:337–347.

9. Delhotal-Landes B, Flouvat B, Liote F et al. Pharmacokinetic interactions between NSAIDs (indomethacin or sulindac) and H$_2$-receptor antagonists (cimetidine or ranitidine) in human volunteers. Clin Pharmacol Ther. 1988;44:442–452.

10. Dammann HG, Simon-Schultz J, Bauermeister W et al. Prevention of NSAID-induced gastric ulcer with prostaglandin analogues. Lancet. 1989;1:52–53.

11. Rietbrock N, Karim A, Nicholson PA. Prevention of NSAID-induced gastric ulcer with prostaglandin analogues. Lancet. 1989;1:844–845.

12. Muller P, Dammann HG, Langer M, Leucht U, Simon B. Ranitidine improves the gastroduodenal tolerability of acemetacin and indomethacin without affecting the pharmacokinetics of both antirheumatics. Z Gastroenterol. 1989;27:83–86.

13. Howes CA, Pullar T, Sourindhrin I et al. Reduced steady-state plasma concentrations of chlorpromazine and indomethacin in patients receiving cimetidine. Eur J Clin Pharmacol. 1983;24:99–102.

14. Corrocher R, Bambara LM, Caramaschi P et al. Effect of ranitidine on the absorption of aspirin. Digestion. 1987;37:178–183.

15. Trnavska Z, Trnavsky K, Smondrk J. The effect of cimetidine on the pharmacokinetics of salicylic acid. Drugs Exp Clin Res. 1985;11:703–707.

16. Paton TW, Walker SE, Leung FYK, Little AH. Effect of cimetidine on bioavailability of enteric-coated aspirin tablets. Clin Pharm. 1983;2:165–166.

17. O'Laughlin JC, Silvoso GR, Ivey KJ. Effects of an H$_2$-blocker on gastric ulcers in patients taking aspirin: a double-blind study. Gastroenterology. 1980;78(No.5 Part 2):1230.

18. Sullivan KM, Small RE, Rock WL et al. Effects of cimetidine or ranitidine on the pharmacokinetics of flurbiprofen. Clin Pharm. 1986;5:586–589.

19. Kreeft J, Bellamy N, Freeman D. Does chronic H$_2$-antagonist administration alter steady-state flurbiprofen pharmacokinetics? Acta Pharmacol Toxicol. 1986;59(Suppl V):Abstract 253:96.

20. Mailhot C, Dahl SL, Ward JR. The effect of cimetidine on serum concentrations of piroxicam. Pharmacotherapy. 1986;6:112–117.

21. Said SA, Foda AM. Influence of cimetidine on the pharmacokinetics of piroxicam in rat and man. Arzneim-Forsch Drug Res. 1989;39:790–792.

22. Dixon JS, Lacey LF, Pickup ME, Langley SJ, Page MC. A lack of pharmacokinetic interaction between ranitidine and piroxicam. Br J Clin Pharmacol. 1991;39:583–586.

23. Verbeeck RK, Corman CL, Wallace SM. Single and multiple dose pharmacokinetics of enteric coated ketoprofen: effect of cimetidine. Eur J Clin Pharmacol. 1988;35:521–527.

24. Farnham DJ. Studies of isoxicam in combination with aspirin, warfarin sodium and cimetidine. Semin Arthritis Rheum. 1982;12(Suppl. 2):179–183.

25. Holford NHG, Altman D, Riegelman S et al. Pharmacokinetic and pharmacodynamic study of cimetidine administered with naproxen. Clin Pharmacol Ther. 1981;29:251–252.

26. Scavone JM, Greenblatt DJ, Matlis R, Harmatz JS. Interaction of oxaprozin with acetaminophen, cimetidine and ranitidine. Eur J Clin Pharmacol. 1986;31:371–374.

27. Karim A, Smith M, Belliel S, Hunt T. Lack of drug-drug interaction between prostaglandin E, analogue misoprostol and NSAIDs. In: Proc Third Interscience World Conf Monte Carlo; 1989 (Abst).

28. Karim A, Rozek LF, Leese PT. Absorption of misoprostol (cytotec), an antiulcer prostaglandin, or aspirin is not affected when given concomitantly to healthy human subjects. Gastroenterology. 1989;92:1742.

29. Nicholson PA, Karim A, Smith M. Pharmacokinetics of misoprostol in the elderly, in patients with renal failure and when co-administered with NSAID or antipyrine, propranolol or diazepam. J Rheumatol. 1990;17(Suppl. 20):33–37.

30. Hsyu P-H, Cox JW, Pullen RH, Gee WL, Euler AR. Pharmacokinetic interactions between arbaprostil and aspirin in humans. Biopharm Drug Disp. 1989;10:411–422.

31. Unsworth J, Sturman S, Lunec J, Blake DR. Renal impairment associated with non-steroidal anti-inflammatory drugs. Ann Rheum Dis. 1987;46:233-236.

32. Dixon JS, Bojar R, Bird HA. Renal impairment in relation to non-steroidal anti-inflammatory drugs. Ann Rheum Dis. 1988;47:260–264.

33. Van Den Ouweland FA, Gribnau FWJ, Van Ginneken CAM, Tan Y, Van De Putte LBA. Naproxen kinetics and disease activity in rheumatoid arthritis: a within-patient study. Clin Pharmacol Ther. 1988;43:79–85.

39
Influence of different anti-inflammatory substances on ethanol- and indomethacin-induced gastrointestinal mucosal damage

Klara Gyires

Department of Pharmacology, Semmelweis University of Medicine,
Nagyvárad tér 4, POB 370, H-1445 Budapest, Hungary

INTRODUCTION

The non-steroidal anti-inflammatory agents, besides their anti-inflammatory and analgesic properties, also cause gastrointestinal mucosal damage. Prostaglandins exert protective action in the gastrointestinal tract, but induce inflammation and pain. Since inflammatory reactions are observed in the early phase of gastric damage [1], substances which inhibit the acute inflammation via non-prostaglandin mechanisms might exert mucosal protective action. Some years ago we reported that pyrido-pyrimidine derivatives possess analgesic and anti-inflammatory properties and protect the gastric mucosa against damages induced by non-steroidal anti-inflammatory substances and necrotizing agents [2–4]. The aim of the present study is to demonstrate with further examples that structurally different compounds with antiphlogistic activity decrease gastric mucosal damage as well.

METHODS

Male and female Sprague–Dawley CFY rats (140–170 g) were used. The animals were acclimatized for at least 4 days before experiments. During this time they had free access to food and water. Room temperature was 21 $\pm 1°C$.

Side-effects of Anti-inflammatory Drugs 3. Rainsford KD, Velo GP (eds),
Inflammation and Drug Therapy Series, Volume V.

Carrageenan oedema test

The method described by Winter et al. [5] was used; 0.1 ml of 1% carrageenan was injected into the subplantar hind paw of the rats. The volume of oedema was measured by plethysmography 3 hours after carrageenan injection. The test compounds were given either orally (p.o.) or subcutaneously (s.c.) 60 or 30 min respectively before carrageenan injection.

Writhing test

The method originally described by Vander Wende [7] modified by Koster and Anderson [6] was employed in mice. The inflammatory pain was induced by an intraperitoneal (i.p.) injection of 0.6% acetic acid and the non-inflammatory pain by 2% $MgSO_4$ i.p. [8]. After the first writhing appeared the mice were kept under observation for 5 minutes and the number of writhings was counted during this period. The test compounds were injected i.p. 30 minutes before the challenge.

Gastric lesion production

The rats were fasted for 24 hours before the experiment and were allowed free access to water. They were kept in cages with a metal grid to avoid coprophagy. The degree of gastric mucosal damage was estimated using a binocular magnifier (2x) by the observer unaware of the treatment the rats received. The lesions were scored as follows: 1 – petechiae, erosions less than 1 mm; 2 – erosions of 1–2 mm; 3 – erosions of 3–4 mm; 4 – erosions of 5–6 mm. Ulcer index was expressed as a sum of partial scores in each group of rats divided by the number of animals.

(a) Acidified ethanol-induced gastric damage

After 24 hours starvation the rats were given 0.5 ml of acidified ethanol (98% ethanol in 200 mmol/l HCL) by gavage and killed 2 hours later. The stomachs were removed and examined for mucosal lesions described above. The test compounds were given orally using a glass gastric probe 40 min prior to ethanol administration.

351

(b) Indomethacin-induced gastric damage

Following 24 hour starvation the rats were given 20 mg/kg of indomethacin orally and were killed 4 hours later. The stomachs were removed and examined for lesions described above. The test compounds were injected orally 1 hour either before or after the administration of indomethacin.

Measurement of increased vascular permeability of gastric mucosa caused by ethanol

The method described by Szabo et al. [1] was used with some modifications. Evans blue 0.5% (in a volume of 2 ml/kg) was given intravenously (i.v.) to the rats 24 hours after starvation. Thirteen min later 1 ml of 100% ethanol was given orally and 2 min later the rats were killed, the glandular stomach was removed, weighed, examined for mucosal lesions, cut into small pieces and was placed in 1% methanolic solution of suramin for 48 hours [9]. During 48 hours the dye was extracted from the gastric tissue and its concentration was measured spectrophotometrically at a wavelength of 610 nm. The test substances were given p.o. 30 min before injection of dye solution.

Indomethacin-induced intestinal lesions

The intestinal lesions were produced by 20 mg/kg of indomethacin given orally. The rats were allowed free access to food and water both before and during experiment. The test compounds were given for 4 consecutive days and indomethacin was administered on the second day of treatment 1 hour after the test substances. Seventy-two hours after the injection of indomethacin the rats were sacrificed and the total small intestine from the pylorus to the caecum was carefully removed, measured for length, incised and examined for the presence and the degree of lesions. The degree of mucosal damage (ulcer index) was estimated according to Tsuromi et al. [10].

Drugs used: cysteamine (Sigma, USA), FPL 55712 (Fisons, England), indomethacin (Chinoin, Hungary), morphine HCl (Alkaloida, Hungary), N-ethylmaleimide (Sigma, USA), rimazolium (Chinoin, Hungary), suramin (Bayer, FRG).

Statistical analysis: the non-parametric Mann–Whitney U test and the Student's two-tailed t-test for unpaired observations were used to evaluate the statistical significance.

RESULTS AND DISCUSSION

Table 1 summarizes the analgesic and anti-inflammatory effect of cysteamine, the SH alkylator, N-ethylmaleimide (NEM), morphine, the pyrido-pyrimidine derivative rimazolium, and for comparison, indomethacin.

The drugs studied inhibited the carrageenan-induced inflammation; the rank order of anti-inflammatory potency was NEM > morphine > indomethacin > cysteamine > rimazolium. The analgesic activity of drugs was studied on inflammatory (acetic-acid induced) and non-inflammatory ($MgSO_4$-induced) pain. The drugs were highly effective against inflammatory pain. However, cysteamine, NEM and indomethacin were less effective against the non-inflammatory pain reaction indicating that their anti-inflammatory property might be involved in their analgesic action.

Since inflammatory phenomena are supposed to be involved in the early phase of gastric damage [1] the ID_{50} values of the drugs obtained against acidified ethanol-induced lesions were compared with the ID_{30} values gained in the carrageenan-oedema test. The rank order of potencies of drugs studied is the same in the two tests. However, the effective doses of morphine, cysteamine, and rimazolium against acidified ethanol-lesions were lower than in the inflammation tests suggesting that the anti-inflammatory property of the drugs is only one of the factors responsible for gastroprotection. Similar conclusions can be drawn from experiments where the gastric lesions and enhanced vascular permeability of gastric mucosa were studied in parallel (Figure 1). In agreement with the results of

Table 1. The analgesic and anti-inflammatory effect of cysteamine, N-ethylmaleimide (NEM), indomethacin, morphine and rimazolium

Compound	ED_{50} $\mu mol/kg$ i.p. (95% confidence limit)		ID_{30} $\mu mol/kg$ (95% confidence limit)
	Acetic acid writing test[a]	*$MgSO_4$*	*Carrageenan oedema*[b]
Cysteamine	88.5 (77.1–107.5)	123.4 (105.5–146.7)	176.9 p.o. (140.8–220)
NEM	7.2 (6.0–8.6)	13.7 (11.2–16.7)	2.0 p.o. (1.5–2.6)
Indomethacin	0.5 (0.4–0.6)	14.0 (11.4–17.0)	3.9 p.o. (3.2–4.6)
Morphine	0.53 (0.4–0.6)	0.4 (0.3–0.48)	2.9 s.c. (2.2–3.7)
Rimazolium	187.8 (152.2–230.2)	104.9 (86.7–125.8)	245.0 (196–306)

[a] mice ($n = 10$)
[b] rat ($n = 7$)

Table 2. The effect of cysteamine, N-ethylmaleimide (NEM), morphine and rimazolium on carrageenan-induced inflammation and acidified ethanol-induced gastric lesions (rats, $n = 7$)

Compound	ID_{30} $\mu mol/kg$ carrageenan oedema	ID_{50} $\mu mol/kg$ p.o. acidified ethanol-lesions
Cysteamine	176.9 p.o. (140.8–220)	98.2 (79.8–119.8)
NEM	2.0 p.o. (1.5–2.6)	4.4 (3.5–5.4)
Morphine	2.9 s.c. (2.25–3.74)	0.26 (0.16–0.31)
Rimazolium	245.0 p.o. (196–306)	110.0 (91–132)

Szabo *et al.* [1], cysteamine, NEM, morphine and, according to our previous data [11], rimazolium, decreased the vascular permeability of gastric mucosa induced in the early phase of ethanol-induced gastric damage. However, the reduction of gastric lesions by these agents was more pronounced suggesting involvement of other factors in gastroprotection. The question arises, whether the inhibition of enhanced vascular permeability by these agents is primary or secondary to lesion development; that is whether the inhibition of mucosal damage is due to gastric mucosal 'vasoprotection' or if the latter is the consequence of mucosal protection.

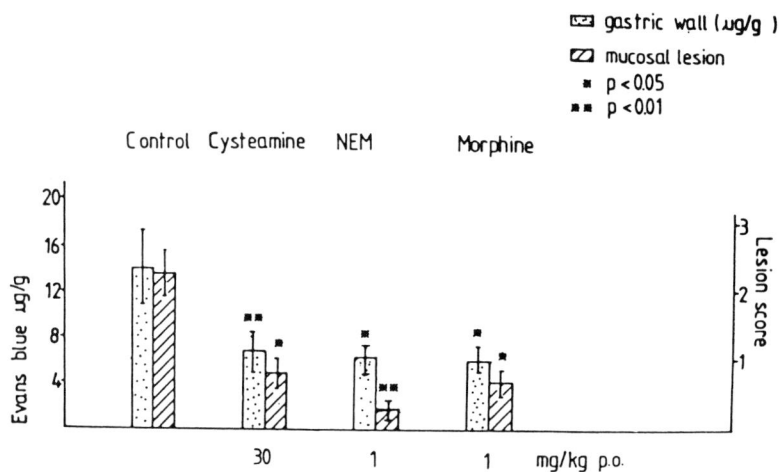

Figure 1. The effect of cysteamine, N-ethylmaleimide (NEM) and morphine on the enhanced vascular permeability and gastric mucosal lesions caused by 100% ethanol 2 min after the ethanol challenge. The values are the mean $\pm$ SEM of 7 rats, *: $p < 0.05$; **: $p < 0.01$

354

We also studied the effect of compounds against indomethacin-induced gastric damage (Figure 2). Pretreating the rats with cysteamine, NEM or morphine inhibited indomethacin-induced mucosal lesions. However, by giving the drugs 1 hour after indomethacin, quite different effects were seen. Cysteamine exerted very pronounced protection, while NEM like morphine [12] aggravated the indomethacin-induced lesions. Macroscopically the type of lesions could be compared to the ethanol-induced mucosal damage. These data suggest that prostaglandins (PGs) are not likely to be involved in the protective action of cysteamine, since cysteamine was effective even when PG generation was abolished by indomethacin. This assumption is supported by the findings of Konturek et al. [13] who failed to find increase in mucosal PG generation in normal or ethanol-treated rats with cysteamine. However, they found SH compounds ineffective against acetylsalicylic acid-induced lesions.

What is the explanation for the dual actions of NEM and morphine i.e. aggravating and protective effects? Previously we [14] suggested that morphine might somehow enhance the liberation of arachidonic acid which would result in an increased PG formation. The enhanced PG

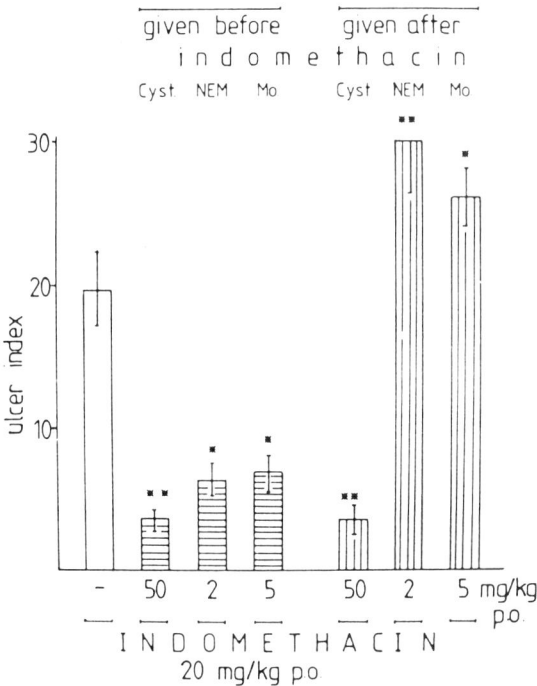

Figure 2. The effect of cysteamine (Cyst.), N-ethylmaleimide (NEM), and morphine (Mo.) on indomethacin-induced lesions (20 mg/kg p.o.) given 1 hour either before or after indomethacin. The values are the mean $\pm$ SEM of 7 rats. *: $p < 0.05$' **: $p < 0.01$; p.o. = per os

production [15] may contribute to protective action of morphine. However, when cyclo-oxygenase is blocked in the presence of indomethacin, arachidonic acid is metabolized by lipoxygenase pathway(s) resulting in the enhanced production of leukotrienes, so causing aggravation of mucosal damage. To test this hypothesis the rats were pretreated with FPL-55712, an antagonist of leukotrienes C_4, F_4, E_4. FPL-55712 was reported to inhibit experimental mucosal damage e.g. stress- or necrotizing-agent induced gastric lesions [16,17]. According to our preliminary data (Table 3) FPL-55712 reduced both the indomethacin-induced lesions and the aggravating action of NEM and morphine. However, the aggravating effect of morphine and NEM expressed as a percentage was about the same in both control and FPL-55712-treated groups. Consequently, our present data do not support the hypothesis that enhanced leukotriene formation is responsible for the increase of mucosal damage, even though Parmar [18] suggested enhanced formation of leukotrienes induced by morphine in the presence of indomethacin.

We also studied the effect of morphine, cysteamine and NEM on intestinal lesions induced by indomethacin. While cysteamine and morphine decreased the lethality but failed to influence the mucosal damage, NEM exerted a very pronounced inhibition both on the development of intestinal lesions and lethality induced by indomethacin.

Summarizing our results: cysteamine, NEM and morphine showed similar profile in analgesic and inflammatory tests and in ulcer models induced by acidified ethanol or indomethacin. However, their gastro-

Table 3. The effect of FPL-55712 on indomethacin-induced gastric damage and the aggravating action of N-ethylmaleimide and morphine (rat, $n = 7$)

Compound	Dose mg/kg p.o.	Ulcer index $\pm$ SEM %	Change in
Indomethacin	20	21.6 ± 3.7	−
Indomethacin + NEM	20 2	41.0 ± 5.6[+a]	$+89$[+a]
Indomethacin + Morphine	20 5	35.5 ± 4.1[+a]	$+64$[+a]
Indomethacin + FPL-55712	20 10	12.2 ± 2.4[+a]	-43[+a]
Indomethacin + FPL-55712 + NEM	20 10 2	21.7 ± 3.5[+b]	$+78$[+b]
Indomethacin + FPL-55712 + Morphine	20 10 5	19.7 ± 2.8[+b]	$+61$[+b]

[+a] $p < 0.05$ compared to indomethacin-treated group
[+b] $p < 0.05$ compared to indomethacin + FPL-55712 treated

Table 4. The effect of cysteamine, morphine and *N*-ethylmaleimide (NEM) on indomethacin-induced intestinal lesions (rat, $n = 10$)

Compound	Dose mg/kg p.o.	Lethality %	Lesion index	Intestinal length (cm)	Body weight gain (+) loss (-) (g)
Control	0	0	0	112±11	+10±2
Indomethacin	20	20	2.0±0.3	82±14	+2±0.3
Indomethacin	20				
+ Morphine	2	20	1.5±0.3	90±15	0
Indomethacin	20	60	3.0±0.5	69±12	-2±0.3
Indomethacin	20				
+ Morphine	10	20	2.1±0.4	79±8	0
Indomethacin	20	60	3.5±0.6	70±9	-5±0.6
Indomethacin	20				
+ Cysteamine	50	60	2.7±0.4	70±8	0
+ Cysteamine	100	40	2.5±0.3	77±9	-2±0.3
Indomethacin	20	20	2.1±0.4	68±7	-4±0.3
Indomethacin	20				
+ NEM	2	0	0.1±0.02[+]	105±12[+]	+7±0.9[+]

[+] $p < 0.05$

protective effects were evident specifically when given 1 hour after indomethacin; cysteamine exerted protective but NEM and morphine aggravating action. To determine whether the protective action of cysteamine against indomethacin-induced gastric damage is due to a specific interaction between cysteamine and indomethacin or that this protective effect is characteristic of other sulphydryl compounds too, we examined the effect of D,L-penicillamine and 2,3-dimercaptosuccinic acid on indomethacin-induced gastric damage given 1 hour after indomethacin. Our preliminary data show that both agents decreased the indomethacin-induced mucosal lesions indicating that the SH group in the molecule is responsible for this protective action.

ACKNOWLEDGEMENT

The author wishes to thank Mrs Szalai and Mrs Barna for technical assistance.

REFERENCES

1. Szabo S, Trier JS, Brown A, Schonoar J. Early vascular injury and increased permeability in gastric mucosal injury caused by ethanol in the rat. Gastroenterology. 1985;88:228–236.

2. Knoll J, Fürst S, Meszaros Z. The pharmacology of 1,6-dimethyl-3-carbethoxy-4-oxo-6,7,8,9-tetrahydro-homopyrimidazol-methylsulphate (Mz144), a new potent non narcotic analgesic. III. Analysis of the central and peripheral effects. Arzneim Forsch. 1971;21:727–733.

3. Gyires K, Fürst S, Miklya I, Budavári I, Knoll J. Analysis of the analgesic and anti-inflammatory effects of rimazolium, a pyrido-pyrimidine derivative, compared with that of prostaglandin-synthesis inhibitors and morphine. Drug Exp Clin Res. 1985;11:493–500.

4. Gyires K, Hermecz I, Knoll J. Comparison of the effect of prostaglandin synthesis inhibitors and pyrido-pyrimidine derivatives. In: Szabo S, Mozsik Gy, eds. New pharmacology of ulcer disease: experimental and new therapeutic approaches. New York: Elsevier;1987:488–504.

5. Winter CA, Risley EA, Nuss GV. Carrageenan-induced edema in the hind paw of the rat as an assay for antiinflammatory drugs. Proc Soc Exp Biol Med. 1965;111:544–547.

6. Koster R, Anderson M, DeBeer EJ. Acetic acid for analgesic screening. Fed Proc. 1959;18:412.

7. Van der Wende C, Margolin S. Analgesic test based upon experimentally induced acute abdominal pain in rats. Fed Proc. 1956;15:494.

8. Gyires K, Torma Z. The use of the writing test in mice for screening different types of analgesics. Arch Int Pharmacodyn Ther. 1984;267:131–140.

9. Jancso-Gabor A, Szolcsanyi J, Jancso N. A simple method for measuring the amount of azovan blue exuded into the skin in response to an inflammatory stimulus. J Pharm Pharmacol. 1967;227:35–41.

10. Tsuromi K, Kyuki K, Fujimura H. Interaction of aspirin and mepirizole in rats as shown by gastrointestinal ulcerogenic and antiinflammatory activities. J Pharmacodyn. 1980;3:659–666.

11. Gyires K, Hermecz I, Knoll J. The effect of some antiulcer agents on the early vascular injury of gastric mucosa induced by ethanol in rats. Acta Phys Hung. 1989;73(2–3):149–154.

12. Gyires K, Furst S, Farczadi E, Marton A. Morphine potentiates the gastroulcerogenic effect of indomethacin in rats. Pharmacology. 1985;30:25–31.

13. Konturek SJ, Brzozowski T, Piastucki I, Radecki T, Szabo S. Gastric cytoprotection by agents altering gastric mucosal sulfhydryl compounds: role of endogenous prostaglandins. In: Samuelsson B, Paoletti R, Ramwell P, eds. Advances in prostaglandins, thromboxane and leukotriene research. Vol. 12. New York: Raven Press;1983:411–416.

14. Gyires K. Morphine inhibits the ethanol-induced gastric mucosal damage in rats. Arch Int Pharmacodyn Ther. 1990;306:170–181.

15. Ferri S, Arrigo-Reina R, Candeletti S, Murari G, Speroni E, Scoto G. Central and peripheral sites of actions for the protective effect of opioids of the rat stomach. Pharmacol Res Commun. 1983;15:409–418.

16. Konturek SJ, Brzozowski T, Drozdowicz D, Garlicki J, Beck G. Role of leukotrienes and platelet activating factor in acute gastric mucosal lesions in rats. Eur J Pharmacol. 1989;164:285–292.

17. Ogle CW, Cho CH. The protective mechanism of FPL55712 against stress-induced gastric ulceration in rats. Agents Actions. 1989;26:350–354.

18. Parmar NS, Tariq M, Ageel AM. Studies on the possible mechanism of morphine-induced potentiation of gastroulcerogenic effect of indomethacin in rats. Arch Int Pharmacodyn Ther. 1987;289:149–160.

40

The role of copper in preventing gastric damage by acetylsalicylic acid

L. Franco, I. Erbetti, P. Bacchini* and G.P. Velo

Istituto di Farmacologia, Università di Verona, Verona, Italy;
*S. Orsola Malpighi Hospital, Bologna, Italy

INTRODUCTION

In a previous paper we evaluated the anti-inflammatory/anti-arthritic activity of a series of bis(2-benzimidazolyl) thioethers (NSN) and their copper(II) chelates [1]. The observation that copper complexes might increase gastric mucus content when given orally, makes these compounds interesting for the potential therapeutic implications. To examine this possibility, the ligand NSN which was found to produce stable 1:1 copper(II) adducts, its copper complex (CuNSN) and $CuCl_2$ were evaluated in experimental gastric ulceration. Since copper is an important co-factor in prostaglandin synthesis [2] and it is well known that prostaglandins (PGs) have a cytoprotective effect on gastric mucosa [3], it was also interesting to study if the prostaglandin system was involved in the potential anti-ulcer action of these compounds.

MATERIALS AND METHODS

Anti-ulcer activity

To test the anti-ulcer activity we produced gastric lesions with acetyl-salicylic acid (ASA) in groups of 7 male Sprague–Dawley rats (weight 180–200 g) fasted 24 hours before the experiment with free access to water.

Each animal received orally 100 mg/kg of ASA and at the same time 50, 100 mg/kg of NSN; 25, 50, 100, 200 mg/kg of CuNSN; 25, 50 mg/kg of $CuCl_2$. These doses are made on a molar basis. Control animals received vehicle alone.

Side-effects of Anti-inflammatory Drugs 3. Rainsford KD, Velo GP (eds),
Inflammation and Drug Therapy Series, Volume V.

After 4 hours the animals were sacrificed and gastric lesions were evaluated, in blind conditions, by use of an arbitrary scale from 0 to 7 after removing the mucus which might mask the appearance of the lesions. Mucous effusion was evaluated by use of an arbitrary scale from 0 to 3.

Assay of the production of PGE_2

The ability of the rat gastric mucosa to generate PGE_2 was evaluated in male Sprague–Dawley rats weighing 175–200 g. The animals were treated orally with CuNSN 100 mg/kg, $CuCl_2$ 25 mg/kg; the control group received vehicle only. One hour after treatment the animals were sacrificed and the gastric mucosa was stripped and prepared for the generation of PGE_2 according to the method described before [4]. Two ml of ice-cold phosphate buffer (0.1 N, pH 7.4) were added to gastric mucosal fragments immediately prior to testing. The samples were then shaken for 60 seconds and incubated for 10 minutes at room temperature. Samples were centrifuged (3000 x g, 2 minutes, 4°C) and the supernatant kept at –20°C until the assay.

PGE_2 in the medium was measured after extraction with Sep-pak C_{18} cartridges (Waters Associated, Milford, USA) and assayed with a highly sensitive PGE_2 ^{125}I RIA kit (Du Pont NEN Division, Germany). Cross reactivity with PGE_1 was 3.7%, and with all other prostaglandins less than 0.4%. After extraction, recovery of the added $[^3H]$-6-keto-$PGF_{1\alpha}$ (151 Ci/mmol) exceeded 80%. The limit of detection was 1 pg per assay tube. Non-specific binding was $\leqslant 8\%$. Intra- and inter-assay variations were 6% and 10% respectively. The results are expressed as nanograms of PGE_2/mg protein. Proteins were determined in the biopsy samples according to Lowry.

RESULTS AND DISCUSSION

Anti-ulcer activity

In agreement with previous results [1] NSN did not show any significant anti-ulcer activity. Also like the early studies [1] CuNSN at all doses produced a significant ($p < 0.01$ and $p < 0.001$ Mann–Whitney U test) reduction in the gastric-lesion severity (Table 1). A significant correlation between inhibition of the gastric lesions and doses of CuNSN was found ($p < 0.01$, Spearman rank correlation r = –0.616). $CuCl_2$, too, produced a statistical significant ($p < 0.001$ Mann–Whitney U test) reduction in gastric-lesion severity and CuNSN and $CuCl_2$ elicited a copious mucous effusion in agreement with earlier studies [2,5] (Table 1).

Table 1. Effect of NSN, CuNSN and CuCl$_2$ on gastric lesions induced by ASA (100 mg/ kg)

Treatment	Oral dose (mg/kg)	No. of animals	Lesion severity	Mucous effusion
Controls	–	15	4.47 ± 0.64	0
NSN	50	7	4.14 ± 0.69	0
NSN	100	7	3.14 ± 1.35	0
CuNSN	25	7	3.57 ± 0.79*	0.36 ± 0.47
CuNSN	50	7	1.86 ± 0.90**	1.40 ± 0.65
CuNSN	100	7	2.14 ± 0.38**	1.80 ± 0.44
CuNSN	200	7	1.71 ± 0.49**	2.80 ± 0.71
CuCl$_2$	25	7	1.71 ± 0.75**	2.10 ± 0.34
CuCl$_2$	50	7	2.14 ± 1.07**	2.70 ± 0.54

Mean ± SD; *$p < 0.01$; **$p < 0.001$ compared to the controls

The histological examination showed necrotic lesions in the stomach of control animals and a normal appearance of the mucosa or little damage in the stomach of treated animals.

PGE$_2$ assay

The output of PGE$_2$ obtained by control rat gastric mucosal fragments incubated *ex vivo* for 10 minutes was 2.87 ± 0.34 ng/mg protein. *Ex vivo* release of PGE$_2$ after previous intragastric administration of CuNSN at the dose of 100 mg/kg, was not significantly different from control values (2.54 ± 1.50 ng/mg protein).

Similar results were seen after intragastric administration of CuCl$_2$ at the dose of 25 mg/kg (Table 2).

The results show that CuNSN and CuCl$_2$ when given orally are effective against the gastric damage induced by ASA and elicit a copious mucous effusion.

PGE$_2$ output indicates that CuNSN and CuCl$_2$ are not able to modify the amounts of PGE$_2$ obtained from incubated rat gastric mucosal pieces, suggesting that mechanisms other than stimulation of prostaglandin

Table 2. Output of PGE$_2$ from rat gastric mucosal fragments incubated *ex vivo* in rat treated orally with CuNSN and CuCl$_2$

Treatment	Oral dose (mg/kg)	No. of animals	ng PGE$_2$/ mg of protein
Controls˙	–	6	2.87 ± 0.34
CuNSN	100	6	2.54 ± 1.50
CuCl$_2$	25	6	2.45 ± 1.10

synthesis are involved. Copper ions are released at low pH in the stomach lumen from complexes, and they are involved in the mucous effusion response [5]. It is likely that the gastric protection of these compounds is due to this effect. Moreover copper complexes may have a superoxide dismutating activity [6] and the reduction of superoxide anions could have the effect of reducing the amount of these active radicals in the stomach tissue.

Acknowledgements

We are most grateful to Professor M. Bressan for giving us the compounds NSN and CuNSN.

REFERENCES

1. Milanino R, Concari E, Conforti A, Marrella M, Franco L, Moretti U, Velo GP, Rainsford KD, Bressan M. Synthesis and anti-inflammatory effects of some bis(2-benzimidazo-lyl)thioethers and their copper(II) chelates, orally administered to rats. Eur J Med Chem. 1988;23:217–224.
2. Rainsford KD. Reactions of the gastric mucosa to orally administered copper and other metal complexes. In: Rainsford KD, Brune K, Whitehouse MW, eds. Trace elements in the pathogenesis and treatment of inflammation. Agents Actions Suppl. 1981;8:369–387.
3. Robert A, Nezamis JE, Lancaster C, Alexander JH. Cytoprotection by prostaglandins in rats. Gastroenterology. 1979;77:433–443.
4. Cavallini G, Franco L, Brocco G, Orlandi PG, Riele A, Manara P, Paveri V, Velo GP. Gastric PGE_2 release in healthy and alcoholic subjects after ethanol stimulation. Ital J Gastroenterol. [in press].
5. Rainsford KD, Whitehouse HW. Gastric mucous effusion elicited by oral copper compounds – potential antiulcer activity. Experientia. 1976;32:1172–1173.
6. Weser U, Schubotz LM. Catalytic reactions of copper complexes with superoxide. In: Rainsford KD, Brune K, Whitehouse HW, eds. Trace elements in the pathogenesis and treatment of inflammation. Agents Actions Suupl. 1981;8:103–120.

41

Effect of NSAID therapy on plasma, whole blood cell (BC), and 24h urine zinc in patients with rheumatoid arthritis (RA)

R. Milanino[1], A. Frigo[2], M. Marrella[1], L.M. Bambara[2], U. Moretti[1], D. Biasi[2], M. Pasqualicchio[1], L. Mainenti[1] and G.P. Velo[1]

[1]Istituto di Farmacologia, and [2]Istituto di Patologia Medica, Università di Verona, Verona, Italy

INTRODUCTION

Some years ago, animal experiments carried out using rat intestinal preparations showed that prostaglandin synthetase inhibitors, such as aspirin and indomethacin, induced a statistically significant decrease of the transfer of zinc from the intestinal lumen to the perfusate [1,2]. On the other hand, the administration of indomethacin and naproxen to healthy volunteers has been found to cause an increase in urinary zinc output [3], indomethacin, but not naproxen, inducing also a fall in plasma zinc concentration [3]. Plasma zinc was found to be significantly lower than normal in RA conditions [4], and the consumption of NSAIDs by RA patients appeared to further decrease the concentration of zinc in their plasma [5]. However, plasma zinc being correlated directly with serum albumin and inversely with serum globulins and erythrocyte sedimentation rate (ESR) [5], the question arises whether the lower plasma zinc level observed in RA patients taking NSAIDs could be related to the severity of their disease rather than to an *in vivo* effect of NSAIDs on the intestinal absorption of zinc.

PATIENTS AND METHODS

Sixty-three patients with classical or definite RA according to the American Rheumatism Association 1988 criteria were studied together with 30 controls matched by sex and age. The mean duration of disease was 6.2 years (range 0.7–28). Apart from NSAIDs, all RA patients were under treatment with other drugs (steroids, gold salts, chloroquine, D-

Side-effects of Anti-inflammatory Drugs 3. Rainsford KD, Velo GP (eds), Inflammation and Drug Therapy Series, Volume V.

penicillamine). The number of tender and swollen joints, Ritchie index, duration of morning stiffness, grip strength, ARA functional and anatomical classification, extra-articular manifestations, ESR, C reactive protein, rheumatoid factor, complete blood count, haematocrit (Ht), haemoglobin concentration (Hb), serum albumin and globulins, serum iron and fibrinogen were used to arbitrarily divide the RA patients in four classes of physician assessment (Phys. Ass.), i.e. 0 in remission, 1 mild, 2 moderate, 3 severe. Biohumoral indices were determined by standard laboratory procedures.

For zinc analysis, fasting blood samples were collected in the early morning using heparinized syringes, and immediately centrifuged to separate the cell fraction from plasma. Zinc determinations in non-haemolytic deproteinized plasma, urine and in acid-digested BC preparations [6] were carried out by flame atomic absorption spectroscopy (Perkin-Elmer 3030 atomic absorption spectrophotometer).

RESULTS

In all the examined RA patients, plasma Zn concentration was found to be lower than that of controls (Table 1), and it was also found to correlate directly with serum albumin, Hb concentration and grip strength, and inversely with ESR, fibrinogen and anatomical stage (data not shown).

Neither the disease (Table 1) nor the assumed drugs (Table 2) appeared to significantly modify the status of zinc in BC and urine, although plasma Zn concentration was found to be significantly lower in RA patients taking NSAIDs compared with patients on different medications (Table 2).

However, some important biohumoral (ESR, Ht, Hb, fibrinogen) and clinical (tender and swollen joints, the Ritchie index, grip strength) parameters have been found significantly worse in RA patients taking NSAIDs compared with non-takers (Table 3). Moreover, if RA patients are stratified according to their Phys. Ass. class plasma Zn concentration does not appear to be significantly depressed by the consumption of NSAIDs (Table 4).

CONCLUSIONS

The data presented in this paper show that rheumatoid arthritis modifies significantly the status of zinc in plasma, suggesting also the existence of an inverse relationship between plasma Zn and the overall severity of the disease.

The use of NSAIDs apparently induces a further decrease of plasma zinc concentration in RA patients taking these drugs compared to patients on different medications. However, RA patients assuming NSAIDs seem

Table 1. Zinc in plasma, whole blood packed cells (BC) and 24h urine, in controls and RA patients

Group (n)	Plasma Zn μmol/L (SD)	BC Zn μmol/L (SD)	24h urine Zn μmol (SD)
Controls (30)	16.0 (1.8)	211.0 (36.0)	7.1 (5.0)
RA patients (63)	13.9 (2.1)**	225.6 (33.1)	7.0 (4.4)

**p < 0.01, Student's t test

Table 2. Zinc status in RA patients taking or not taking NSAIDs

Parameter (units)	RA patients taking NSAIDs[a] mean (SD)	RA patients non-taking NSAIDs[b] mean (SD)
Plasma Zn (μmol/L)	13.5 (2.2)	14.8 (1.7)*
BC Zn (μmol/L packed cells)	224.0 (35.0)	229.3 (28.8)
24h urine (μmol)	6.4 (3.1)	8.3 (6.3)

[a]n = 44, [b]n = 19
*p < 0.05, Student's t test

Table 3. Some biohumoral and clinical parameters in RA patients taking or not taking NSAIDs

Parameter (units)	RA patients taking NSAIDs[a] mean (SD)	RA patients not taking NSAIDs[b] mean (SD)
ESR (mm/h)	41.1 (20.7)	16.8 (13.0)**
Ht (%)	36.6 (4.0)	39.4 (5.4)*
Hb (g/L)	118.0 (15)	128.0 (17)*
Fibrinogen (g/L)	4.0 (1.3)	2.9 (1.7)**
Tender joints (n)	21.2 (10.1)	12.3 (11.1)**
Swollen joints (n)	11.5 (8.0)	7.3 (5.2)**
Ritchie's index	18.6 (8.1)	11.0 (8.9)**
Grip strength (average)	81.0 (36.1)	135.2 (60.2)**

[a]n = 44, [b]n = 19
*p < 0.05, **p < 0.01, Student's t test

Table 4. Plasma zinc (μmol/l) in RA patients taking or not taking NSAIDs stratified according to their physician assessment

Phys. Ass. classes	taking NSAIDs mean (SD) n	not taking NSAIDs mean (SD) n
0 to 1	14.4 (2.5) 9	15.7 (1.7) 9
2 to 3	13.3 (2.2) 35	14.0 (1.3)* 10

*p < 0.05, Student's t test versus classes 0 + 1

365

to be affected by a more serious disease as shown by some important biochemical and clinical indices. Moreover, within the same classes of physician assessment, the consumption of NSAIDs does not modify significantly plasma zinc levels.

In conclusion, our results seem to suggest that the lower plasma zinc concentration observed in RA patients taking NSAIDs could be related to the severity of their disease rather than to an effect of NSAID therapy on intestinal zinc absorption.

REFERENCES

1. Smith KT, Cousins RJ, Silbon BL, Failla ML. Zinc absorption and metabolism by isolated, vascularly perfused rat intestine. J Nutr. 1978;108:1849–1857.
2. Song MK, Adham NF. Role of prostaglandin E2 in zinc absorption in the rat. Am J Physiol. 1978;234:E99–E105.
3. Elling H, Kiilerich S, Christiansen C, Gylding-Sabroe J. The effect of indomethacin and naproxen on zinc metabolism. Scand J Rheumatol. 1978;7:145–146.
4. Niedermeier W, Griggs JH. Trace metal composition of synovial fluid and blood serum of patients with rheumatoid arthritis. J Chron Dis. 1971;23:527–536.
5. Balogh Z, El-Ghobarey AF, Fell GS, Brown DH, Dunlop J, Dick GS. Plasma zinc and its relationship to clinical symptoms and drug treatment in rheumatoid arthritis. Ann Rheum Dis. 1980;39:329–332.
6. Marrella M, Milanino R. Simple and reproducible method for acid extraction of copper and zinc from rat tissue for determination by flame atomic absorption spectroscopy. Atom Spectrosc. 1986;7:40–42.

Index

Side-effects of Anti-inflammatory Drugs 3. Rainsford KD, Velo GP (eds), Inflammation and Drug Therapy Series, Volume V.

New Journal . . .

INFLAMMOPHARMACOLOGY

AN INTERNATIONAL INTERDISCIPLINARY JOURNAL PUBLISHING TOPICAL REVIEWS AND RESEARCH ARTICLES ON INFLAMMATION AND PHARMACOLOGY

EDITOR-IN-CHIEF: Professor K.D. Rainsford, Department of Biomedical Sciences, McMaster University Health Sciences Centre, Hamilton, Ontario L8N 3Z5, Canada

---

Inflammopharmacology publishes papers on all aspects of inflammation and its pharmacological control emphasizing comparisons of (a) different inflammatory states, and (b) the action, therapeutic efficacy and safety of drugs employed in the treatment of inflammatory conditions. The comparative aspects of the types of inflammatory conditions include gastrointestinal disease (e.g. ulcerative colitis, Crohn's disease), parasitic diseases, toxicological manifestations of the effects of drugs and environmental agents, and arthritic conditions. There is no other single journal available at present which covers all the major aspects of the subject. The emphasis on comparative aspects of drug actions is meant to highlight their efficacy and toxicity profiles as well as variability in their clinical response and safety.

In summary the Journal covers:
- Experimental development of *in vitro* systems and *in vivo* animal models
- Assay methodologies
- Biochemical, immunological and pharmacological studies
- Clinical pharmacology and therapeutics
- Drug-induced side-effects – their incidence and mechanisms
- Comparative drug studies and trials
- Novel approaches towards the therapy of inflammatory conditions, including brief but clearly scientifically conducted reports on therapies with as yet undefined materials (e.g. natural products, immunological agents) which may be considered to give leads or encouragement to others to further define the active ingredients and explore their actions.

Publication programme, 1991: Volume 1 (4 issues).
Subscription prices, per volume (4 issues): Dfl 328.–/US$170.00 inclusive of postage.
Subscriptions should be sent to: **Kluwer Academic Publishers Group, PO Box 322, 3300 AH Dordrecht, The Netherlands** or at **PO Box 358, Accord Station, Hingham, MA 02018-0358, USA**, or to any subscription agent.